Diabetes

TRANSLATIONAL MEDICINE SERIES

Diabetes

Translating Research into Practice

Edited by

Carla J. Greenbaum
Benaroya Research Institute
Seattle, Washington, USA

Leonard C. Harrison
The Walter and Eliza Hall Institute of Medical Research
Parkville, Victoria, Australia

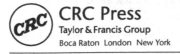

CRC Press
Taylor & Francis Group
Boca Raton London New York

CRC Press is an imprint of the
Taylor & Francis Group, an **informa** business

CRC Press
Taylor & Francis Group
6000 Broken Sound Parkway NW, Suite 300
Boca Raton, FL 33487-2742

First issued in paperback 2019

© 2008 by Taylor & Francis Group, LLC
CRC Press is an imprint of Taylor & Francis Group, an Informa business

No claim to original U.S. Government works

ISBN-13: 978-1-4200-4371-6 (hbk)
ISBN-13: 978-0-367-38701-3 (pbk)

Library of Congress Cataloging-in-Publication Data

Diabetes: translating research into practice / edited by Carla J. Greenbaum,
Leonard C. Harrison.
       p. ; cm. – (Translational medicine series; 9)
    Includes bibliographical references and index.
    ISBN-13: 978-1-4200-4371-6 (hardcover : alk. paper)
    ISBN-10: 1-4200-4371-4 (hardcover : alk. paper)
  1. Diabetes.   I. Greenbaum, Carla J.   II. Harrison, Leonard C.   III. Series.
    [DNLM: 1. Diabetes Mellitus. WK 810 D5425 2008]
    RC660.D552 2008
    616.4'62 – dc22   2008013276

Visit the Taylor & Francis Web site at
http://www.taylorandfrancis.com

and the CRC Press Web site at
http://www.crcpress.com

Preface

"To study the phenomenon of disease without books is to sail an uncharted sea, while to study books without patients is not to go to sea at all."

Sir William Osler

Galen, Maimonides, Jenner, and Osler tour the modern academic medical center, agape at the application of medicine in 2008. Their wonderment at the pandemonium confronting them on the wards turns to complete incomprehension as they eavesdrop on a seminar titled, "Translational Medicine." A white-haired, casually dressed lecturer explains to a room full of distracted and tired looking, multihued men and women that scientific discoveries must be "translated" to medical care to improve the health of individuals. When a member of the audience interjects, "This won't get my grant funded," there is a murmur of agreement from a fidgety audience looking for an excuse to leave. How is it possible, these wise men wonder, that people speak of the need to reconnect science and health—how did the disconnect happen in the first place?

The answer (though not the solution) is simple. Even these giants of medicine's past could not possibly grasp the enormity of new scientific information and the complexities of social, cultural, and economic factors impacting on the delivery of medical care and the health of the community—the reality of modern medicine. Information requires analysis and conversion to knowledge, and knowledge requires reduction to practice. A casual PubMed search with "diabetes" as a keyword reveals more than 17,000 articles during the past year alone! Even the most vigilant, sleep-deprived doctor could not keep up.

The need for translational medicine is another way of saying that we must cross boundaries, talk with one another despite differences in training and outlook, and periodically lift our heads to look broadly at the question of health. Conceptually, it means that what is learned in basic science must challenge extant paradigms, lead to new insights into the bases of ill-health, and deliver potentially new approaches to diagnosis, prevention, and treatment to be tested clinically. What is learned through clinical testing must be efficaciously translated to patients and the community. The loop then must be both closed and perpetuated so that clinical observations inform basic science questions.

A small part in making this a reality is literally in translating because, like a fledgling foreign language student, the clinician has only a rudimentary understanding of the language of the basic scientist, and the basic scientist working in "omics" often does not understand the language of clinical care. The language barrier is not the only, or even the most important, block to translational medicine. There are significant institutional barriers including historical specialty-based divisions of academia and academic centers, as well as mechanisms of funding, career planning, regulatory requirements, and intellectual property issues. In the United States, the NIH RoadMap initiative is trying to change this environment, by promoting collaborative efforts to bring medical science and health together again, and similar efforts are underway elsewhere.

These ruminations on translational medicine are the genesis of this book. It is aimed both at the scientist, who wants to better understand the big picture, and the clinician, who wants to understand where new diagnostics and therapeutics come from. Authors were asked to try to bridge the language gap—not write the standard "review," which would be rapidly outdated, but provide a succinct overview and rationale of their subject and its relevance to human health. We hope this experiment works to broaden the reader's perspective and encourage creative, collaborative thinking and the work needed to translate research to practice.

Perhaps, if our august predecessors visit again in decades hence, their incredulity will be at how translational medicine has changed the lives of people with diabetes.

Carla J. Greenbaum
Leonard C. Harrison

Contents

Contributors

Peter Achenbach   Diabetes Research Institute, Munich, Germany

Benedikt A. Aulinger   Department of Medicine, Division of Endocrinology, Vontz Center for Molecular Studies, University of Cincinnati, Cincinnati, Ohio, U.S.A.

Tandy Aye   Department of Pediatric Endocrinology, Stanford Medical Center, Stanford, California, U.S.A.

Polly J. Bingley   Diabetes and Metabolism, Department of Clinical Science at North Bristol, University of Bristol, Bristol, U.K.

Ezio Bonifacio   CRTD, Dresden University of Technology, Dresden, Germany

Michael Brownlee   JDRF Einstein Centre for Diabetic Complications, Diabetes and Metabolism Division, Baker Heart Research Institute, Melbourne, Victoria, Australia

Bruce Buckingham   Department of Pediatric Endocrinology, Stanford Medical Center, Stanford, California, U.S.A.

Ranjan Chakrabarti   Metabolic Disorder Group, Dr. Reddy's Laboratories Ltd., Discovery Research, Hyderabad, India

Mark E. Cooper   JDRF Einstein Centre for Diabetic Complications, Diabetes and Metabolism Division, Baker Heart Research Institute, Melbourne, Victoria, Australia

David A. D'Alessio   Department of Medicine, Division of Endocrinology, Vontz Center for Molecular Studies, University of Cincinnati, Cincinnati, Ohio, U.S.A.

Shirley Elkassaby   The Walter and Eliza Hall Institute of Medical Research, Parkville, Victoria, Australia

Mark A. Febbraio   Cellular and Molecular Metabolism Laboratory, Baker Heart Research Institute, Prahran, Victoria, Australia

Spiros Fourlanos   The Walter and Eliza Hall Institute of Medical Research, Parkville, Victoria, Australia

Thomas W. Gardner   Departments of Ophthalmology and Cellular and Molecular Physiology, Pennsylvania State College of Medicine, Hershey, Pennsylvania, U.S.A.

Carla J. Greenbaum   Diabetes Program, Benaroya Research Institute, Seattle, Washington, U.S.A.

David M. Harlan   Diabetes Branch, NIDDK, National Institutes of Health (DHHS), and Professor of Medicine, Uniformed Services University of the Health Sciences, Bethesda, Maryland, U.S.A.

Leonard C. Harrison   The Walter and Eliza Hall Institute of Medical Research, Parkville, Victoria, Australia

Andrea Hevener   David Geffen School of Medicine, Division of Endocrinology, Diabetes and Hypertension, University of California, Los Angeles, California, U.S.A.

Gregory R. Jackson   Departments of Ophthalmology and Cellular and Molecular Physiology, Pennsylvania State College of Medicine, Hershey, Pennsylvania, U.S.A.

Mahfuzul Khan   Endocrinology Training Program, Diabetes Branch, NIDDK, National Institutes of Health (DHHS), Bethesda, Maryland, U.S.A.

Graeme I. Lancaster   Cellular and Molecular Metabolism Laboratory, Baker Heart Research Institute, Prahran, Victoria, Australia

Parimal Misra   Metabolic Disorder Group, Dr. Reddy's Laboratories Ltd., Discovery Research, Hyderabad, India

David A. Quillen   Departments of Ophthalmology and Cellular and Molecular Physiology, Pennsylvania State College of Medicine, Hershey, Pennsylvania, U.S.A.

Stephen S. Rich   Center for Public Health Genomics and Departments of Public Health Sciences and Medicine, University of Virginia School of Medicine, Charlottesville, Virginia, U.S.A.

Michèle M. Sale   Center for Public Health Genomics and Departments of Medicine and Biochemistry & Molecular Genetics, University of Virginia School of Medicine, Charlottesville, Virginia, U.S.A.

Marzieh Salehi   Department of Medicine, Division of Endocrinology, Vontz Center for Molecular Studies, University of Cincinnati, Cincinnati, Ohio, U.S.A.

Ingrid U. Scott   Departments of Ophthalmology and Cellular and Molecular Physiology, Pennsylvania State College of Medicine, Hershey, Pennsylvania, U.S.A.

Jonathan E. Shaw   International Diabetes Institute, Melbourne, Victoria, Australia

John M. Wentworth   The Walter and Eliza Hall Institute of Medical Research, Parkville, Victoria, Australia

Paul Z. Zimmet   International Diabetes Institute, Melbourne, Victoria, Australia

1

Reappraising the Stereotypes of Diabetes

Leonard C. Harrison, John M. Wentworth, Shirley Elkassaby, and Spiros Fourlanos
The Walter and Eliza Hall Institute of Medical Research, Parkville, Victoria, Australia

Carla J. Greenbaum
Diabetes Program, Benaroya Research Institute, Seattle, Washington, U.S.A.

INTRODUCTION

Diabetes is defined by a persistently elevated blood glucose concentration, leading to complications that can be acute and long term. Acutely, marked hyperglycemia impairs water and electrolyte balance and energy utilization, leading to polyuria, polydipsia, dehydration, weight loss, and eventually, cerebral dysfunction and coma. Chronically, hyperglycemia impairs a variety of cell functions, leading in particular to complications in blood vessels and nerves. Diabetes is a syndrome, i.e., a combination of symptoms and signs caused by hyperglycemia, which may be the outcome of one or more different underlying mechanisms. A small proportion of diabetes is "secondary," accounted by well-defined genetic or acquired disorders. However, the vast majority of diabetes is classified stereotypically as type 1 diabetes (T1D, formerly called juvenile-onset or insulin-dependent diabetes) and type 2 diabetes (T2D, formerly called adult-onset or insulin-independent diabetes), which accounts for approximately 85% of all diabetes.

Insulin is the central endocrine regulator of glucose metabolism. The concentration of blood glucose reflects a balance between insulin secretion and insulin action. Over the last century, the view emerged that T1D is due to defective insulin secretion, more recently attributed to autoimmune-mediated destruction of pancreatic β-cells, whereas T2D is due to defective insulin action ("insulin resistance") or perhaps more correctly to defective glucose utilization through pathways that are sensitive to insulin. However, like many classification schemes, this one ignores the middle ground where, as is now apparent, an increasing number of people with diabetes are congregated. In this chapter, we argue that the dichotomous view is an oversimplification that impedes our understanding of diabetes, and its treatment and prevention in the 21st century. We are not the first to say this (1). It is time to deconstruct the type 1 and type 2 stereotypes to enable clinicians and scientists to deal more adequately with the epidemic of diabetes, to understand the nature of environment–gene interactions responsible for diabetes, and to devise new strategies to prevent diabetes and its long-term complications. This paradigm shift has important implications for human welfare.

THE SPECTRUM OF DIABETES

Insulin secretion and insulin action are continuous, normally distributed variables that interact to determine glycemia. In diabetes, hyperglycemia reflects deficits in one or both of these parameters. To understand their relative contributions is to understand the natural history of diabetes before and after diagnosis. The prevailing paradigm sees insulin secretion and insulin action at opposite extremes of their distribution functions to define two types of diabetes. We should not think of the diabetes syndrome as two diseases, but consider how genes and environment interact to impair mechanisms of both insulin secretion and insulin action. Impaired β-cell function is well documented in T2D (2–4) and insulin resistance has recently been shown to be a risk factor for the development of T1D (5–7). Also, insulin action should not be thought of as occurring only in "the periphery," because insulin signalling modulates insulin secretion (8).

With the increasing incidence of both T1D and T2D, "hybrid" or "overlap" diabetes with clinical and pathogenetic features of both the types has become more obvious. In younger individuals, it is no longer uncommon to see obesity and insulin resistance, hypertension and dyslipidemia together with pancreatic islet autoantibodies and accelerated β-cell failure, and a family history of both T1D and T2D. In the pediatric population, this has been called "double diabetes" (9) or latent autoimmune diabetes in youth (10), and in the adult population "type 1.5 diabetes" or latent autoimmune diabetes in adults (LADA) (11). Individuals with hybrid diabetes generally have weaker immunogenetic markers of classic T1D, i.e., lower risk human leukocyte antigen (HLA) genes and islet autoantibodies of lower avidity to fewer antigens, predominantly to glutamic acid decarboxylase.

WHAT IS THE RISE OF DIABETES TELLING US?

The steady increase in the incidence of both T1D (12) and T2D (13) can only be explained by an effect of environment to increase the penetrance of genes that predispose to both the types of diabetes. Insulin resistance, short for impaired insulin action relative to a reference population or control group, is now recognized as a feature of both T1D and T2D. Along with other features of the "metabolic syndrome," insulin resistance in T2D is associated with evidence for low-grade systemic inflammation (14–17). We suggest that the environmental agents responsible for the increasing incidence of diabetes are "proinflammatory" and impact innate immune inflammatory pathways to engender insulin resistance. How they act at the molecular and cellular levels should be a high priority for research funding so as to strengthen the case for public health initiatives and new drug development.

The contribution of environment to the rising incidence of diabetes is dramatically illustrated by the changing contribution of human leukocyte antigen (HLA) susceptibility genes to new cases of T1D over time. Although T1D is a polygenic disease, HLA genes, which code for molecules that bind and present peptide antigens to T cells, account for approximately half the genetic risk (18). The proportion of children with the highest risk HLA phenotype (DR3,4; DQ2,8) was shown to be significantly lower in a U.K. cohort diagnosed between 1985 and 2002 compared to a cohort diagnosed between 1920 and 1946 (19). On the other hand, the proportion of children with lower risk phenotypes (DR4/X and DR3/X) was higher in the recent cohort. These findings were consistent with a Finnish study (20) in which children who developed T1D between 1939 and 1965 carried a higher proportion of high-risk HLA genes compared to those diagnosed between 1990 and 2001. In both studies, the baseline comparator populations were diagnosed more than 50 years ago, when survival from T1D was significantly less than it is today, raising the possibility of bias-based selection. We analyzed HLA-DRB1 genes known to confer risk for T1D in relation to year of birth and age at diagnosis over the last five decades (21). As shown in Fig. 1, the proportion, but not the incidence, of children with the highest risk DRB1 genotype (DR3,4) has progressively decreased. The increase in the incidence of T1D is entirely accounted for by children with lower risk genotypes (e.g. DR4/X and DR3/X) who previously might not have developed diabetes, at least in childhood. Age at diagnosis across the decades for children with the highest risk DRB1 genotype has not changed, but for children with lower risk HLA genotypes has decreased significantly since the 1980s (21). We propose that the incidence and age of diagnosis of high-risk children is stable because adaptive, antigen-specific T cell–mediated immunity responsible for β-cell destruction is already optimal with HLA-DR3,4, whereas lower risk genotypes can be complemented by innate immunity promoted (along with insulin resistance) by a proinflammatory environment.

These temporal changes not only underscore the impact of environment, but also illustrate that while the contribution of genes to T1D has changed, it has not lessened over time. They indicate that studies of polygenic disorders like diabetes need to consider year of birth and diagnosis, in dissecting the relative influences of genes and environment. Furthermore, they show that the HLA profile of classic, juvenile-onset T1D has broadened and is now similar to that of adults with

a)

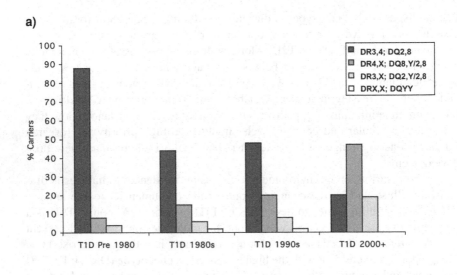

b)

	1985		2002	
	Incidence 11.3/100,000		Incidence 23.2/100,000	
Genotype	Carriers	Cases	Carriers	Cases
DR3,4-DQ2,8	44%	5.0	20%	4.6
DR4,X-DQ8,Y or 2,8	15%	1.7	**47%**	**10.9**
DR3,X-DQ2,Y or 2,8	4%	0.5	**18%**	**4.2**
DRX,X-DQY,Y	2%	0.2	0%	0

Figure 1   The rising incidence of T1D is accounted for by individuals with lower risk HLA genotypes.

autoimmune diabetes or LADA (11). People diagnosed today with LADA were born 30 or more years ago when the incidence of T1D was less than half of what it is today and the contribution of environment much less. Born today, they would develop diabetes in childhood and be diagnosed as having T1D.

Why are more and more children with lower genetic susceptibility for T1D falling under the shadow of a diabetogenic environment? Multiple candidate environmental agents have changed over the last half-century (Fig. 2). At the same time, the prevalence of obesity has increased dramatically. If the increase in obesity, well known as a marker of insulin resistance, mirrors the changing environment, then one might also expect to observe an interaction between obesity and genes in T1D. In a preliminary study of 50 adults presenting consecutively with autoimmune diabetes, we (SF and LCH) observed that the frequency of the high-risk HLA phenotypes DR3,4 and DQ2,8 was significantly lower in the presence

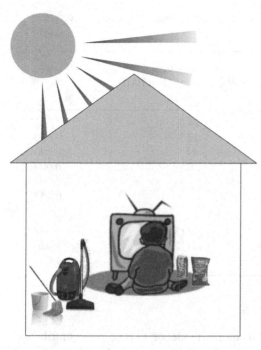

How has the environment changed?

Infections
  ('hygiene hypothesis')

Food
  calories, composition

Exercise

Climate
  ambient temp
  UVR-vitamin D

Sleep

Pharmaceuticals

Modifiers: culture, education, wealth,
access to technology, family size,
maternal age, ...

Figure 2 Multiple factors contribute to the modern day diabetogenic environment.

of obesity and insulin resistance (Table 1). This implies that obesity and insulin resistance can overcome a lower genetic risk for adaptive immunity. Recent studies demonstrate that adipose tissue in obesity is richly endowed with activated macrophages, which may be the source of factors that mediate insulin resistance (22–25). However, obesity per se might not be the cause of insulin resistance: some obese individuals are not insulin resistant and some nonobese individuals are insulin resistant. Moreover, short-term changes in total caloric intake or diet composition can alter insulin sensitivity before an apparent change in adipose tissue mass (26). The degree of obesity associated with insulin resistance may reflect the nature of the diet, e.g., the saturated fat content, rather than total energy consumption, and some environmental conditions, e.g., vitamin D deficiency, may promote insulin resistance independent of adipose tissue accumulation.

Evidence that insulin resistance contributes to the pathogenesis of T1D came from a prospective study of prediabetic children with pancreatic islet autoantibodies who were followed to diabetes (5). The presence of insulin resistance, measured indirectly as HOMA-R, particularly when standardized for insulin secretion, was an independent risk factor for progression from preclinical to clinical disease. This finding was confirmed in post hoc analyses of data from the DPT-1 oral insulin (6) and ENDIT nicotinamide (7) trials for the prevention of T1D. Subsequently, contrary to the usual order of research findings from mouse to man, insulin resistance

Table 1 Interaction of HLA and Obesity in 50 Adults Presenting Consecutively with
Autoimmune Diabetes

	Obese (> median BMI), $n = 25$	Nonobese (< median BMI), $n = 25$	p
BMI	31.7	24.5	
Age	41.9	48.3	0.600
Waist circumference	105	89	<0.0001
Waist–hip ratio	0.94	0.89	<0.0001
HOMA-R[a]	2.5	1.4	0.007
Number of islet antibodies	1.0	1.0	0.953
HLA Class II genes[b]			
DR3,4; DQ2,8	2 (8%)	13 (52%)	0.002
DRX,4; DQY,8	11 (44%)	3 (12%)	0.026
DR3/X; DQ2/Y	5 (20)	5 (20)	1.0

[a]HOMA-R is a measure of insulin resistance.
[b]X is a non-3 or -4 allele and Y is a non-2 or -8.

was shown to be a feature in the NOD mouse model of T1D (27). A contribution
of insulin resistance to the development of T1D has important implications: for
prevention by environment modification and drugs that improve insulin action,
and for stratification of subjects in prevention trials.

A UNIFIED INFLAMMATORY BASIS OF DIABETES

Most of the genes or genetic loci known to be associated with T1D (28) are
involved in one way or another with immune function. Most encode proteins
involved in adaptive immunity, i.e., at the immune synapse between a linear antigenic peptide bound to an HLA molecule and the cognate T-cell receptor. These
elements of adaptive immunity distinguish T1D from T2D. Crucial to understanding the common ground between T1D from T2D is that the initiation and
maintenance of adaptive immunity depends absolutely on the prior activation of
innate immune cells and pathways. Innate immunity, orchestrated by a range of
cells including macrophages, neutrophils, NK cells, mast cells, eosinophils, and
others that express receptors of lesser specificity than the antigen receptors on T or
B cells, elicits strong inflammatory responses mediated by free radicals, cytokines,
and chemokines. Circulating markers of activated innate immune inflammatory
pathways that are associated with T2D include acute-phase proteins (C-reactive
protein, haptoglobin), cytokines (TNF-α, IL-1, IL-6, IL-8, IL-18), and chemokines
(MCP-1, MIF) (14–17). The concentrations of these inflammatory markers mirror
changes in insulin action and glucose tolerance, secondary to environmental modification, e.g., by diet (29,30). As suggested, innate immune activation promoted

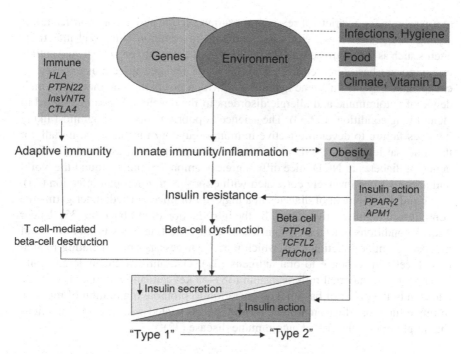

Figure 3 Gene–environment interactions promote inflammatory mechanisms of diabetes.

by a proinflammatory environment may lead to insulin resistance and complement weaker adaptive immunity, leading to hybrid diabetes. Insulin resistance is present across the spectrum of diabetes, with HLA and other adaptive immune genes being superimposed to determine the autoimmune features of T1D (Fig. 3).

HOW HAS THE ENVIRONMENT CHANGED?

The health of individuals in developed and developing nations depends on understanding how environment has wrought the epidemic of diabetes. The environment for the modern children is different in many ways from that of their grandparents. As depicted in Fig. 2, the modern child lives inside a clean, oversized house, in a controlled climate, devoid of the sun and fresh air, watching television or playing computer games, exercising less, and consuming proinflammatory foods. Many social, cultural, educational, technological, and economic factors have contributed to this scenario. Some examples of candidate environmental agents are discussed next.

Infections

The infectious environment has changed in several ways. Parasitic infections of infancy such a pinworm are no longer endemic (31). Newborns are less exposed to microbiota for a variety of reasons (caesarian section and hospital births, fewer siblings, cleaner houses), exposure of infants to common childhood infectious agents such as enteroviruses may be delayed until entry into preschool, and antibiotic exposure has increased (32). The impact of reduced infectious exposure is encapsulated by the "hygiene hypothesis," which posits that the increasing incidence of autoimmune and allergic disorders in the developed world is related to clean living conditions (32,33). The science is poorly understood but most likely involves failure to develop effective immunoregulatory mechanisms, initially at the mucosal level. The NOD mouse model of diabetes is illustrative. The incidence of diabetes in NOD mice differs greatly among colonies around the world and appears to be inversely correlated with exposure to microbial infection (34). The rapid development of diabetes in a majority of mice housed under germ-free conditions is significantly reduced by the introduction of gut bacteria (35). Under "dirty" conditions, bacterial colonization of the intestine leads to maturation of mucosal immune function (36), which may be necessary for generating regulatory T cells in response to oral antigens (37). One antigen encountered orally by neonates in maternal milk is insulin (38)—a key autoantigen in T1D (39). In addition to the effect of bacterial colonization to promote maturation of mucosal immune function, dirty environments may be associated with specific infections that might reduce the risk of autoimmune disease (32).

Food

Apart from total energy intake, specific foods or dietary constituents, e.g., saturated fats including trans-fatty acids (40), fructose (41), and advanced glycation end-products (42), may modify inflammatory pathways and/or metabolism (Fig. 4) and engender insulin resistance. The effects of dietary constituents on the biochemistry of mitochondria, the NF-κB pathway, and the endoplasmic reticulum is currently the focus of much attention (24) and should lead to a stronger rationale for preventative health measures and the development of new drugs for diabetes and its complications. Ultimately, the quantity and quality of the food we consume is determined by complex cultural and political factors, but these are not beyond the influence of clinicians and scientists concerned for the global environment.

Vitamin D

The primary source of vitamin D in humans is ultraviolet B light induced synthesis in the skin. In the absence of dietary supplementation, lack of exposure to sunlight leads to vitamin D deficiency. The significant prevalence of vitamin D deficiency is now recognized, not just in those living furthest away from the equator but in any population in which people avoid sunlight for fear of skin cancer, cover their skin for cultural or religious reasons, or receive less light due to global dimming from pollutants. A critical co-contributory factor is the progressive reduction in the recommended daily allowance of vitamin D over the last 50 years from

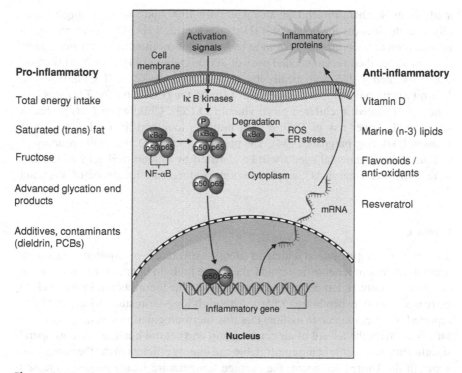

Figure 4 Foods modify cellular pathways of inflammation.

at least 5,000 IU to the present 400 IU, which happens to be the minimum dose sufficient to prevent rickets, following adequate prenatal intake (43,44). However, in addition to its role in calcium and bone metabolism, vitamin D is a pleiotropic steroid required at higher levels for anti-inflammatory, anti-apoptotic, and immunoregulatory effects (45,46).

Several lines of evidence link vitamin D deficiency to both T1D and T2D. Vitamin D–deficient rats have reduced insulin secretion in response to a glucose load, which is corrected by administration of 1,25-dihydroxyvitamin D3 (calcitriol), the active form (47). Small pilot trials in both nondiabetic and diabetic humans have demonstrated that vitamin D supplementation improves β-cell function (48–50), and an independent association was documented between serum 25-hydroxyvitamin D3 and glucose tolerance in humans (51). Vitamin D may have a separate role to promote insulin action. In a large Caucasian population, a negative association was found (51) between serum 25-hydroxyD3 and HOMA-R, a well-validated index of insulin resistance. Consistent with this observation, a study of 164 healthy adults found a positive correlation between serum 25-hydroxyD3 and insulin sensitivity measured by hyperinsulinemic euglycemic clamp (52). Three European epidemiological studies have demonstrated an inverse relationship between vitamin D intake and the incidence of T1D. In a 1966 birth cohort study from Northern Finland, an area with only 1900 hours direct sunlight annually and the highest incidence of T1D in the world, T1D status was related to prerecorded data on infants 7–24 months of age given vitamin D less than, more than, or at the then recommended dose of 2000 IU daily (44). The 2000 IU dose was associated with a dramatically low relative risk of 0.12 (95% CI 0.03–0.47). In a multinational European case–control study, the odds ratio for T1D was significantly reduced in children given vitamin D (53). Children in Norway had a significantly lower risk of T1D, if their mothers took cod liver oil (a source of vitamin D) during pregnancy (54). The place of vitamin D within the panoply of candidate environmental agents will be clarified by randomized controlled trials to test whether vitamin D3 supplementation reduces the incidence of T1D and T2D.

Climate

The ambient temperature at which no energy expenditure is required to maintain normal body temperature is termed thermoneutral. In humans fed *ad libitum* exposure to ambient temperatures above or below the thermoneutral zone leads to increased energy expenditure (55,56). Although long-term studies have not been reported, it is reasonable to assume that this thermoregulation translates to lower fat stores. With the advent of air conditioning and central heating, we now spend significantly more time being comfortable and energy efficient in the thermoneutral zone. In the United Kingdom, the average temperature inside houses increased from 13°C to 18°C between 1970 and 2000 (57). We have created conditions in which we expend less energy, even when we are inactive.

Sleep

Changing work and leisure practices have reduced the average duration of sleep across all ages. In United States, the average duration of sleep of adults has fallen from more than 9 to just more than 7 hours in the last few decades (58). Prospective studies of children and young adults followed, respectively, for years found an inverse relationship between sleep duration and weight gain (59,60). Moreover, self-reported overnight sleep duration of less than 6 hours was shown to be an independent predictor of diabetes (61,62). This is consistent with the finding that experimental sleep deprivation for six consecutive nights impairs glucose tolerance in healthy adults (63). In rats, sleep deprivation induced hyperphagia (64). Similarly, experimental sleep reduction in humans increased appetite and was associated with orexigenic changes in circulating concentrations of leptin (decreased) and ghrelin (increased) (65). In the minds of clinicians, sleep ranks well below diet and exercise as a modifiable lifestyle factor, yet it may be the easiest for people to change. This mindset highlights a need for clinical trials to test whether promoting sleep prevents obesity and diabetes.

IMPLICATIONS OF REAPPRAISING THE STEREOTYPES OF DIABETES

The reappraisal of diabetes stereotypes has important conceptual and practical implications. The frequent pronouncement that T2D is an avoidable life-style disease and that T1D is an unavoidable genetic disease is patently false. Any means of avoiding or reducing exposure to the modern day diabetogenic environment should benefit diabetes across the spectrum. Identification of the many genes contributing to T1D and T2D proceeds apace, but the challenge for scientists will be to integrate genetic data and a knowledge of how environmental agents impact molecular and biochemical pathways to impair insulin secretion and action. Given the combinatorial possibilities, there will be many roads to hyperglycemia, with more and more decimals appearing between 1 and 2, and a corresponding range of pharmacogenomic-based therapies. The new paradigm has implications currently for preventing and treating all forms of diabetes, starting with environment modification and extending to anti-inflammatory drugs. The latter approach is not new. Salicylates were first documented to improve glucose tolerance over a century ago (66,67) and more recently have been shown to inhibit signaling in the NF-κB pathway at the level of the I-κB kinase complex β, leading to a decrease in proinflammatory mediators and insulin resistance (68). Modern interest in T2D as a disorder of low-grade inflammation dates from the observation that TNF-α is expressed by adipose tissue of obese mice (69). Mice deficient in TNF-α have increased insulin sensitivity (70), and administration of TNF-α to humans causes insulin resistance (71). However, initial trials of TNF-α antagonists did not reveal significant benefit in T2D; (72) although, subsequently, analysis of subjects with rheumatoid arthritis undergoing treatment with monoclonal antibody to TNF-α revealed improved insulin sensitivity (73). TNF-α is only one of many proinflammatory mediators overexpressed in T2D and IL-1β is another. Treatment of T2D subjects with an IL-1β antagonist improved insulin secretion and glucose tolerance (74). Completely restoring glucose homeostasis is likely to require approaches directed not just at a single target but a network of inflammatory mediators or their pathways.

Although as scientists we must be "splitters," as clinicians we must still be "lumpers" because diabetes type is less important than correcting hyperglycemia to prevent complications. From the clinician's perspective, controlling hyperglycemia with whatever works is the primary goal. Despite controversies over the years about the benefits of exogenous insulin, no particular method of controlling glycemia appears to be better than another in regard to preventing long-term complications. The possible exception, from the UKPDS trial, is that treatment of overweight T2D subjects with metformin was associated with decrease in cardiovascular disease and death, independent of glycemic control (75). The choice of treatment may nevertheless be influenced by the knowledge that a patient is insulin deficient or markedly insulin resistant. A patient with no detectable meal-stimulated C-peptide will require insulin therapy; a patient with insulin resistance associated with reversible obesity is unlikely to require insulin; a patient with insulin resistance and islet autoantibodies is likely to require insulin in the foreseeable future. Clinicians are ideally placed to discern disease heterogeneity, and thus inform the science of dissecting mechanisms that underlie the spectrum of diabetes.

REFERENCES

1. Gale EAM. Declassifying diabetes. Diabetologia 2006; 49:1989–1995.
2. Leahy JL. Natural history of beta-cell dysfunction in NIDDM. Diabetes Care 1990; 13:992–1010.
3. Del Prato S, Marchetti P. Beta- and alpha-cell dysfunction in type 2 diabetes. Horm Metab Res 2004; 36:775–781.
4. Kitabchi AE, Temprosa M, Knowler WC, et al. Role of insulin secretion and sensitivity in the evolution of type 2 diabetes in the diabetes prevention program: Effects of lifestyle intervention and metformin. Diabetes Care 2005; 54:2404–2414.
5. Fourlanos S, Narendran P, Byrnes GB, et al. Insulin resistance is a risk factor for progression to type 1 diabetes. Diabetologia 2004; 47:1661–1667.
6. Xu P, Cuthbertson D, Greenbaum C, et al. Role of insulin resistance in predicting progression to type 1 diabetes. Diabetes Care 2007; 30:2314–2320.
7. Bingley PJ, Mahon JL, Gale EAM. European Nicotinamide Diabetes Intervention Trial Group: Insulin resistance and progression to type 1 diabetes in the European Nicotinamide Diabetes Intervention Trial (ENDIT). Diabetes Care 2008; 31:146–150.
8. White MF. Regulating insulin signaling and β-cell function through IRS proteins. Can J Physiol Pharmacol 2006; 84:725–737.
9. Libman IM, Becker DJ. Coexistence of type 1 and type 2 diabetes mellitus: 'Double' diabetes? Pediatr Diabetes 2003; 4:110–113.
10. Reinehr T, Schober E, Wiegand S, et al. Beta-cell autoantibodies in children with type 2 diabetes mellitus: Subgroup or misclassification? Arch Dis Child 2006; 91:473–477.
11. Fourlanos S, Dotta F, Greenbaum CJ, et al. Latent autoimmune diabetes in adults (LADA) should be less latent. Diabetologia 2005; 48:2206–2212.
12. Gale EAM. The rise of childhood type 1 diabetes in the 20th century. Diabetes 2002; 51:3353–3361.
13. Fox CS, Pencina MJ, Meigs JB, et al. Trends in the incidence of type 2 diabetes mellitus from the 1970s to the 1990s: The Framingham Heart Study. Circulation 2006; 113:2914–2918.
14. Pickup JC. Inflammation and activated innate immunity in the pathogenesis of type 2 diabetes. Diabetes Care 2004; 27:813–823.
15. Kolb H, Mandrup-Poulsen T. An immune origin of type 2 diabetes? Diabetologia 2005; 48:1038–1050.
16. Wellen KE, Hotamisligil GS. Inflammation, stress, and diabetes. J Clin Invest 2005; 115:1111–1119.
17. Hotamisligil GS. Inflammation and metabolic disorders. Nature 2006; 444:860–867.
18. Eisenbarth GS, Pugliese A. Type 1 diabetes mellitus of man: Genetic susceptibility and resistance. In: Type 1 Diabetes: Molecular, Cellular and Clinical Immunology,

2.5ed. (online). Eisenbarth GS, Ed. Denver, CO: The Barbara Davis Center for Childhood Diabetes, 2007, 2403–2407. Available at: http://www.uchsc.edu/misc/diabetes/eisenbook.html.

19. Gillespie KM, S.C. B, A.H. B, et al. The rising incidence of childhood type 1 diabetes and reduced contribution of high-risk HLA haplotypes. Lancet 2004; 364:1699–1700.

20. Hermann R, Knip M, Veijola R, et al. Temporal changes in the frequencies of HLA genotypes in patients with type 1 diabetes—indication of an increased environmental pressure? Diabetologia 2003; 46:420–425.

21. Fourlanos S, Varney MD, Tait BD, et al. Lower-risk HLA genotypes account for the rising incidence of type 1 diabetes. Diabetes Care, *in press*.

22. Weisberg SP, McCann D, Desai M, et al. Obesity is associated with macrophage accumulation in adipose tissue. J Clin Invest 2003; 112:1796–1808.

23. Xu H, Barnes GT, Yang Q, et al. Chronic inflammation in fat plays a crucial role in the development of obesity-related insulin resistance. J Clin Invest 2003; 112: 1821–1830.

24. Özcan U, Cao Q, Yilmaz E, et al. Endoplasmic reticulum stress links obesity, insulin action, and type 2 diabetes. Science 2004; 306:457–461.

25. Lumeng CN, DeYoung SM, Bodzin JL, Saltiel AR. Increased inflammatory properties of adipose tissue macrophages recruited during diet-induced obesity. Diabetes 2007; 56:16–23.

26. Lovejoy JC. The influence of dietary fat on insulin resistance. Current Diabetes Reports 2002; 2:435–440.

27. Chaparro RJ, Konigshofer Y, Beilhack GF, et al. Non-obese diabetic mice express aspects of both type 1 and type 2 diabetes. Proc Natl Acad Sci U.S.A. 2006; 103:12475–12480.

28. Todd JA, Walker NM, Cooper JD, et al. Robust associations of four new chromosome regions from genome-wide analyses of type 1 diabetes. Nat Genet 2007; 39:857–864.

29. Bruun JM, Helge JW, Richelsen B, Stallknecht B. Diet and exercise reduce low-grade inflammation and macrophage infiltration in adipose tissue but not in skeletal muscle in severely obese subjects. Am J Physiol Endocrinol Metab 2006; 290:E961–E967.

30. Qi L, van Dam RM, Liu S, et al. Whole-grain, bran, and cereal fiber intakes and markers of systemic inflammation in diabetic women. Diabetes Care 2006; 29:207–211.

31. Gale EAM. A missing link in the hygiene hypothesis? Diabetologia 2002; 45:588–594.

32. Bach JF. The effect of infections on susceptibility to autoimmune and allergic diseases. New Engl J Med 2002; 347:911–920.

33. Strachan DP. Hay fever, hygiene, and household size. BMJ 1989; 299:1259–1260.

34. Pozzilli P, Signore A, Williams AJ, Beales PE. NOD mouse colonies around the world—recent facts and figures. Immunol Today 1993; 14:193–196.

35. Funda DP, Fundova P, Harrison LC. Microflora-dependency of selected diabetes-preventive diets: Germ-free and ex-germ-free monocolonized NOD mice as models for studying environmental factors in type 1 diabetes. In: 13th International Congress of Immunology, Rio de Janiero, Brazil, 2007; p. MS11.14

36. Macpherson AJ, Harris NL. Interactions between commensal intestinal bacteria and the immune system. Nat Rev Immunol 2004; 4:478–485.

37. Locke NR, Stankovic S, Funda DP, Harrison LC. TCR gamma–delta intraepithelial lymphocytes are required for self-tolerance. J Immunol 2006; 176;6553–6559.

38. Shehadeh N, Shamir R, Berant M, Etzioni A. Insulin in human milk and the prevention of type 1 diabetes. Pediatr Diabetes 2001; 2:175–177.
39. Narendran P, Mannering SI, Harrison LC. Proinsulin—a pathogenic autoantigen in type 1 diabetes. Autoimmun Rev 2003; 2:204–210.
40. Odegaard AO, Pereira MA. Trans fatty acids, insulin resistance, and type 2 diabetes. Nutr Rev 2006; 64:364–372.
41. Elliott SS, Keim NL, Stern JS, et al. Fructose, weight gain, and the insulin resistance syndrome. Am J Clin Nutr 2002; 76:911–922.
42. Yamagishi S, Ueda S, Okuda S. Food-derived advanced glycation end products (AGEs). A novel therapeutic target for various disorders. Curr Pharm Des 2007; 13;2832–2836.
43. Vieth R. Vitamin D supplementation, 25-hydroxyvitamin D concentrations, and safety. Am J Clin Nutr 1999; 69:842–856.
44. Hypponen E, Laara E, Reunanen A, et al. Intake of vitamin D and risk of type 1 diabetes: A birth-cohort study. Lancet 2001; 362:1389–1400.
45. Holick MF. Vitamin D: Importance in the prevention of cancers, type 1 diabetes, heart disease, and osteoporosis. Am J Clin Nutr 2004; 79:362–371.
46. Campbell MJ, Adorini L. The vitamin D receptor as a therapeutic target. Expert Opin Ther Targets 2006; 10:735–748.
47. Norman AW, Frankel JB, Heldt AM, Grodsky GM. Vitamin D deficiency inhibits pancreatic secretion of insulin. Science 1980; 209:823–825.
48. Inomata S, Kadowaki S, Yamatani T, et al. Effect of 1 alpha (OH)-vitamin D3 on insulin secretion in diabetes mellitus. Bone Miner 1986; 1:187–192.
49. Kumar S, Davies M, Zakaria Y, et al. Improvement in glucose tolerance and β-cell function in a patient with vitamin D deficiency during treatment with vitamin D. Postgrad Med J 1994; 70:440–443.
50. Borissova AM, Tankova T, Kirilov G, et al. The effect of vitamin D3 on insulin secretion and peripheral insulin sensitivity in type 2 diabetic patients. Int J Clin Pract 2003; 57:258–261.
51. Scragg R, Sowers M, Bell C. Serum 25-hydroxyvitamin D3, diabetes, and ethnicity in the Third National Health and Nutrition Examination Survey. Diabetes Care 2004; 27:2813–2818.
52. Chiu KC, Chu A, Go VL, Saad MF. Hypovitaminosis D is associated with insulin resistance and β-cell dysfunction. Am J Clin Nutr 2004; 79:820–825.
53. The Eurodiab Substudy 2 Study Group:. Vitamin D supplement in early childhood and risk for type 1 (insulin-dependent) diabetes mellitus. Diabetologia 1999; 42:51–54.
54. Stene LC, Ulriksen J, Magnus P, Joner G. Use of cod-liver oil during pregnancy associated with lower risk of type 1 diabetes in the offspring. Diabetologia 2000; 43:1093–1098.
55. Westerterp-Plantenga MC, van Marken Lichtenbelt WD, Cilissen C, Top S. Energy metabolism in women during short exposure to the thermoneutral zone. Physiol Behav 2002; 75:227–235.
56. Keith SW, Redden DT, Katzmarzyk PT, et al. Putative contributors to the secular increase in obesity: Exploring the roads less traveled. Int J Obes (Lond) 2006; 30:1585–1594.
57. English House Condition Survey. Housing research summary: English House Condition Survey 1996. Minister OotDP, Ed., The Stationary Office, UK, 2000.

58. Bonnet MH, Arand DL. We are chronically sleep deprived. Sleep 1995; 18: 908–911.
59. Agras WS, Hammer LD, McNicholas F, Kraemer HC. Risk factors for childhood overweight: A prospective study from birth to 9.5 years. J Pediatr 2004; 145:20–25.
60. Hasler G, Buysse D, Klaghofer R, et al. The association between short sleep duration and obesity in young adults: A 13-year prospective study. Sleep 2004; 27:602–603.
61. Ayas NT, White DP, Al-Delaimy WK, et al. A prospective study of self-reported sleep duration and incident diabetes in women. Diabetes Care 2003; 26:380–384.
62. Yaggi HK, Araujo AB, McKinlay JB. Sleep duration as a risk factor for the development of type 2 diabetes. Diabetes Care 2006; 29:657–661.
63. Spiegel K, Leproult R, Van Cauter E. Impact of sleep debt on metabolic and endocrine function. Lancet 1999; 354:1435–1439.
64. Everson CA. Functional consequences of sustained sleep deprivation in the rat. Behav Brain Res 1995; 69:43–54.
65. Spiegel K, Tasali E, Penev P, Van Cauter E. Sleep curtailment in healthy young men is associated with decreased leptin levels, elevated ghrelin levels and increased hunger and appetite. Ann Intern Med 2004; 141:846–850.
66. Ebstein W. Zur therapie des diabetes mellitus, insbesondere über die anwendeng der salicylauren natron bei demselben. Berl Klin Wochenschr 1876; 13;337–340.
67. Williamson R. On the treatment of glycosuria and diabetes mellitus with sodium salicylate. Br Med J 1901; 1:760–762.
68. Yuan M, Konstantopoulos N, Lee J, Hansen L, et al. Reversal of obesity- and diet-induced insulin resistance with salicylates or targeted disruption of Ikk β. Science 2001; 293;1673–1677.
69. Hotamisligil GS, Shargill NS, Spiegelman BM. Adipose expression of tumor necrosis factor-α: Direct role in obesity-linked insulin resistance. Science 1993; 259:87–91.
70. Uysal KT, Wiesbrock SM, Marino MW, Hotamisligil GS. Protection from obesity-induced insulin resistance in mice lacking TNF-α function. Nature 1997; 389:610–614.
71. Krogh-Madsen R, Plomgaard P, Moller K, et al. Influence of TNF-α and IL-6 infusions on insulin sensitivity and expression of IL-18 in humans. Am J Physiol Endocrinol Metab 2006; 291:E108–14.
72. Ofei F, Hurel S, Newkirk J, et al. Effects of an engineered human anti-TNF-α antibody (CDP571) on insulin sensitivity and glycemic control in patients with NIDDM. Diabetes 1996; 45:881–85.
73. Kiortsis DN, Mavridis AK, Vasakos S, et al. Effects of infliximab treatment on insulin resistance in patients with rheumatoid arthritis and ankylosing spondylitis. Ann Rheum Dis 2005; 64:765–766.
74. Larsen CM, Faulenbach M, Vaag A, et al. Interleukin-1-receptor antagonist in type 2 diabetes mellitus. New Engl J Med 2007; 356:1517–1526.
75. UK Prospective Diabetes Study (UKPDS) Group. Effect of intensive blood-glucose control with metformin on complications in overweight patients with type 2 diabetes (UKPDS 34). Lancet 1998; 352:854–865.

2

How Can We Use Genetic Information in the Clinic?

Michèle M. Sale

Center for Public Health Genomics and Departments of Medicine and Biochemistry & Molecular Genetics, University of Virginia School of Medicine, Charlottesville, Virginia, U.S.A.

Stephen S. Rich

Center for Public Health Genomics and Departments of Public Health Sciences and Medicine, University of Virginia School of Medicine, Charlottesville, Virginia, U.S.A.

INTRODUCTION

It is commonly stated that genomics approaches and knowledge will be rapidly transferred to the clinic. While there is growing evidence that genomics research is increasing our knowledge of common diseases, in particular diabetes, the evidence that genomic information is having an immediate and major impact on clinical practice is less obvious. Molecular diagnosis is now possible for more than 80% of patients with monogenic (single gene) forms of diabetes, and this knowledge can be used to inform treatment decisions (1). Other more common forms of diabetes have more complex genetic (and environmental) contributions to risk, making prediction, prevention, and treatment less clear. This chapter will provide a summary of current knowledge of the genetic contribution to several diabetes phenotypes, the prospects for applying genetic information in the clinical setting, and identify some of the barriers to the application of this information in translational research and personalized medicine.

TERMS AND TOOLS FOR GENETIC STUDIES

Definitions

Association analysis: Within a population of individuals, a mutation may occur within a gene that alters the risk of a disease. The "variant" allele will be in close proximity to another genetic marker locus, so that the allele of the marker that is physically adjacent to the variant will tend to be transmitted together over time. This concept, linkage disequilibrium, is the basis for analysis of genetic markers in a set of "cases " (individuals with disease) and "controls" (individuals without disease). Association analysis tests whether a genetic marker has a significantly different frequency in cases from controls and, therefore, suggests that the disease-modifying variant is near the marker.

HapMap: The International HapMap Project developed a "map" of the human genome that utilized SNP genotyping to provide a description of common patterns of human variation. The HapMap provides a resource for identifying genes affecting traits and diseases in human populations by listing the known SNPs and their relationships to other SNPs.

Linkage analysis: Genetic linkage occurs when two loci are physically close to one another, so that the probability of recombination occurring among the loci is less than that observed when the two loci are on different chromosomes. In general, there is decreasing frequency of recombination with decreasing genetic distance. For discovery of genes contributing to risk of disease, linkage analysis uses this concept to map a disease locus to a genetic marker locus using a family-based approach (in order to estimate the frequency of recombination). Linkage analysis can be performed either assuming a genetic transmission model of the disease (parametric) or under no assumptions of the disease (nonparametric).

Methylation: A chemical reaction that occurs in vertebrate DNA at sites associated with genes (CpG islands), particularly at gene promoters, results in significant effects on gene activity or expression.

Modes of inheritance: Patterns that appear in families, whereby a trait is transmitted from one generation to the next. An autosomal dominant mode of inheritance is observed when an individual possesses one copy of a variant allele and one normal allele (e.g., Huntington's disease); in contrast, an autosomal recessive mode of inheritance requires that the individual has two copies of a variant allele to express a phenotype (e.g., cystic fibrosis).

Mutations: Permanent alterations in DNA that often have no major effect and, due to their rarity, are lost in the population in which they arise; however, mutations may remain in the population (as a SNP) by either providing a selective advantage or due to chance (if they have a relatively "neutral" effect on survival). With changing environmental conditions, the effect of mutations on survival can change, so that what was once neutral or beneficial can become deleterious (as postulated for the "thrifty gene" model of diabetes).

SNP (pronounced "snip"): Single nucleotide polymorphism, a common type of variation that occurs in human DNA approximately once in every

1000 bases. SNPs serve as genetic markers to identify causal variants that affect human variation or disease risk.

Types of Studies

One common method of discovery of novel genetic risk factors (or disease-related genes) is through a genome-wide linkage scan of affected sibling pairs. This has led to the discovery of a number of genes with relatively large effect of somewhat low prevalence. Another method to identify genetic factors is through a candidate gene association study in which frequencies of candidate gene polymorphisms are compared among diabetes cases and diabetes-free controls. Candidate gene studies based upon known biological pathways have resulted in equivocal outcomes, in part due to the complexity of the pathways being investigated. Recently, the resources of the HapMap have permitted analysis of the entire genome by association (genome-wide association scan). Based upon this approach (either with tagged SNPs or nonsynonymous SNPs), several novel disease susceptibility genes have been identified. The first gene complement factor H (*CFH*), contributes to risk of age-related macular degeneration (2,3). The second gene, interferon-induced helicase region, *IFIH1*, contributes to risk of (T1D)(4). The third gene, interleukin 23 receptor, *IL23R*, affects risk of inflammatory bowel disease (5). All three of these genes were newly identified and, importantly, provided insights on novel pathways and therapeutic targets.

MONOGENIC FORMS OF DIABETES

Maturity Onset Diabetes of the Young

Maturity onset diabetes of the young (MODY) was originally described as a nonketotic form of diabetes with autosomal dominant inheritance and onset before the age of 25 years (6,7). Despite a similar MODY phenotype, genetic research has revealed several molecular causes of MODY. The extensive genetic heterogeneity accompanied by a wide phenotypic spectrum within specific MODY groups (based upon genetic variant) has made it more appropriate to use the WHO/ADA genetic subgroup classification (8).

The most common form of MODY, MODY3, is caused by mutations of the hepatic transcription factor 1 gene *TCF1*, also known as hepatocyte nuclear factor-1α (*HNF1A*) (9). *TCF1* has been found to bind to regulatory regions of at least 222 target genes in hepatocytes and 106 genes in pancreatic islets (10). *TCF1* dimerization produces an intermolecular 4-helix bundle, which is destabilized by MODY3 mutations (11) and is thought to be responsible for the resulting metabolic dysregulation. Affected individual are not insulin-dependent but may show a large glucose increment in response to an oral glucose tolerance test in the early stages. Severe hyperglycemia after puberty often leads to an incorrect diagnosis of type 1 diabetes. Frequently, patients can be treated with diet, but will show postprandial hyperglycemia following a high carbohydrate meal, since they are unable to secrete sufficient insulin (12). Progressive deterioration of glycemic control usually results in the need for pharmacological treatment. Patients are usually very responsive to sulfonylurea drugs and sensitivity is often retained for many years (13,14), although dose titration is needed to avoid hypoglycemic episodes. Glycemic control achieved with sulfonylureas is often better than with insulin, possibly because the β-cell defect is upstream of the sulphonylurea receptor; although insulin therapy may eventually be required, if β-cell deterioration progresses (14,15). MODY3 patients are at increased risk of diabetic retinopathy and nephropathy, but the frequency of cardiovascular disease is not increased (16,17).

The second most common form of MODY, MODY1, is due to mutations of the hepatocyte nuclear factor-4α gene (*HNF4A*). Like *TCF1*, *HNF4A* is a transcription factor that regulates several hepatic genes, including *TCF1* (6), and MODY mutations disrupt dimerization and transcriptional activity (18). Clinically, MODY1 is similar to MODY3, except that patients do not have the glycosuria and low renal threshold frequently seen in MODY3 patients (19,20). Patients with these transcription factor mutations have a range of extra-pancreatic complications and it can be difficult to tease apart organ-specific effects (9), although, as with other forms of diabetes, the severity of complications is generally impacted by the degree of glucose control. As with MODY3, patients usually respond well to low doses of sulfonylureas (21).

MODY2 is due to a heterozygous mutation in the glucokinase gene. Affected individuals have persistent mild fasting hyperglycemia, rarely requiring pharmacological treatment (usually dietary restrictions are sufficient). Parents may have a diagnosis of type 2 diabetes or, if undiagnosed, one parent will usually show mildly elevated fasting blood glucose (19). Glucokinase serves as the glucose "sensor" of insulin-producing β-cells. Affected individuals have a higher "set point", but rarely show significant deterioration of hyperglycemia (19) with only a 7 mmol/L increase in fasting glucose. Individuals with MODY2 have little response to oral hypoglycemic agents or insulin, since these exogenous agents reduce endogenous insulin secretion resulting in the same degree of hyperglycemia (22). Patients typically have HbA$_{1c}$ levels within or just above the normal range (22,23) and seldom experience microvascular or macrovascular complications, even when untreated (24).

MODY5 is caused by mutations in the gene for transcription factor 2 (*TCF2*), also known as hepatocyte nuclear factor-1β (*HNF1B*) (25). Although only identified in a small number of families, additional mechanisms of gene disruption have recently been identified, such as gene rearrangement (26) and exonic duplication (27). Investigation of patients with diabetes and slowly progressive nondiabetic nephropathy (28) suggests that this form of MODY may be more frequent than previously suspected (17). It is associated with pancreatic atrophy, renal developmental disorders such as renal cysts and renal dysplasia (28), genital tract malformations, and abnormal liver function tests (17). Clinical manifestation is related to the pattern of expression of *TCF2* in pancreas, urinary and genital tracts, and liver and biliary ducts during development (29,30). MODY5 patients are not sensitive to sulfonylureas and usually require insulin treatment (31).

The remaining known MODY subtypes have a much lower prevalence. Only a few families have been reported with MODY4, caused by mutations in the gene for insulin promoter factor 1 (*IPF1*) (32) and MODY6, due to mutations in neurogenic differentiation 1 (*NEUROD1*) gene (33,34). *IPF1* is a key regulator of insulin and somatostatin transcription (35–37) and glucose homeostasis (38), and is also critical for both exocrine and endocrine pancreas development (39,40). Missense and truncation mutations diminish or abolish its activity (41–43). *NEUROD1* forms a heterodimer with the ubiquitous helix–loop–helix protein E47, which regulates insulin gene expression by binding to the insulin promoter (44). As with *IPF1*, *NEUROD1* mutations that disrupt critical binding domains or result in premature protein termination have been noted (33). The Kruppel-like factor gene 11 (*KLF11* or *TIEG2*) gene was identified in a collection of families with type 2 diabetes with early onset of disease; *KLF11* acts as a glucose-inducible regulator of the insulin gene (45). Variants of *KLF11* impair transcriptional activity resulting in reduced insulin expression, suggesting this form of diabetes is MODY-like (MODY7) (45).

MODY8 has been described as a syndrome of diabetes and pancreatic exocrine dysfunction present in a small number of families, caused by mutations in the gene for carboxyl ester lipase, a major component of pancreatic juice which is responsible for the duodenal hydrolysis of cholesterol esters and retinyl esters prior to absorption (46). The symptoms (abdominal pain and loose stools) of this syndrome may be underreported in diabetes patients. A study of 1021 patients with typical type 1 or type 2 diabetes indicated the prevalence of fecal elastase deficiency may be as high as 23% (47), suggesting that systematic screening of exocrine dysfunction in the general diabetes population could identify additional subjects with this syndrome.

Neonatal Diabetes

Neonatal diabetes, generally defined as diabetes before the age of 6 months, has an incidence of 1 in 400,000 live births (48) and represents less than 1% of patients typically diagnosed with type 1 diabetes (49). It is classified clinically as either transient neonatal diabetes mellitus (TNDM) or permanent neonatal diabetes mellitus (PNDM), although the distinction is rarely evident at the time of diagnosis.

Most TNDM cases (79%) are due to an imprinting abnormality of the chromosome 6q24 region, containing *ZAC* and *HYMA1* genes. In simple terms, imprinted genes are switched off by the addition of a methyl group(s) generally in the promoter region, preventing gene transcription. The most common cause of TNDM is paternal duplication of this region, or paternal uniparental disomy where the child inherits two copies of this region of chromosome 6 from the father, with no contribution from the mother (50–52). Paternal uniparental isodisomy, paternal gene duplication, or differential methylation (imprinting) can result in a similar effect—overexpression of paternal copy(ies). In other cases, more localized methylation abnormalities have been noted (53). All of these situations lead to overexpression of ZAC and/or HYMA1 within the TNDM locus. Although it is not entirely clear at this point as to which gene is responsible, overexpression of zac1 in rat INS-1 cells impairs glucose-stimulated insulin secretion (54) and overexpression of the entire TNDM locus has been shown to reduce IPF1 expression in the embryonic mouse pancreas (55). Diabetes is usually diagnosed in the first week and may be associated with macroglossia (23% of cases) (51). Although TNDM resolves at a median of 12 weeks (51), approximately 60% will relapse, most often during adolescence (56). Initial insulin treatment can be reduced or ceased if diabetes resolves, and relapsed patients can frequently be treated with diet alone although they may require insulin therapy later in life (50).

Perhaps the best example of genetic information informing appropriate treatment is seen in patients with PNDM. Heterozygous activating mutations of the gene for the ATP-sensitive–inwardly-rectifying potassium channel subunit Kir6.2 (KCNJ11) cause 30% to 58% of cases of diabetes diagnosed in those younger than 6 months of age (57). In the β-cell, glucose metabolism increases intracellular ATP production from ADP. The increased ATP/ADP ratio leads to the closure of ATP-sensitive potassium channels and membrane depolarization. Subsequent activation of voltage-dependent calcium channels and influx of calcium result in insulin granule exocytosis (58). Patients with KCNJ11 mutations have K_{ATP} channels with decreased sensitivity to ATP (59–63), resulting in channels that remain open in the presence of glucose, consequently reducing insulin secretion (63,64) (Fig. 1). The majority of cases (80% to 90%) are due to de novo mutations (48), and cannot be identified on the basis of family history. Neurological features are observed in 20% of patients, and may be present as part of the developmental delay, epilepsy, and neonatal diabetes (DEND) syndrome, although a proportion of these patients have moderate development delay in the absence of epilepsy (63). KCNJ11 is expressed in β-cells, pituitary tissue, skeletal muscle, brain, and vascular and nonvascular smooth muscle and channels act by coupling metabolic activity, such as secretion or muscle contraction, to membrane potential (65). Mutations associated with severe disease bias the channel conformation toward the open state (61). Since patients present with hyperglycemia, undetectable C-peptide, and frequently (30%) ketoacidosis, they are often initially treated with insulin (63). However, a study of 49 patients showed that 90% could successfully be treated with sulfonylureas, with improved glycemic control and decreased HbA_{1c} levels maintained for at least 1 year of follow-up (57). The response to treatment also reflects the particular mutation carried by the patient. Subjects with the Q52R, I296L, and L164P mutations of the KCNJ11 gene show only modest responses to the sulfonylurea drug tolbutamide (61,62), and result in the more severe DEND syndrome (64), whereas those with the V59M mutation result in a less severe syndrome (64,66–68) and a greater degree of ATP sensitivity (69). The more common KCNJ11 R201H mutation has a 40-fold reduction in ATP

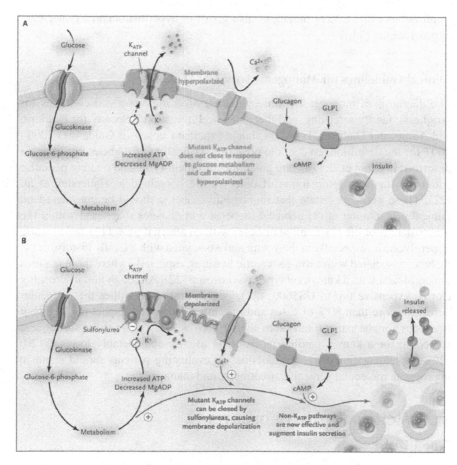

Figure 1   Proposed model of the action of sulfonylurea on β-cells expressing mutations in the Kir6.2 subunit of the K_{ATP} channel. *Source*: From Ref. 57.

sensitivity in the homozygous state (64), while G43R, G53S, and I182V have an approximately four-fold reduction in sensitivity to ATP (59). Understanding the functional characteristics of the mutation can help predict, to some extent, the likely success of sulfonylurea therapy.

The β-cell K_{ATP} channel is an octameric complex of 4 Kir6.2 units and 4 sulfonylurea receptor 1 (SUR1) units (70,71); the latter is encoded by the ATP-binding cassette C8 gene (*ABCC8*). While binding of ATP to Kir6.2 brings about channel closure, sulfonylurea drugs bind to the cytosolic nucleotide binding domains of SUR1 (72). Mutations in *ABCC8* are the most common cause of hyperinsulinemia of infancy (48), in which insulin is oversecreted even in the presence of hypoglycemia. Mutations can result in the absence of SUR1 on the membrane's surface, or to reduce surface expression of K_{ATP} channels (73). A small number of *KCNJ11* mutations also result in hyperinsulinemia, rather than hyperglycemia (74,75).

Clinical Guidelines for Monogenic Forms of Diabetes

The diagnosis of monogenic forms of diabetes has important consequences for prognosis, family screening, and therapy. The International Society for Pediatric and Adolescent Diabetes (ISPAD) Clinical Practice Consensus Guidelines 2006–2007 for the definition, epidemiology, and classification of diabetes mellitus are described in Craig et al. (76), and guidelines for identifying and treating pediatric patients with monogenic forms of diabetes are contained in Hattersley et al. (22). These guidelines state that monogenic diabetes should be considered on clinical presentation of (1) neonatal diabetes and diabetes diagnosed within the first 6 months of life (2), familial diabetes with an affected parent (3), mild fasting hyperglycemia, especially in the young and associated with a family history, or (4) diabetes associated with extra-pancreatic features, especially where these features are consistent with a known subtype or syndrome (22). Although initial screening can be expensive (up to US$600) (22), genetic testing identifies the molecular defect in more than 80% of cases and this information can impact management decisions for the patient and often their relatives (1). The cost for subsequent screening for a known familial mutation is usually considerably lower ($120) (22). Implementation of these guidelines in evaluating patients should result in appropriate molecular screening, treatment, and management.

MULTIFACTORIAL FORMS OF DIABETES

Type 1 Diabetes

T1D is associated with immune-mediated destruction of β-cells. As a result, there is a complete dependence upon exogenous insulin in order to regulate blood glucose levels. T1D is the third most prevalent chronic disease of childhood, affecting 0.3% of the general population by the age of 20 years and with a lifetime risk of nearly 1% (77). It is estimated that approximately 1.4 million individuals in the U.S.A. (10–20 million worldwide) have T1D (78). In most cases, a preclinical period marked by the presence of autoantibodies to pancreatic β-cell antigens (GAD$_{65}$, insulin, IA-2, zinc transporter 8) precedes the onset of hyperglycemia. This preclinical period provides a window of opportunity for secondary prevention (see chap. 6 for further information). T1D is strongly clustered in families with an overall genetic risk ratio (λ_S) of approximately 15 (79). To date, only four T1D susceptibility loci have been identified with convincing and reproducible statistical support: genes in the human major histocompatibility complex (the HLA class I and class II genes), insulin (*INS*), *CTLA4-ICOS*, and *PTPN22* genes. Additional genes and regions have been identified through genome-wide approaches, but have yet to be replicated.

Major Histocompatibility Complex (MHC)

At least one region (comprised of multiple loci) that contributes strongly to the familial clustering of T1D resides within the major histocompatibility complex (MHC) on chromosome 6p21. Genetic, functional, structural, and model studies, all suggest that the HLA class II genes (HLA-DRB1 and HLA-DQB1) likely represent the primary determinants of T1D risk. The frequency of HLA class II susceptibility alleles also correlates well with the population incidence of T1D (80). These studies suggest that the MHC (IDDM1) may account for about 40% of the observed familial clustering of T1D, with a locus-specific genetic risk ratio (λ_S) of approximately 3 (81). High-density genotyping within the MHC has identified a non-HLA candidate gene, inositol 1,4,5-triphosphate receptor 3 (*ITPR3*), as a strong candidate contributing to T1D risk (82). *ITPR3* mRNA and *ITPR3* protein are rapidly upregulated in pancreatic β-cells following stimulation with glucose and the protein is then rapidly degraded in proteasomes. Further, the double *ITPR2/ITPR3* knockout mouse is reported to be hypoglycemic and lean and to have impaired exocrine function. Thus, multiple genes in the MHC (HLA and non-HLA) may contribute to T1D risk.

Insulin

Early studies (83,84) established an association of T1D with the "class I" allele of a variable number of tandem repeats (VNTR) 5′ of the insulin gene (*INS*), with an increase in the homozygote frequency in T1D. T1D risk appears to be largely a dominant trait with the VNTR class III alleles encoding protection from disease. While the biological mechanism underlying the genetic risk has yet to be resolved, variation defined by the VNTR may affect the steady-state level of insulin mRNA in the thymus, thereby influencing immune tolerance to insulin and its precursors, now the favored autoantigens in T1D. Specifically, the class III VNTR alleles are associated with higher levels of insulin mRNA in the thymus, which may account for the associated reduction in risk (or protection) for T1D. The role of insulin in promoting β-cell destruction in T1D and the interaction of variation at the insulin locus with HLA to modify risk of T1D have yet to be fully resolved (85).

CTLA4

The IDDM12 locus lies within the 2q31-q33 region and has been attributed to SNPs in the 3′ UTR of *CTLA4* (86); however, the modest λ_S value predicted for the associated SNPs at *CTLA4* seem unlikely to fully account for the magnitude of the observed evidence for linkage. In the nonobese diabetic (NOD) mouse model of spontaneous autoimmune diabetes, much work in this homologous area has focused on both the *CTLA4* and the functionally polymorphic *NRAMP1* gene (87). Thus, this gene-rich region has yet to be completely resolved with respect to contribution to T1D risk.

PTPN22

Recently, evidence for association of T1D with alleles in the *PTPN22* locus at
1p13 has been reported (88) and replicated in multiple populations. *PTPN22*
encodes a lymphoid-specific tyrosine phosphatase and is also associated with
other autoimmune diseases, including thyroid disease, rheumatoid arthritis, and
systemic lupus erythematosus. The function of this phosphatase in signaling is
currently being explored. The biochemical basis by which *PTPN22* contributes to
the development of human autoimmune diseases may provide insight into common
pathogenic mechanisms and therapeutic targets/interventions.

Other Candidate Genes

T1D susceptibility genes have been identified using both family and case-control
approaches, but relatively few candidates have withstood replication in different
populations. Previously reported loci include *IDDM4* (11q13), *IDDM6* (18q12-
q21), *IDDM9* (3q22-q25), *IDDM11* (14q24-q31), *IDDM16* (14q32), *IDDM17*
(10q25), and *IDDM18* (5q33). While these proposed T1D susceptibility loci may
represent false-positive results, it is possible that they have small effects more
readily detected in certain populations due to variation in allele frequencies or
other factors, including population-specific genetic or environmental effects.

Results from Genome-Wide Association Scans

A genome-wide nonsynonymous SNP scan has been used in a search for additional T1D susceptibility genes (4). The third most associated SNP from this scan
was rs1990760 (A946T) from the interferon induced with helicase C domain 1
(*IFIH1*) gene on chromosome 2q24.3. *IFIH1* is an early type I interferon (IFN)
β-responsive gene, which may contribute to the apoptosis of virally infected cells
in anti-viral immune responses, thus making it a sensor or pathogen recognition
receptor for viral infection. This genetic association between T1D and *IFIH1*,
although yet to be replicated, could provide a molecular relationship between the
development of this autoimmune disease and viral infection. As more intensive
genome-wide scans are in progress, additional candidate genes will be uncovered,
requiring extensive replication and biological examination on their role in the
pathogenesis of T1D.

Recently, the Wellcome Trust Case-Control Consortium (WTCCC) conducted a first-stage genome-wide association scan (89). The scan used 2000 cases
for each of seven diseases and a common set of 3000 controls, genotyped for
500,000 SNPs that spanned the human genome. Two of the seven diseases in the
WTCCC were T1D and T2D. For both T1D and T2D, previously recognized susceptibility loci were confirmed and novel candidate genes were identified. For T1D,
the strongest asssociations were observed for SNPs in the MHC, *PTPN22*, *INS*,
CTLA4, *CD25/IL7R*, and *IFIH1* (90). Several new chromosomal regions exhibited
statistically significant ($P \leq 5 \times 10^{-7}$) associations with T1D. Confirmatory evidence of association resulted in identification of novel, putative susceptibility loci

(*CD226* in 18q22, *ERBB3* in 12q13, *KIAA0350* in 16p13, and *C12orf30* in 12q24) (90). While these findings warrant further replication and study, the number of potential T1D susceptibility genes has now increased to at least 10 in this (U.K. Caucasian) population. Nonetheless, these results further support the hypothesis that genes contributing to risk of T1D act in diverse pathways that involve immune recognition of antigens, T cell development, and immune regulation, all in response to (as yet unidentified) environmental triggers.

Type 2 Diabetes

A limited number of genetic variants have shown association with type 2 diabetes (T2D) across multiple populations. Some MODY and PNDM genes have been shown to contribute to typical, later-onset T1D, including *KCNJ11* (91–93), *HNF4 A* (94,95), and *TCF1* (96,97); although recent large-scale population studies of over 4000 patients and controls suggest that these genes may contribute only modestly, if at all, to the common form of T2D (98). Other confirmed diabetes genes include the genes for calpain 10 (*CAPN10*) (99,100) and peroxisome proliferator-activated receptor γ (*PPARG*) (101,102). The original observation of an association between the protein tyrosine phosphatase 1B gene (*PTPN1*) and T2D (103) and insulin sensitivity (104) has been supported by results from other European-origin populations (105–107), although no association with T2D was seen in a study of Scandanavian, Polish, U.S.A., and Québec case-control populations (108). Given the critical role of *PTP1B* in insulin signaling, small molecule inhibitors of PTP1B have been directly targeted for their therapeutic potential for some time (109), and interest in this area continues to increase (110–112).

Recently, association between the transcription factor 7-like 2 (*TCF7L2*) gene and T2D, first reported by Grant et al. (113) in Icelandic, Danish, and European American populations, has been confirmed in multiple populations of European, African, and East Asian ancestry. Grant et al. (113) suggested that *TCF7L2* may be affecting risk of T2D through regulation of GLP-1. Three prospective studies of *TCF7L2* variants have been reported. In the Diabetes Prevention Program (114), a multi-ethnic cohort, the hazard ratio between the two homozygous extremes for rs7903146, TT genotype versus CC genotype, was 1.55 (95% CI: 1.20–2.01, $P \leq 0.001$). Similarly, in the prospective Second Northwick Park Heart Study (NPHSII), a study of U.K. men with European ancestry, the TT versus CC genotype hazard ratio was 1.87 (0.99–3.53, $P \leq 0.01$) (115). A study of the French DESIR (data from an epidemiological study on the insulin resistance syndrome) cohort found the rs7903146 T allele predicted hyperglycemia (T2D and impaired fasting glucose combined), with a hazard ratio of 1.21 (1.05–1.39, $P = 0.008$) (116). The population attributable risk of certain variants, such as *TCF7L2* rs7903146, is relatively high, estimated from unselected prospective studies to be 17% to 18% for diabetes (114,115) and 10% for hyperglycemia (116).

Recent whole genome association studies confirmed known associations with *TCF7L2* (117–119), *PPARG* (89,119,120), and *KCNJ11* (89,119,120). A number of novel loci have been identified and many have been replicated across multiple populations. Consistently observed associations included SNPs in the gene for solute carrier family 30 (zinc transporter), member 8 (*SLC30A8*) on 8q24 (117,119–121), a zinc transporter, which is expressed exclusively in insulin-producing β-cells (117). Associations with insulin-like factor 2 mRNA binding protein 2 (*IGF2BP2*, also known as IMP-2) intron 2 on 3q27 (89,119–121), and CDK5 regulatory subunit associated protein 1-like 1 (*CDKAL1*) on 6p22.3 were also seen by several groups (118–121). *IGF2BP2* binds to the 5' UTR of the insulin-like growth factor 2 (IGF2) mRNA and regulates IGF2 translation (122). The function of *CDKAL1* is unknown, although CDK5 has been shown to have a role in loss of β-cell function under glucotoxic conditions (123), and inhibition of CDK5 protects β-cells in conditions of glucotoxicity (124). Regions containing hematopoietically expressed homeobox and insulin degrading enzyme (117,119–121), and a region on 9p approximately 125kb from the genes encoding *CDKN2A* and *CDKN2B*, were also associated in more than one study (89,119,120). Both *CDKN2A* and *CDKN2B* are expressed in islets (119), and *CDKN2A* plays a role in pancreatic islet regenerative capacity (125). Associations with the fat-mass and obesity associated (*FTO*) gene, mediated by adiposity, were also detected (89,119,121).

Considerable further work is necessary to determine the actual genes and SNPs responsible for these association signals, and how these influence diabetes risk. It should be noted that all investigations to date have been in populations of European ancestry, apart from the study of Steinthorsdottir et al. (118), who also investigated replication of several loci in Hong Kong Han Chinese and West Africans, and in general the odds ratios for associated alleles do not exceed 1.48, with most in the 1.10 to 1.25 range.

PREDICTION OF DIABETES RISK

One of the most promising applications of genetics is a diabetes risk profile. Identifying the genetic bases of T1D and T2D offers the prospect of approaching each patient as a biologically-defined individual, rather than as a reflection of a population-based risk estimate. This approach would radically alter the manner in which surveillance could be instituted, intervention (and the time of its initiation) employed, and pharmacologic interventions selected.

Prediction of Type 1 Diabetes

T1D is thought to be due to an autoimmune process promoted by environmental factors in genetically-susceptible individuals. The estimated extent of genetic susceptibility to the total risk of T1D is 30% to 50%, suggesting that the risk in any individual is equally due to genes and environment. From the 50% genetic susceptibility, nearly 50% of that (or 25% of the total risk) appears to be attributed to genes in the MHC. In order to augment this relatively low predictive power, there have been extensive searches for biomarkers of T1D risk. The most informative biomarkers identified to date are autoantibodies to islet antigens (insulin, GAD65, IA2/ICA512, Zn transporter 8). Combining these autoantibodies with HLA genotypes is relatively effective for predicting eventual development of T1D in otherwise healthy individuals (126), particularly in siblings of individuals with T1D. In a recent clinical trial (ENDIT) (127), 549 ICA-positive individuals with a family history of T1D were recruited from 20 countries. A total of 159 developed T1D within 5 years. Independent predictors of conversion to T1D were age, first-phase insulin response, baseline glucose tolerance and the number of additional antibody markers, but not specific antibody type or HLA genotype. This study suggested that at-risk individuals less than the age of 25 years with a positive family history of T1D and with two or more additional antibodies at baseline had a 62% risk of T1D occurring within 5 years. Whether additional genetic information would increase prediction, or whether the same criteria could be used in a general population (without a sibling with T1D), remains to be determined. Recent studies have also revealed that insulin resistance, a major component of the pathogenesis of T2D, is a significant risk factor for progression of autoantibody-positive, at-risk relatives to clinical T1D (128,129).

Prediction of Type 2 Diabetes

The presence of impaired glucose tolerance (IGT) combined with genetic information can be used to identify individuals at greatest risk of progression to T2D. The Finnish Diabetes Prevention Study investigated the effect of several polymorphisms on transition from IGT to T2D, including variants in cytokines (130), genes involved in insulin secretion (131), regulation of insulin secretion (132), or insulin signaling pathways (133), as well as the hepatic lipase gene (*LIPC*) (134). From these studies, polymorphisms significantly associated with conversion from IGT to diabetes were *TNFA* -308A (OR 1.80; 1.05–3.09, $P = 0.034$) (130), *ABCC8* 1273AGA (OR 2.0; 1.19–3.36, $P = 0.009$) (131); *SLC2A2* (encoding GLUT2) rs5393 (OR 3.04, 1.34–6.88, $P = 0.008$) (132); and *LIPC*-250GG (OR 1.80; 1.05–3.10; $P = 0.034$) (134). Additive results were also seen for *TNFA* -308A and *IL6* -174CC (OR 2.2, 1.02–4.85, $P = 0.045$) (130); and an *ABCC8* 3-SNP haplotype and *KCNJ11* 23K (OR 5.68, 1.75–18.32, $P = 0.004$) (131). In the Study to Prevent Non-Insulin Dependent Diabetes Mellitus (STOP-NIDDM) trial, designed to investigate the ability of acarbose to prevent T2D in a population with IGT, the *PPARG* 12PP genotype predicted conversion to diabetes in women in the acarbose treatment group (OR 2.89, 1.20–6.96, $P = 0.018$) (135), and adiponectin (*ADIPOQ*) +45G was associated with increased risk (OR 1.8, 1.12–3.00, $P = 0.015$) (136). Carriers of the PPAR-γ coativator 1α (*PPARGC1A*) 482S allele were responsive to acarbose treatment (135), while *ADIPOQ* +45G and +276T haplotype carriers in the placebo group had a higher risk of diabetes (OR 4.5, 1.78–11.3, $P = -0.001$) (136).

Weedon et al. (137) have shown that combinations of three known common variants (*KCNJ11* 23L, *PPARG* 12P, and *TCF7L2* rs7903146T) multiply the odds of T2D, and similar investigations of the effects of multiple variants in prospectively-followed cohorts are underway. Given the relatively high population attributable risk of certain variants, such as *TCF7L2* rs7903146, estimated from unselected prospective studies to be 17% to 18% for diabetes (114,115) and 10% for hyperglycemia (116), and future identification of additional diabetogenic contributors, it is likely that the predictive value of such genetic tests is likely to improve over time.

WHERE WILL WE BE IN FIVE YEARS?

Enormous changes in genetic, statistical, and bioinformatics technologies suggest many novel genes and biological pathways will be identified during the next 5 years that influence an individual's risk for T2D. These advances will not only be limited to the human genomic arena but will also include animal models of disease, innovative imaging of target tissues, and functional approaches to gene expression profiling. Within the context of human genetic research in T2D, several important advances are on the horizon.

As described, the molecular basis for diabetes risk is known for some rare Mendelian syndromes and a few candidate genes. Unfortunately, most individuals presenting with T2D also have other (inherited) risk factors, including obesity, hypertension, and components of the metabolic syndrome. Thus, individuals with T2D often lack distinctive phenotypes and would be expected to show incomplete penetrance, which makes gene discovery more complex.

Personalized Medicine

Two additional outcomes from the discovery of novel genes and pathways will emerge. The first—personalized medicine—stems from multiple advances in technology (biological and informatic). The primary goals for personalized medicine include integrating multiple data sources (genetic, clinical, pharmacologic, epidemiologic, imaging) into an individualized "risk profile", targeted to the individual. This requires not only detailed information that relates measured characteristics of an individual to clinical outcomes, but also the most effective (in terms of clinical outcome and cost) treatments, while maintaining privacy of a person's identity and personal data. The second is directly related to expected advances in technology—human genome sequencing. The goal of a single coverage of the human genome for $1000 may not be achieved in 5 years, but targeted sequencing will permit discovery of significant genetic variation at the individual level. The vast amount of data produced by the human DNA sequence will require new methods of analysis and informatics to determine which of the variants in a sequence may be disease-related.

Barriers to Personalized Medicine

With new technology, implementation in a health care environment may not be immediately obvious. Personalized medicine requires integration of several areas of health care that have typically been isolated. Key issues in personalized medicine are data availability and data flow. Much of the key health care information is maintained in electronic medical records; in many cases, this may be available for outpatients but may not be accessible. Further, utilization of existing data would require authorization (consent) by the patient. This may be appropriate for research (in terms of de-identification) but not for clinical practice. Finally, the collection of critical medical information into a comprehensive database is a formidable and costly task. Genetic information represents only one component of data in the realm of personalized medicine. It should meet the standards of ethics and scientific merit and significant clinical benefit (138).

REFERENCES

1. Gloyn AL, Ellard S. Defining the genetic aetiology of monogenic diabetes can improve treatment. Expert Opin Pharmacother 2006, 7(13):1759–1767.
2. Klein RJ, Zeiss C, Chew EY, et al. Complement factor H polymorphism in age-related macular degeneration. Science 2005; 308(5720):385–389.
3. Edwards AO, Ritter R III, Abel KJ, et al. Complement factor H polymorphism and age-related macular degeneration. Science 2005; 308(5720):421–424.
4. Smyth DJ, Cooper JD, Bailey R, et al. A genome-wide association study of nonsynonymous SNPs identifies a type 1 diabetes locus in the interferon-induced helicase (IFIH1) region. Nat Genet 2006; 38(6):617–619.
5. Duerr RH, Taylor KD, Brant SR, et al.A genome-wide association study identifies IL23R as an inflammatory bowel disease gene. Science 2006; 314(5804):1461–1463.
6. Fajans SS, Bell GI, Polonsky KS. Molecular mechanisms and clinical pathophysiology of maturity-onset diabetes of the young.N Engl J Med 2001; 345(13):971–980.
7. Owen K, Hattersley AT. Maturity-onset diabetes of the young: From clinical description to molecular genetic characterization. Best Pract Res Clin Endocrinol Metab 2001; 15(3):309–323.
8. American Diabetes Association Position Statement. Diagnosis and classification of diabetes mellitus. Diabetes Care 2004; 27(Suppl 1):S5–S10.
9. Stride A, Hattersley AT. Different genes, different diabetes: Lessons from maturity-onset diabetes of the young. Ann Med 2002; 34(3):207–216.
10. Odom DT, Zizlsperger N, Gordon DB, et al. Control of pancreas and liver gene expression by HNF transcription factors. Science 2004; 303(5662):1378–1381.
11. Hua QX, Zhao M, Narayana N, et al. Diabetes-associated mutations in a beta-cell transcription factor destabilize an antiparallel "mini-zipper" in a dimerization interface. Proc Natl Acad Sci U S A 2000; 97(5):1999–2004.
12. Byrne MM, Sturis J, Menzel S, et al. Altered insulin secretory responses to glucose in diabetic and nondiabetic subjects with mutations in the diabetes susceptibility gene MODY3 on chromosome 12. Diabetes 1996; 45(11):1503–1510.

13. Isomaa B, Henricsson M, Lehto M, et al. Chronic diabetic complications in patients with MODY3 diabetes. Diabetologia 1998; 41(4):467–473.
14. Shepherd M, Pearson ER, Houghton J, et al. No deterioration in glycemic control in HNF-1alpha maturity-onset diabetes of the young following transfer from long-term insulin to sulphonylureas. Diabetes Care 2003; 26(11):3191–3192.
15. Pearson ER, Starkey BJ, Powell RJ, et al. Genetic cause of hyperglycaemia and response to treatment in diabetes. Lancet 2003; 362(9392):1275–1281.
16. Timsit J, Bellanne-Chantelot C, Dubois-Laforgue D, et al. Diagnosis and management of maturity-onset diabetes of the young. Treat Endocrinol 2005; 4(1):9–18.
17. Olek K. Maturity-onset diabetes of the young: An update. Clin Lab 2006; 52(11–12):593–598.
18. Stoffel M, Duncan SA. The maturity-onset diabetes of the young (MODY1) transcription factor HNF4alpha regulates expression of genes required for glucose transport and metabolism. Proc Natl Acad Sci USA 1997; 94(24):13209–13214.
19. Stride A, Vaxillaire M, Tuomi T, et al. The genetic abnormality in the beta cell determines the response to an oral glucose load. Diabetologia 2002; 45(3):427–435.
20. Pearson ER, Pruhova S, Tack CJ, et al. Molecular genetics and phenotypic characteristics of MODY caused by hepatocyte nuclear factor 4alpha mutations in a large European collection. Diabetologia 2005; 48(5):878–885.
21. Fajans SS, Brown MB. Administration of sulfonylureas can increase glucose-induced insulin secretion for decades in patients with maturity-onset diabetes of the young. Diabetes Care 1993; 16(9):1254–1261.
22. Hattersley A, Bruining J, Shield J, et al. ISPAD Clinical Practice Consensus Guidelines 2006–2007. The diagnosis and management of monogenic diabetes in children. Pediatr Diabetes 2006; 7(6):352–360.
23. Page RC, Hattersley AT, Levy JC, et al. Clinical characteristics of subjects with a missense mutation in glucokinase. Diabet Med 1995; 12(3):209–217.
24. Velho G, Blanche H, Vaxillaire M, et al. Identification of 14 new glucokinase mutations and description of the clinical profile of 42 MODY-2 families. Diabetologia 1997; 40(2):217–224.
25. Bingham C, Hattersley AT. Renal cysts and diabetes syndrome resulting from mutations in hepatocyte nuclear factor-1beta. Nephrol Dial Transplant 2004; 19(11):2703–2708.
26. Bellanne-Chantelot C, Clauin S, Chauveau D, et al. Large genomic rearrangements in the hepatocyte nuclear factor-1beta (TCF2) gene are the most frequent cause of maturity-onset diabetes of the young type 5. Diabetes 2005; 54(11):3126–3132.
27. Carette C, Vaury C, Barthelemy A, et al. Exonic duplication of the HNF-1{beta} gene (TCF2) as a cause of MODY5. J Clin Endocrinol Metab 2007; 92(7):2844–2847.
28. Bellanne-Chantelot C, Chauveau D, Gautier JF, et al. Clinical spectrum associated with hepatocyte nuclear factor-1beta mutations. Ann Intern Med 2004; 140(7):510–517.
29. Kolatsi-Joannou M, Bingham C, Ellard S, et al. Hepatocyte nuclear factor-1beta: A new kindred with renal cysts and diabetes and gene expression in normal human development. J Am Soc Nephrol 2001; 12(10):2175–2180.
30. Edghill EL, Bingham C, Slingerland AS, et al. Hepatocyte nuclear factor-1 beta mutations cause neonatal diabetes and intrauterine growth retardation: Support for

a critical role of HNF-1beta in human pancreatic development. Diabet Med 2006; 23(12):1301–1306.

31. Pearson ER, Badman MK, Lockwood CR, et al. Contrasting diabetes phenotypes associated with hepatocyte nuclear factor-1alpha and -1beta mutations. Diabetes Care 2004; 27(5):1102–1107.

32. Stoffers DA, Ferrer J, Clarke WL, et al. Early-onset type-II diabetes mellitus (MODY4) linked to IPF1. Nat Genet 1997; 17(2):138–139.

33. Malecki MT, Jhala US, Antonellis A, et al. Mutations in NEUROD1 are associated with the development of type 2 diabetes mellitus. Nat Genet 1999; 23(3):323–328.

34. Kristinsson SY, Thorolfsdottir ET, Talseth B, et al. MODY in Iceland is associated with mutations in HNF-1alpha and a novel mutation in NeuroD1. Diabetologia 2001; 44(11):2098–2103.

35. Ohlsson H, Karlsson K, Edlund T. IPF1, a homeodomain-containing transactivator of the insulin gene. Embo J 1993; 12(11):4251–4259.

36. Leonard J, Peers B, Johnson T, et al. Characterization of somatostatin transactivating factor-1, a novel homeobox factor that stimulates somatostatin expression in pancreatic islet cells. Mol Endocrinol 1993; 7(10):1275–1283.

37. Miller CP, McGehee RE Jr, Habener JF. IDX-1: A new homeodomain transcription factor expressed in rat pancreatic islets and duodenum that transactivates the somatostatin gene. Embo J 1994; 13(5):1145–1156.

38. Hart AW, Baeza N, Apelqvist A, et al. Attenuation of FGF signalling in mouse beta-cells leads to diabetes. Nature 2000; 408(6814):864–868.

39. Jonsson J, Carlsson L, Edlund T, et al. Insulin-promoter-factor 1 is required for pancreas development in mice. Nature 1994; 371(6498):606–609.

40. Jonsson J, Ahlgren U, Edlund T, et al. IPF1, a homeodomain protein with a dual function in pancreas development. Int J Dev Biol 1995; 39(5):789–798.

41. Stoffers DA, Zinkin NT, Stanojevic V, et al. Pancreatic agenesis attributable to a single nucleotide deletion in the human IPF1 gene coding sequence. Nat Genet 1997; 15(1):106–110.

42. Macfarlane WM, Frayling TM, Ellard S, et al. Missense mutations in the insulin promoter factor-1 gene predispose to type 2 diabetes. J Clin Invest 1999; 104(9):R33–R39.

43. Hani EH, Stoffers DA, Chevre JC, et al. Defective mutations in the insulin promoter factor-1 (IPF-1) gene in late-onset type 2 diabetes mellitus. J Clin Invest 1999; 104(9):R41–R48.

44. Naya FJ, Stellrecht CM, Tsai MJ. Tissue-specific regulation of the insulin gene by a novel basic helix-loop-helix transcription factor. Genes Dev 1995; 9(8):1009–1019.

45. Neve B, Fernandez-Zapico ME, Ashkenazi-Katalan V, et al. Role of transcription factor KLF11 and its diabetes-associated gene variants in pancreatic beta-cell function. Proc Natl Acad Sci USA 2005; 102(13):4807–4812.

46. Raeder H, Johansson S, Holm PI, et al. Mutations in the CEL VNTR cause a syndrome of diabetes and pancreatic exocrine dysfunction. Nat Genet 2006; 38(1):54–62.

47. Hardt PD, Hauenschild A, Nalop J, et al. High prevalence of exocrine pancreatic insufficiency in diabetes mellitus. A multicenter study screening fecal elastase 1 concentrations in 1021 diabetic patients. Pancreatology 2003; 3(5):395–402.

48. Gloyn AL, Siddiqui J, Ellard S. Mutations in the genes encoding the pancreatic beta-cell KATP channel subunits Kir6.2 (KCNJ11) and SUR1 (ABCC8) in diabetes mellitus and hyperinsulinism. Hum Mutat 2006; 27(3):220–231.

49. Iafusco D, Stazi MA, Cotichini R, et al. Permanent diabetes mellitus in the first year of life. Diabetologia 2002; 45(6):798–804.

50. Polak M, Shield J. Neonatal and very-early-onset diabetes mellitus. Semin Neonatol 2004; 9(1):59–65.

51. Temple IK, Gardner RJ, Mackay DJ, et al. Transient neonatal diabetes: Widening the understanding of the etiopathogenesis of diabetes. Diabetes 2000; 49(8):1359–1366.

52. Mackay DJ, Coupe AM, Shield JP, et al. Relaxation of imprinted expression of ZAC and HYMAI in a patient with transient neonatal diabetes mellitus. Hum Genet 2002; 110(2):139–144.

53. Gardner RJ, Mackay DJ, Mungall AJ, et al. An imprinted locus associated with transient neonatal diabetes mellitus. Hum Mol Genet 2000; 9(4):589–596.

54. Polychronakos C, Xiaoyu D. Graded overexpression of ZAC impairs glucose stimulated insulin secretion in beta-cells. In: American Diabetes Association Scientific Sessions, 2006. Abstract no.190–0R.

55. Ma D, Shield JP, Dean W, et al. Impaired glucose homeostasis in transgenic mice expressing the human transient neonatal diabetes mellitus locus, TNDM. J Clin Invest 2004; 114(3):339–348.

56. Shield JP. Neonatal diabetes: How research unravelling the genetic puzzle has both widened our understanding of pancreatic development whilst improving children's quality of life. Horm Res 2007; 67(2):77–83.

57. Pearson ER, Flechtner I, Njolstad PR, et al. Switching from insulin to oral sulfonylureas in patients with diabetes due to Kir6.2 mutations. N Engl J Med 2006; 355(5):467–477.

58. Ashcroft FM, Harrison DE, Ashcroft SJ. Glucose induces closure of single potassium channels in isolated rat pancreatic beta-cells. Nature 1984; 312(5993):446–448.

59. Gloyn AL, Reimann F, Girard C, et al. Relapsing diabetes can result from moderately activating mutations in KCNJ11. Hum Mol Genet 2005; 14(7):925–934.

60. Gloyn AL, Cummings EA, Edghill EL, et al. Permanent neonatal diabetes due to paternal germline mosaicism for an activating mutation of the KCNJ11 Gene encoding the Kir6.2 subunit of the beta-cell potassium adenosine triphosphate channel. J Clin Endocrinol Metab 2004; 89(8):3932–3935.

61. Proks P, Antcliff JF, Lippiat J, et al. Molecular basis of Kir6.2 mutations associated with neonatal diabetes or neonatal diabetes plus neurological features. Proc Natl Acad Sci U S A 2004; 101(50):17539–17544.

62. Proks P, Girard C, Haider S, et al. A gating mutation at the internal mouth of the Kir6.2 pore is associated with DEND syndrome. EMBO Rep 2005; 6(5):470–475.

63. Hattersley AT, Ashcroft FM. Activating mutations in Kir6.2 and neonatal diabetes: New clinical syndromes, new scientific insights, and new therapy. Diabetes 2005; 54(9):2503–2513.

64. Gloyn AL, Pearson ER, Antcliff JF, et al. Activating mutations in the gene encoding the ATP-sensitive potassium-channel subunit Kir6.2 and permanent neonatal diabetes. N Engl J Med 2004; 350(18):1838–1849.

65. Inagaki N, Gonoi T, Clement JPt, et al. Reconstitution of IKATP: An inward rectifier subunit plus the sulfonylurea receptor. Science 1995; 270(5239):1166–1170.
66. Massa O, Iafusco D, D'Amato E, et al. KCNJ11 activating mutations in Italian patients with permanent neonatal diabetes. Hum Mutat 2005; 25(1):22–27.
67. Sagen JV, Raeder H, Hathout E, et al. Permanent neonatal diabetes due to mutations in KCNJ11 encoding Kir6.2: patient characteristics and initial response to sulfonylurea therapy. Diabetes 2004; 53(10):2713–2718.
68. Vaxillaire M, Populaire C, Busiah K, et al. Kir6.2 mutations are a common cause of permanent neonatal diabetes in a large cohort of French patients. Diabetes 2004; 53(10):2719–2722.
69. Proks P, Girard C, Ashcroft FM. Functional effects of KCNJ11 mutations causing neonatal diabetes: Enhanced activation by MgATP. Hum Mol Genet 2005; 14(18):2717–2726.
70. Clement JPt, Kunjilwar K, Gonzalez G, et al. Association and stoichiometry of K(ATP) channel subunits. Neuron 1997; 18(5):827–838.
71. Inagaki N, Gonoi T, Seino S. Subunit stoichiometry of the pancreatic beta-cell ATP-sensitive K+ channel. FEBS Lett 1997; 409(2):232–236.
72. Ashcroft FM. Mechanisms of the glycaemic effects of sulfonylureas. Horm Metab Res 1996; 28(9):456–463.
73. Ashcroft FM. ATP-sensitive potassium channelopathies: Focus on insulin secretion. J Clin Invest 2005; 115(8):2047–2058.
74. Nestorowicz A, Wilson BA, Schoor KP, et al. Mutations in the sulfonylurea receptor gene are associated with familial hyperinsulinism in Ashkenazi Jews. Hum Mol Genet 1996; 5(11):1813–1822.
75. Marthinet E, Bloc A, Oka Y, et al. Severe congenital hyperinsulinism caused by a mutation in the Kir6.2 subunit of the adenosine triphosphate-sensitive potassium channel impairing trafficking and function. J Clin Endocrinol Metab 2005; 90(9):5401–5406.
76. Craig ME, Hattersley A, Donaghue K. ISPAD Clinical Practice Consensus Guidelines 2006–2007. Definition, epidemiology and classification. Pediatr Diabetes 2006; 7(6):343–351.
77. Rewers M, LaPorte RE, King H, et al. Trends in the prevalence and incidence of diabetes: Insulin-dependent diabetes mellitus in childhood. World Health Stat Q 1988; 41(3–4):179–189.
78. Libman I, Songer T, LaPorte R. How many people in the U.S. have IDDM? Diabetes Care 1993; 16(5):841–842.
79. Pociot F, McDermott MF. Genetics of type 1 diabetes mellitus. Genes Immun 2002; 3(5):235–249.
80. Ronningen KS, Keiding N, Green A. Correlations between the incidence of childhood-onset type I diabetes in Europe and HLA genotypes. Diabetologia 2001; 44(Suppl 3):B51–B59.
81. Rich SS. Mapping genes in diabetes. Genetic epidemiological perspective. Diabetes 1990; 39(11):1315–1319.
82. Roach JC, Deutsch K, Li S, et al. Genetic mapping at 3-kilobase resolution reveals inositol 1,4,5-triphosphate receptor 3 as a risk factor for type 1 diabetes in Sweden. Am J Hum Genet 2006; 79(4):614–627.

83. Bennett ST, Lucassen AM, Gough SC, et al. Susceptibility to human type 1 diabetes at IDDM2 is determined by tandem repeat variation at the insulin gene minisatellite locus. Nat Genet 1995; 9(3):284–292.

84. Julier C, Lucassen A, Villedieu P, et al. Multiple DNA variant association analysis: Application to the insulin gene region in type I diabetes. Am J Hum Genet 1994; 55(6):1247–1254.

85. Marchand L, Polychronakos C. Evaluation of polymorphic splicing in the mechanism of the association of the insulin gene with diabetes. Diabetes 2007; 56 (3):709–713.

86. Ueda H, Howson JM, Esposito L, et al. Association of the T-cell regulatory gene CTLA4 with susceptibility to autoimmune disease. Nature 2003; 423(6939):506–511.

87. Wicker LS, Chamberlain G, Hunter K, et al. Fine mapping, gene content, comparative sequencing, and expression analyses support Ctla4 and Nramp1 as candidates for Idd5.1 and Idd5.2 in the nonobese diabetic mouse. J Immunol 2004; 173(1):164–173.

88. Bottini N, Musumeci L, Alonso A, et al. A functional variant of lymphoid tyrosine phosphatase is associated with type I diabetes. Nat Genet 2004; 36(4):337–338.

89. The Wellcome Trust Case Control Consortium. Genome-wide association study of 14,000 cases of seven common diseases and 3000 shared controls. Nature 2007; 447(7145):661–678.

90. Todd JA, Walker NM, Cooper JD, et al. Robust associations of four new chromosome regions from genome-wide analyses of type 1 diabetes. Nat Genet 2007; 39(7):857–864.

91. Nielsen EM, Hansen L, Carstensen B, et al. The E23K variant of Kir6.2 associates with impaired post-OGTT serum insulin response and increased risk of type 2 diabetes. Diabetes 2003; 52(2):573–577.

92. Gloyn AL, Weedon MN, Owen KR, et al. Large-scale association studies of variants in genes encoding the pancreatic beta-cell KATP channel subunits Kir6.2 (KCNJ11) and SUR1 (ABCC8) confirm that the KCNJ11 E23K variant is associated with type 2 diabetes. Diabetes 2003; 52(2):568–572.

93. van Dam RM, Hoebee B, Seidell JC, et al. Common variants in the ATP-sensitive K+ channel genes KCNJ11 (Kir6.2) and ABCC8 (SUR1) in relation to glucose intolerance: Population-based studies and meta-analyses. Diabet Med 2005; 22(5):590–598.

94. Love-Gregory LD, Wasson J, Ma J, et al. A common polymorphism in the upstream promoter region of the hepatocyte nuclear factor-4 alpha gene on chromosome 20q is associated with type 2 diabetes and appears to contribute to the evidence for linkage in an ashkenazi jewish population. Diabetes 2004; 53(4):1134–1140.

95. Silander K, Mohlke KL, Scott LJ, et al. Genetic variation near the hepatocyte nuclear factor-4 alpha gene predicts susceptibility to type 2 diabetes. Diabetes 2004; 53(4):1141–1149.

96. Weedon MN, Owen KR, Shields B, et al. A large-scale association analysis of common variation of the HNF1alpha gene with type 2 diabetes in the U.K. Caucasian population. Diabetes 2005; 54(8):2487–2491.

97. Winckler W, Burtt NP, Holmkvist J, et al. Association of common variation in the HNF1alpha gene region with risk of type 2 diabetes. Diabetes 2005; 54(8):2336–2342.

98. Winckler W, Weedon MN, Graham RR, et al. Evaluation of common variants in the six known maturity-onset diabetes of the young (MODY) genes for association with type 2 diabetes. Diabetes 2007; 56(3):685–693.

99. Horikawa Y, Oda N, Cox NJ, et al. Genetic variation in the gene encoding calpain-10 is associated with type 2 diabetes mellitus. Nat Genet 2000; 26(2):163–175.

100. Cox NJ, Hayes MG, Roe CA, et al. Linkage of calpain 10 to type 2 diabetes: the biological rationale. Diabetes 2004; 53(Suppl 1):S19–S25.

101. Deeb SS, Fajas L, Nemoto M, et al. A Pro12Ala substitution in PPARgamma2 associated with decreased receptor activity, lower body mass index and improved insulin sensitivity. Nat Genet 1998; 20(3):284–287.

102. Altshuler D, Hirschhorn JN, Klannemark M, et al. The common PPARgamma Pro12Ala polymorphism is associated with decreased risk of type 2 diabetes. Nat Genet 2000; 26(1):76–80.

103. Bento JL, Palmer ND, Mychaleckyj JC, et al. Association of protein tyrosine phosphatase 1B gene polymorphisms with type 2 diabetes. Diabetes 2004; 53(11):3007–3012.

104. Palmer ND, Bento JL, Mychaleckyj JC, et al. Association of protein tyrosine phosphatase 1B gene polymorphisms with measures of glucose homeostasis in Hispanic Americans: The insulin resistance atherosclerosis study (IRAS) family study. Diabetes 2004; 53(11):3013–3019.

105. Ukkola O, Rankinen T, Lakka T, et al. Protein tyrosine phosphatase 1B variant associated with fat distribution and insulin metabolism. Obes Res 2005; 13(5):829–834.

106. Spencer-Jones NJ, Wang X, Snieder H, et al. Protein tyrosine phosphatase-1B gene PTPN1: Selection of tagging single nucleotide polymorphisms and association with body fat, insulin sensitivity, and the metabolic syndrome in a normal female population. Diabetes 2005; 54(11):3296–3304.

107. Cheyssac C, Lecoeur C, Dechaume A, et al. Analysis of common PTPN1 gene variants in type 2 diabetes, obesity and associated phenotypes in the French population. BMC Med Genet 2006; 7:44.

108. Florez JC, Agapakis CM, Burtt NP, et al. Association testing of the protein tyrosine phosphatase 1B gene (PTPN1) with type 2 diabetes in 7883 people. Diabetes 2005; 54(6):1884–1891.

109. Tobin JF, Tam S. Recent advances in the development of small molecule inhibitors of PTP1B for the treatment of insulin resistance and type 2 diabetes. Curr Opin Drug Discov Devel 2002; 5(4):500–512.

110. Rao GS, Ramachandran MV, Bajaj JS. In silico structure-based design of a potent and selective small peptide inhibitor of protein tyrosine phosphatase 1B, a novel therapeutic target for obesity and type 2 diabetes mellitus: A computer modeling approach. J Biomol Struct Dyn 2006; 23(4):377–384.

111. Lee S, Wang Q. Recent development of small molecular specific inhibitor of protein tyrosine phosphatase 1B. Med Res Rev. 2007; 27(4):553–573.

112. Ala PJ, Gonneville L, Hillman M, et al. Structural insights into the design of non-peptidic isothiazolidinone-containing inhibitors of protein tyrosine phosphatase 1B. J Biol Chem. 2006; 281(49):38013–38021.

113. Grant SF, Thorleifsson G, Reynisdottir I, et al. Variant of transcription factor 7-like 2 (TCF7L2) gene confers risk of type 2 diabetes. Nat Genet 2006; 38(3):320–323.

114. Florez JC, Jablonski KA, Bayley N, et al. TCF7L2 polymorphisms and progression to diabetes in the Diabetes Prevention Program. N Engl J Med 2006; 355(3):241–250.

115. Humphries SE, Gable D, Cooper JA, et al. Common variants in the TCF7L2 gene and predisposition to type 2 diabetes in UK European Whites, Indian Asians and Afro-Caribbean men and women. J Mol Med. 2006; 84(12):1005–1014.

116. Cauchi S, Meyre D, Choquet H, et al. TCF7L2 Variation Predicts Hyperglycemia Incidence in a French General Population: The Data From an Epidemiological Study on the Insulin Resistance Syndrome (DESIR) Study. Diabetes 2006; 55(11):3189–3192.

117. Sladek R, Rocheleau G, Rung J, et al. A genome-wide association study identifies novel risk loci for type 2 diabetes. Nature 2007; 445(7130):881–885.

118. Steinthorsdottir V, Thorleifsson G, Reynisdottir I, et al. A variant in CDKAL1 influences insulin response and risk of type 2 diabetes. Nat Genet 2007; 39(6):770–775.

119. Scott LJ, Mohlke KL, Bonnycastle LL, et al. A genome-wide association study of type 2 diabetes in Finns detects multiple susceptibility variants. Science 2007; 316(5829):1341–1345.

120. Saxena R, Voight BF, Lyssenko V, et al. Genome-wide association analysis identifies loci for type 2 diabetes and triglyceride levels. Science 2007; 316(5829):1331–1336.

121. Zeggini E, Weedon MN, Lindgren CM, et al. Replication of genome-wide association signals in UK samples reveals risk loci for type 2 diabetes. Science 2007; 316(5829):1336–1341.

122. Nielsen FC, Nielsen J, Christiansen J. A family of IGF-II mRNA binding proteins (IMP) involved in RNA trafficking. Scand J Clin Lab Invest Suppl 2001; 234:93–99.

123. Wei FY, Nagashima K, Ohshima T, et al. Cdk5-dependent regulation of glucose-stimulated insulin secretion. Nat Med 2005; 11(10):1104–1108.

124. Ubeda M, Rukstalis JM, Habener JF. Inhibition of cyclin-dependent kinase 5 activity protects pancreatic beta-cells from glucotoxicity. J Biol Chem 2006; 281(39):28858–28864.

125. Krishnamurthy J, Ramsey MR, Ligon KL, et al. p16INK4a induces an age-dependent decline in islet regenerative potential. Nature 2006; 443(7110):453–457.

126. Wasserfall CH, Atkinson MA. Autoantibody markers for the diagnosis and prediction of type 1 diabetes. Autoimmun Rev 2006; 5(6):424–428.

127. Bingley PJ, Gale EA. Progression to type 1 diabetes in islet cell antibody-positive relatives in the European Nicotinamide Diabetes Intervention Trial: the role of additional immune, genetic and metabolic markers of risk. Diabetologia 2006; 49(5):881–890.

128. Fourlanos S, Narendran P, Byrnes GB, Colman PG, Harrison LC. Insulin resistance is a risk factor for progression to type 1 diabetes. Diabetologia 2004 Oct; 47(10):1661–1667.

129. Xu P, Cuthbertson D, Greenbaum C, et al. Role of insulin resistance in predicting progression to type 1 diabetes. Diabetes Care 2007 Sep; 30(9):2314–2320.

130. Kubaszek A, Pihlajamaki J, Komarovski V, et al. Promoter polymorphisms of the TNF-alpha (G-308A) and IL-6 (C-174G) genes predict the conversion from impaired glucose tolerance to type 2 diabetes: The Finnish Diabetes Prevention Study. Diabetes 2003; 52(7):1872–1876.

131. Laukkanen O, Pihlajamaki J, Lindstrom J, et al. Polymorphisms of the SUR1 (ABCC8) and Kir6.2 (KCNJ11) genes predict the conversion from impaired glucose tolerance to type 2 diabetes. The Finnish Diabetes Prevention Study. J Clin Endocrinol Metab 2004; 89(12):6286–6290.

132. Laukkanen O, Lindstrom J, Eriksson J, et al. Polymorphisms in the SLC2A2 (GLUT2) gene are associated with the conversion from impaired glucose tolerance to type 2 diabetes: The Finnish Diabetes Prevention Study. Diabetes 2005; 54(7):2256–2260.

133. Laukkanen O, Pihlajamaki J, Lindstrom J, et al. Common polymorphisms in the genes regulating the early insulin signalling pathway: effects on weight change and the conversion from impaired glucose tolerance to Type 2 diabetes. The Finnish Diabetes Prevention Study. Diabetologia 2004; 47(5):871–877.

134. Todorova B, Kubaszek A, Pihlajamaki J, et al. The G-250A promoter polymorphism of the hepatic lipase gene predicts the conversion from impaired glucose tolerance to type 2 diabetes mellitus: The Finnish Diabetes Prevention Study. J Clin Endocrinol Metab 2004; 89(5):2019–2023.

135. Andrulionyte L, Zacharova J, Chiasson JL, et al. Common polymorphisms of the PPAR-gamma2 (Pro12Ala) and PGC-1alpha (Gly482Ser) genes are associated with the conversion from impaired glucose tolerance to type 2 diabetes in the STOP-NIDDM trial. Diabetologia 2004; 47(12):2176–2184.

136. Zacharova J, Chiasson JL, Laakso M. The common polymorphisms (single nucleotide polymorphism [SNP] +45 and SNP +276) of the adiponectin gene predict the conversion from impaired glucose tolerance to type 2 diabetes: The STOP-NIDDM trial. Diabetes 2005; 54(3):893–899.

137. Weedon MN, McCarthy MI, Hitman G, et al. Combining Information from Common Type 2 Diabetes Risk Polymorphisms Improves Disease Prediction. PLoS Med 2006; 3(10):e374.

138. Knoppers BM, Joly Y, Simard J, et al. The emergence of an ethical duty to disclose genetic research results: international perspectives. Eur J Hum Genet 2006; 14(11):1170–1178.

3

Early Detection and Prediction of Type 2 Diabetes

Jonathan E. Shaw and Paul Z. Zimmet

International Diabetes Institute, Melbourne, Victoria, Australia

INTRODUCTION

Diabetes is now estimated to affect 246 million people worldwide, with this figure expected to rise to 380 million by the year 2025 (1). The rising numbers of people with diabetes, fuelled by an increasing prevalence of obesity, may soon start to reverse the reductions in cardiovascular disease (CVD) mortality that have resulted from improved control of risk factors (smoking, hypertension and dyslipidemia), and better treatment of acute CVD events, over recent decades.

Approximately 90% of those with diabetes have type 2 diabetes but substantial proportions of those with type 2 diabetes are undiagnosed. Data from Australia, typical of many other developed countries, show that 50% of all those with diabetes are undiagnosed (2), with much higher figures reported in developing countries (3). As a result of the often long time interval between actual disease onset and the time of clinical diagnosis, up to 50% of patients will have evidence of diabetic complications by the time of diagnosis.

Screening for the presence of undiagnosed diabetes thus seems to be a logical next step, and ought to reduce the risk of both microvascular and macrovascular complications of diabetes by allowing treatment to commence earlier in the natural history of disease. The argument is supported by strong evidence in recent years that the risk of developing type 2 diabetes can be reduced substantially, by both lifestyle and pharmacological interventions among those at high risk (4). This reinforces the need to identify those at risk of developing type 2 diabetes, as well as those who already have the disease. However, it should also be emphasized

41

that, like any intervention, screening for preclinical disease must be adequately evaluated before introduction to routine practice.

This chapter will describe the evidence for and against the use of screening programs for type 2 diabetes, and will then detail the methods and algorithms available for screening.

TO SCREEN OR NOT TO SCREEN

Screening for a disease can only be justified when the following conditions regarding the disease are met:

- It represents an important health problem.
- It is present at a high enough prevalence (within the total or a specific target population) to make screening cost-effective.
- It has a relatively long asymptomatic phase, during which cases can be identified by screening that would not normally come to light.
- It is amenable to interventions that have a proven, beneficial effect on clinically meaningful outcomes.

Furthermore, the test for the disease must be safe, acceptable to the target population, and must have adequate sensitivity and specificity. Ideally, any screening program should be assessed in randomized controlled trials, measuring health outcomes and costs in screened and unscreened populations. While screening programs for certain cancers have been proven in randomized controlled trials to reduce morbidity and mortality, such studies have not been undertaken in type 2 diabetes. Thus, definitive proof for the value of screening for type 2 diabetes is not available. In the absence of such information, screening may be thought to be worthwhile, if all or most of the above conditions are fulfilled. Some of the relevant data for type 2 diabetes are outlined below.

1. Type 2 diabetes affects up to 9% (5) of the adult population (older than 20 years) in the developed world, with higher rates in parts of the developing world. Approximately, 50% of the cases are undiagnosed in Europid groups but many more are undiagnosed in most developing countries and in underprivileged, minority groups in developed countries (3).
2. Diabetic complications are common at the time of clinical diagnosis and less frequent among people diagnosed during screening surveys. It has been estimated that type 2 diabetes begins 4 to 7 years before the time of clinical diagnosis (6).
3. The U.K. Prospective Diabetes Study (UKPDS) demonstrated that aggressive blood glucose and blood pressure–lowering therapy in newly diagnosed (after clinical presentation) people with diabetes reduces the risk of long-term complications (7,8).
4. Studies of people with impaired glucose tolerance, who are at high risk of developing diabetes, show that lifestyle intervention reduces the risk

of developing diabetes by about 60%, while pharmacological interventions reduce the risk by 25% to 60% (4).

5. Hyperglycemia is an important cardiovascular risk factor. The risk is apparent among people with diabetes, impaired glucose tolerance (IGT), impaired fasting glucose (IFG) (9,10), and even high-normal fasting plasma glucose (FPG 4.7–6.0 mmol/L) (11), and the absolute risk of CVD is significantly increased by the presence of diabetes. Ample evidence now clearly shows that treatment with angiotensin converting enzyme inhibitors and statins reduces mortality and morbidity in people with diabetes (12). This indicates that knowledge of an individual's diabetes status is important as a basis on which treatment to prevent CVD is instituted.

The above summary stands as strong circumstantial evidence in favour of screening for type 2 diabetes. However, screening programs are large and costly, and like all interventions, have the potential to cause harm. Some of the potential disadvantages are summarized below.

1. Screening programs for diabetes typically involve several steps: identifying those who need blood testing, undertaking initial blood tests in those found to be at risk, and repeating blood tests for borderline cases or for confirming the diagnosis. Since up to 50% of all adults may need to have blood tests, and one or more of the steps involve visits to doctors and absence from work as well, the costs of a national program are substantial. While those in favour of screening point to evidence suggesting that in the long run the cost of the program would be outweighed by savings resulting from early treatment and prevention of costly complications, others argue that the costs of a screening program cannot be justified in the absence of trial data, confirming the net benefit of the intervention.

2. Misclassification of some screened individuals is inevitable, as no screening test is perfectly sensitive or specific. False-negative screenees (i.e., those who really have the condition but are classified as normal) may be falsely reassured by the negative test, and not seek help even when symptoms manifest. For certain diseases, false negatives may have disastrous consequences. For example, a missed diagnosis of phenylketonuria will lead to irreparable brain damage. False-negative screenees in diabetes screening programs are less likely to come to great harm. On the other hand, false-positive screenees (i.e., those whose tests are positive on the screening, but do not have the disease) may suffer through the inconvenience, expense, and anxiety of undergoing unnecessary further diagnostic tests.

3. The major consequence of type 2 diabetes is CVD, with far more people with type 2 diabetes suffering clinical complications from CVD than from any of the microvascular complications. However, the evidence that CVD can be prevented by lowering blood glucose is not strong. A small substudy of the UKPDS showed CVD benefits for therapy with metformin (13), and a large trial of thiazolidinedione, pioglitazone, showed CVD benefits, but the results

of this trial have been hotly debated (14). The strong evidence for the CVD benefits of blood pressure lowering and cholesterol lowering have led some to propose that screening for diabetes may not be necessary, if there is adequate screening and treatment for hypertension and dyslipidemia.

Despite the lack of clinical trial data, most authorities now recommend some form of screening for those at high risk of developing type 2 diabetes. This is based on the assumption that the benefits reported for interventions among people with clinically diagnosed diabetes are likely to apply also to those with diabetes diagnosed through screening, and that these benefits outweigh possible adverse effects of screening.

HOW TO SCREEN FOR TYPE 2 DIABETES

Screening for type 2 diabetes (or for those at high risk of developing it) almost always involves a two-stage process, in which simple, preliminary screening tools are used to identify those whose risk is high enough to justify undergoing blood glucose testing, followed by screening, and diagnostic blood testing, if indicated. The alternative would be to subject the whole population to a screening blood test, as, for example, in screening newborns for hypothyroidism and phenylketonuria. The latter is significantly more costly and involves blood testing for a large proportion of the population, whose risk for type 2 diabetes is manifestly very low, e. g. those under the age of 40, of normal body weight, and from a low-risk ethnic group. Nevertheless, it needs to be appreciated that the only way of identifying all individuals with undiagnosed diabetes and all those at high risk of developing diabetes is to perform an oral glucose tolerance test (OGTT) on all the members of the population, and to repeat this at regular intervals. All other approaches will miss a proportion of cases, which typically would be at least 25%.

In setting the threshold for a positive screening test leading to further investigation, there will always be a trade-off between the sensitivity of the test (the proportion of all cases that can be correctly identified) and its specificity (the proportion of all noncases that can be correctly identified). For any screening test, increasing its sensitivity will inevitably lead to a reduction in its specificity. Thus, if age were to be used as the single screening criterion to identify those who should have blood glucose testing, sensitivity would increase as the age threshold fell. However, as the age threshold falls into younger and younger age groups, ensuring that a higher and higher proportion of cases screen positive, the number of false positives also rises, and specificity falls.

In the screening algorithms used for type 2 diabetes, the thresholds at which the test is called positive can, like age, be varied continuously, yielding combinations of sensitivity and specificity ranging from one end of the spectrum (sensitivity 100%, specificity 0%) to the other (sensitivity 0%, specificity 100%). Clearly, neither end of this spectrum is desirable, but thresholds in between yield combinations of sensitivity and specificity that vary *between* different tests. At

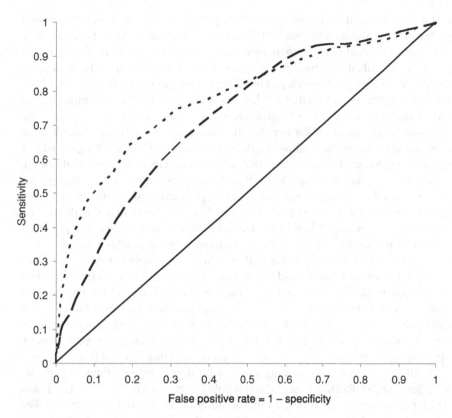

Figure 1 Receiver operating characteristics curves for two tests, showing the sensitivity and specificity of a range of thresholds for each test. The dotted line comes closer to the ideal point at the top left-hand corner and has a larger area under the curve, hence, indicating the superior test.

a sensitivity of 70%, one test may have a specificity of 60% while another may have, at the same sensitivity, a specificity of 90%, making it a superior screening test. These concepts are illustrated in Figure 1, which shows the receiver operating characteristics (ROC) curves (plots of sensitivity against specificity at all possible thresholds of a test), for two different tests.

Preliminary Screening Tools

Over recent years, a number of preliminary screening tools have been developed to identify, in a simple manner, those at high risk for diabetes, who can then go on to have blood glucose testing and/or be entered directly into a lifestyle intervention program. These tools have been developed using data from large epidemiological studies or from clinical trials, in which diabetes was established in all individuals by blood testing (usually, the OGTT). It needs to be appreciated that a screening tool developed in one study population will never perform as well (in terms of sensitivity and specificity) as in another population, and that this drop in performance is always much greater when the tool is used in a different ethnic group. This is illustrated by looking at a potential threshold for body mass index (BMI). A screening tool developed in a Europid population is likely to find that a BMI of 25 kg/m^2 is a useful threshold, below which very few cases of undiagnosed type 2 diabetes occur (i.e., sensitivity is high). However, when using the same threshold in an Asian-Indian population, among whom diabetes is much more common at lower levels of adiposity, the sensitivity of a BMI of 25 kg/m^2 will be considerably lower. The message is that before a particular screening tool is used, its performance must be established in the relevant populations (outside the specific one in which the tool was developed) i.e., in a population of similar ethnicity and diabetes risk to the population in question. The sensitivity and specificity of a screening tool developed in Europid Germans cannot be assumed to apply when used in Hispanics, Pacific Islanders, Asian-Indians, or other ethnic groups.

Some preliminary screening tools are based on simple parameters, such as age, diet, height, and weight, and hence lend themselves to be used by the general public. Others also include biomedical measurements, such as blood pressure or lipid levels and are designed for use by medical practitioners. Such tools rely for their public health impact on the fact that, in most developed countries a very high proportion of adults attend a primary care physician every year, making opportunistic screening an appealing method of detecting those at risk.

Of the preliminary screening tools so far developed, the Finnish Diabetes Risk Score (FINDRISK) (Table 1) has probably been the most studied (15). It was developed in a population-based Finnish study of 35- to 64-year-olds followed for 10 years, and contains only those demographic, lifestyle, and anthropometric factors that can be easily measured by the general public without any medical assistance. The score attached to each variable reflects the strength of its independent relationship with the development of diabetes over the following 10 years, and depending on the desired sensitivity of the screening process (often governed by local financial constraints with regard to resources available to manage those positive screenees), a threshold can be selected for the total score above which further action is taken. The score has been studied in a variety of populations and shown to have acceptable properties both for identifying those at high risk for future diabetes as well as those with current undiagnosed diabetes.

The Diabetes Prediction Model was developed from the San Antonio Heart Study, which comprised a mixed population of Hispanic and non-Hispanic white participants (16). The model requires the results of blood lipids, blood pressure, and fasting glucose, to predict the risk of developing diabetes over the subsequent 7. 5 years, and has been validated in other populations.

Other tools have been developed for use in Asian-Indian populations, among whom it appears that variation in risk between different subgroups implies that specific sets of tools will need to be developed for this large and diverse population (17).

Table 1 FINDRISK Score for Identifying Those at High Risk of Developing Diabetes (15)[a]

---

1. Age
   a. Less than 45 yr = 0
   a. 45–54 yr = 2
   b. 55–64 yr = 3
   c. More than 64 yr = 4
2. BMI
   a. Less than 25 kg/m^2 = 0
   b. 25–30 kg/m^2 = 1
   c. More than 30 kg/m^2 = 3
3. Waist circumference
   a. Women <80 cm, men <94 cm = 0
   b. Women 80–88 cm, men 94–102 cm = 3
   c. Women >88 cm, men >102 cm = 4
4. Do you usually have daily at least 30 minutes of physical activity at work and/or during leisure time (including normal daily activity)?
   a. Yes = 0
   b. No = 2
5. How often do you eat vegetables, fruit or berries?
   a. Every day = 0
   b. Not every day = 1
6. Have you ever taken antihypertensive medication regularly?
   a. No = 0
   b. Yes = 2
7. Have you ever been found to have high blood glucose (e. g., in a health examination, during an illness, during pregnancy)?
   a. No = 0
   b. Yes = 5
8. Has any of the members of your immediate family or other relatives been diagnosed with diabetes (type 1 or type 2)?
   a. No = 0
   b. Yes: Grandparent, aunt, uncle, or first cousin (but no own parent, brother, sister, or child) = 3
   c. Yes: Parent, brother, sister, or own child = 5

---

[a]The number of points for each item in the score is shown.
Total risk score:

<7	Low, estimated 1 in 100 will develop diabetes.
7–11	Slightly elevated, estimated 1 in 25 will develop diabetes
12–14	Moderate, estimated 1 in 6 will develop diabetes
15–20	High, estimated 1 in 3 will develop diabetes
>20	Very high, estimated 1 in 2 will develop diabetes

Table 2   Australian Guidelines to Identify High-Risk Groups for
Screening for Type 2 Diabetes

Age $\geq$55 (age $\geq$35 for high risk ethnic groups)
IGT or IFG (current or previous)
Previous gestational diabetes
Women with polycystic ovary syndrome who are obese
All people with clinical CVD (myocardial infarction, angina or stroke)
Any two of:
   Age $\geq$45 (35 in high risk ethnic groups)
   Obesity (BMI > 30)
   1st degree relative with type 2 diabetes
   Hypertension

Source: From Ref. 18.

The tools described above have been derived from statistical (usually regression) analyses, linking independently associated variables with the development of or presence of diabetes. The weighting of each individual parameter reflects its strength of association with diabetes. However, others have taken a simpler approach, at least for developing tools to identify those, most likely to have undiagnosed diabetes. The Australian National Health and Medical Research Council promotes a screening tool comprised of high-risk categories (18) (Table 2). No score needs to be calculated, and anyone falling into any of the individual categories is recommended to have blood glucose testing. While such tools lack statistical sophistication and are likely to perform less well than the aforementioned scores, their simplicity may facilitate their widespread use.

Screening and Diagnostic Blood Tests

After presumptively identifying those at high risk for diabetes, the next step is to measure glycemia. This usually involves blood glucose testing, but urine glucose testing and the potential use of HbA1c will also be discussed. Since diabetes is defined on the basis of blood glucose values and screening for diabetes risk also involves blood glucose measurement, diabetes is unusual in that the same test can either be a screening or a diagnostic test. This is unlike other conditions in which the screening and diagnostic tests are very different, e. g., measurement of prostate-specific antigen and prostatic biopsy, respectively, for screening and diagnosis of prostate cancer, and may cause confusion in discussing the screening process for diabetes.

Urine Glucose Testing

Urine testing has no place as a screening tool, where there is a means available (including reflectance meters) to measure blood glucose. Urine testing neither has acceptable sensitivity nor specificity. Its use can be advocated only when blood testing is either not available or is particularly expensive. Even in the latter situation, however, costs involved in confirmatory testing in positive screenees (depending on the level accepted as positive) may eventually outweigh initial savings. The renal threshold for glucose varies with age (higher), sex (lower in men), pregnancy (lower), and ethnic group, as well as demonstrating wide variability between individuals. Hence, the validity of urine glucose as a screening test is highly questionable. Furthermore, sensitivity and specificity will vary depending on the level of glycosuria deemed significant, the state of hydration of subjects, and the type of test strips used.

One of the crucial limitations of urine glucose testing is that glycosuria only appears when the blood glucose value exceeds the renal threshold, which is usually around 10 mmol/L. Since this is substantially higher than the fasting plasma glucose diagnostic cut-point for diabetes of 7.0 mmol/L, it stands to reason that a substantial proportion of those with undiagnosed diabetes will not have glycosuria, and thus, cannot be identified by this type of screening.

Glycated Hemoglobin

Glycated hemoglobin (HbA1c) is the "gold standard" for assessing long-term glycemic control in those with established diabetes. Since it reflects average glycemia over the previous two to three months, unlike fasting blood glucose or the OGTT, does not need any special preparation of the individual to undertake the test and can be done at any time of the day, it has significant potential as an aid to either screening for or diagnosing diabetes. However, there are important limitations. The most commonly quoted limitation is its lack of sensitivity compared to either FPG or the OGTT. This, of course, is simply a matter of definition, as diabetes is defined by blood glucose values and therefore no other test can be as good as blood glucose in approximating to blood glucose. A number of studies have, however, shown that HbA1c bears the same relationship with the microvascular complications of diabetes as does blood glucose, raising the possibility that at some stage diabetes might be defined by HbA1c instead of (or perhaps as well as) blood glucose. At that point, the performance of HbA1c as a screening test would instantaneously improve.

Despite the potential attraction of HbA1c as both a screening and a diagnostic tool, technical problems remain. Significant progress has been made in the last decade in the standardization of results from the different types of HbA1c assay, but variation remains between methods and among laboratories using the same method. A cut-point developed in one laboratory may not directly apply to other laboratories. Furthermore, the cost of the assay means that it would not be available to large parts of the world.

Nevertheless, studies that have examined the utility of combining HbA1c with FPG as an efficient means of screening for diabetes and limiting the number of OGTTs required, have shown encouraging results. A study from Hong Kong (19) showed that, of all subjects with FPG $\geq$5. 6 mmol/L, undiagnosed diabetes (by 2 hour glucose in the OGTT) was present in only 14% of those with a "low-risk"

HbA1c (less than 5. 5%) compared to 60% of those with HbA1c $\geq$5. 5%. Of all those with FPG <5. 6 mmol/L, only 4% had undiagnosed diabetes. The addition of HbA1c would have reduced the number of OGTTs required by 19%, would have identified a small proportion of screenees as not needing further testing even though 14% had diabetes, and would have reduced the total number of screenees found to have diabetes by only 5%. Therefore, there may be some value in using HbA1c as part of the screening process, although cost/benefit assessments need to be undertaken.

Blood Glucose and the OGTT

Abnormal glucose tolerance is defined in terms of raised blood glucose levels. The diagnostic level depends on the nature of the specimen (venous or capillary, whole blood or plasma) and whether the blood is collected randomly (in relation to eating habit and time of the day), in a fasting state or at specified intervals following a standard glucose load (20,21).

FPG is often considered the ideal first screen for glucose intolerance. It is simple and cheap, although requiring an overnight fast (with the consequent cost and inconvenient implications of a further medical visit). Although used as a screening test, it may directly identify 60% to 70% of people with undiagnosed diabetes, without recourse to the OGTT (22). Furthermore, it can also identify people with IFG. Its limitations are that 30% to 40% of people with undiagnosed diabetes have a "nondiabetic" fasting glucose, and an even higher proportion of those with IGT have a completely normal fasting glucose. In one study, the median FPG of those with IGT was 5.4 mmol/L (23). The properties of FPG (at the threshold of $\geq$6.1 mmol/L, i. e., the lower limit of IFG, rather than diabetes) as a screening tool for diabetes (diagnosed by the OGTT) have been reported in a number of studies (Table 3). From these data, the median sensitivity for diabetes was 78%, and the median specificity was 91%. Thus, it is clear that using the FPG threshold of 6.1 mmol/L will result in approximately 20% of those with undiagnosed diabetes being missed. In order to improve this, a lower threshold (e. g., 5.5 mmol/L) could be used to select people who should be assessed further with an OGTT. This, of course, would necessarily lower the specificity of the test and increase the numbers of individuals required to have the OGTT.

Random (or casual) blood glucose testing is the easiest and simplest form of blood glucose testing, since it requires no preparation. There are however limited data (24,25) on the properties of random blood glucose testing (measured by reflectance meter in both studies) as a screening tool for diabetes (Table 4). Interestingly, in one of the studies (25) the performance of the test was related to postprandial interval, and diabetes prediction was better with earlier measurement (1–2 hours postprandially). On the basis of the two studies, and by comparing tables 4 and 5, it can be seen that in order to achieve a sensitivity of 80% to 90%, the specificity of a random blood is likely to be considerably lower than that of a fasting value. There is, however, one caveat. The design of the studies of random blood glucose measurements, necessarily involved random testing and OGTTs to

Table 3 Characteristics of FPG Measurement as a Screening Test for Type 2 Diabetes in Various Populations[a]

Population	Number	Sensitivity (%)	Specificity (%)	Predictive value (%)	
				Positive test	Negative test
U.S.A. (NHANES) (28)	2844	84	90	30	84
Holland (29)	2540	88	88	30	91
U.S.A. (elderly) (30)	4515	71	87	47	63
Hong Kong (31)	1486	58	98	36	92
Australia (2)	11,247	72	91	17	89
Mauritius (32)	3,528	85	92	37	82
Japan Brazil (33)	647	92	92	72	83

[a] Fasting plasma glucose value of 6.1 mmol/L (110 mg/dL) or more constitutes a positive screening test. Type 2 diabetes is defined as a fasting plasma glucose value of 7.0 mmol/L (126 mg/dL) or more, or a plasma glucose value of 11.1 mmol/L (200 mg/dL) or more, 2 hours following a 75 g OGTT.

be performed on different days. However, the studies of FPG involved only a single OGTT, in which, classification by fasting glucose is compared to classification by the fasting and 2 hour values combined. Given the day-to-day variation in blood glucose, these design differences would tend to favour the single-day studies of fasting glucose.

It has been suggested that a random plasma glucose of 5. 6 to 11. 0 mmol/L represents an uncertain range, in which diabetes can be neither diagnosed nor confidently excluded (21). Such a result should be followed by an OGTT or fasting glucose, although it should be noted that the lower limit of 5. 6 mmol/L has been selected rather arbitrarily. Overall, the limited data on random glucose

Table 4 The Performance of a Random Whole Blood Glucose as a Screen for Diabetes

Engelgau et al., 1995 (24)	
At sensitivity of 90%[a]:	Median specificity 48–52% (according to age group)
At specificity of 90%:	Median sensitivity 49–52%
Optimal:	Median sensitivity 73–76%
	Median specificity 76–78%
Qiao et al., 1995 (25)	
Cut-off 5.8 mmol/L	Sensitivity 63%, specificity 85%[b]
Cut-off 5.2 mmol/L	Sensitivity 78%, specificity 62%[b]

[a] The cut-off value of random whole blood glucose for a sensitivity of 90% was 4.4–6.7, depending on age and postprandial interval.
[b] Sensitivities and specificities were less in women than men at all thresholds.

testing would indicate that it is inferior to FPG and should only be used when there are difficulties in arranging a fasting test (e. g., work commitments or availability of glucose testing). While a random glucose has significant limitations in screening asymptomatic individuals, it is generally unequivocal in individuals with clear symptoms of diabetes.

The 75 g OGTT is the gold standard for the diagnosis of diabetes. It should be noted that while many laboratories commonly measure and report 1-hour plasma glucose values, these cannot be used for diagnostic purposes; indeed, diagnostic thresholds for this time point are not available although laboratories may quote "normal ranges". The prevalence of diabetes by the FPG is approximately the same as that by the 2-hour plasma glucose (though, this varies by age, obesity, and ethnicity), but the individuals identified as diabetic by the two thresholds are not necessarily the same (22). At least in terms of CVD and mortality, those who are diabetic on the 2-hour value are at increased risk compared to those with normal glucose tolerance (26).

Unfortunately, the OGTT has poor intraindividual repeatability, particularly in the IFG and IGT ranges and over short time periods. Clinicians should therefore repeat the OGTT on asymptomatic positive screenees before a final diagnosis is made. It also appears that there may be ethnic differences in the stability of an OGTT diagnosis of type 2 diabetes over time (27). Nevertheless, at least in Americans, the 2-hour–diagnostic level for type 2 diabetes selects individuals who, in the main, remain clearly diabetic when retested some years later (27). It is the standard practice that a diagnosis is only confirmed when both the first and repeat tests are above the diagnostic threshold, but it would probably be more logical to make a diagnosis in those whose mean value (from two tests) is over the diagnostic cut-point.

RECOMMENDED SCREENING ALGORITHM

Taking into account the discussion above on screening for undiagnosed type 2 diabetes and identifying those at high risk, the following broad algorithm can be recommended:

1. Preliminary screening with a tool such as FINDRISK, which can be performed by the general public as well as by health care professionals.
2. Measurement of FPG in those found to be at high risk using the preliminary screening tool
3. Follow-up on the basis of the FPG:

FPG <5.5 mmol/L—No further blood testing
FPG 5. 5 to 6.9 mmol/L—Proceed to OGTT
FPG ≥7.0 mmol/L—Repeat FPG to confirm the clinical diagnosis of diabetes.

Irrespective of the blood glucose test results, all those found to be at high risk on the preliminary screening should be offered lifestyle intervention, because even if their current blood glucose values are normal, they remain at risk of developing diabetes.

SUMMARY

Type 2 diabetes is common and serious but typically asymptomatic in its early stages. As interventions are available that reduce morbidity and mortality, as well as the risk of developing diabetes, there is a strong argument for screening the population to identify those at highest risk.

Screening programs should begin with simple tools that are effective in identifying those at highest risk and can be used by the general public. Those found to be at high risk should undergo further screening and diagnostic blood glucose testing to accurately characterize their glucose tolerance status, and should commence a lifestyle intervention program (relevant whether they currently have diabetes or are at risk).

It should be recognized that hard, trial evidence for the benefit of screening is not yet available and that the diagnostic process for diabetes is often complex and clumsy, with the need for two and sometimes three separate blood tests to make and confirm the diagnosis. The attention of researchers should be focussed on tackling these issues. In the meantime, the likely benefits of currently recommended screening programs should encourage their implementation by individuals, healthcare professionals, and healthcare providers.

REFERENCES

1. Sicree R, Shaw J, Zimmet P. Diabetes and impaired glucose tolerance. In: Gan D, ed. Diabetes Atlas, 3rd ed. Brussels: International Diabetes Federation; 2006:10–149.
2. Dunstan DW, Zimmet PZ, Welborn TA, et al. The rising prevalence of diabetes and impaired glucose tolerance: The Australian Diabetes, Obesity and Lifestyle Study. Diabetes Care 2002; 25(5):829–834.
3. Sadikot SM, Nigam A, Das S, et al. The burden of diabetes and impaired glucose tolerance in India using the WHO 1999 criteria: Prevalence of diabetes in India study (PODIS). Diabetes Res Clin Pract 2004; 66(3):301–307.
4. Alberti KG, Zimmet P, Shaw J. International Diabetes Federation: A consensus on Type 2 diabetes prevention. Diabet Med 2007; 24(5):451–463.
5. Cowie CC, Rust KF, Byrd-Holt DD, et al. Prevalence of diabetes and impaired fasting glucose in adults in the U. S. population National Health And Nutrition Examination Survey 1999–2002. Diabetes Care 2006; 29(6):1263–1268.
6. Harris MI, Klein R, Welborn TA, Knuiman MW. Onset of NIDDM occurs at least 4 to 7 years before clinical diagnosis. Diabetes Care 1992; 15:815–819.
7. UKPDS (United Kingdom Prospective Diabetes Study Group). Intensive blood glucose control with sulphonylureas or insulin compared with conventional treatment and risk of complications in patients with type 2 diabetes (UKPDS 33). Lancet 1998; 352:837–853.

8. UKPDS (United Kingdom Prospective Diabetes Study Group). Tight blood pressure control and risk of macrovascular and microvascular complications in type 2 diabetes (UKPDS 38). Bmj 1998; 317(7160):703–713.

9. Coutinho M, Gerstein H, Wang Y, Yusuf S. The relationship between glucose and incident cardiovascular events: A metagression analysis of published data from 20 studies of 95,783 individuals followed for 12. 4 years. Diabetes Care 1999; 22:233–240.

10. Barr EL, Zimmet PZ, Welborn TA, et al. Risk of cardiovascular and all-cause mortality in individuals with diabetes mellitus, impaired fasting glucose, and impaired glucose tolerance: The Australian Diabetes, Obesity, and Lifestyle Study (AusDiab). Circulation 2007; 116(2):151–157.

11. Bjornholt JV, Erikssen G, Aaser E, et al. Fasting blood glucose: An underestimated risk factor for cardiovascular death. Results from a 22-year–follow-up of healthy nondiabetic men. Diabetes Care 1999; 22(1):45–49.

12. Yusuf S, Sleight P, Pogue J, et al. Effects of an angiotensin-converting-enzyme inhibitor, ramipril, on cardiovascular events in high-risk patients. The Heart Outcomes Prevention Evaluation Study Investigators. N Engl J Med 2000; 342(3):145–153.

13. UKPDS: United Kingdom Prospective Diabetes Study Group. Effect of intensive blood-glucose control with metformin on complications in overweight patients with Type 2 diabetes: (UKPDS 34). Lancet 1998; 352:854–865.

14. Dormandy JA, Charbonnel B, Eckland DJ, et al. Secondary prevention of macrovascular events in patients with type 2 diabetes in the PROactive Study (PROspective pioglitAzone Clinical Trial In macroVascular Events): A randomised controlled trial. Lancet 2005; 366(9493):1279–1289.

15. Lindstrom J, Tuomilehto J. The diabetes risk score: A practical tool to predict type 2 diabetes risk. Diabetes Care 2003; 26(3):725–731.

16. Stern MP, Williams K, Haffner SM. Identification of persons at high risk for type 2 diabetes mellitus: Do we need the oral glucose tolerance test? Ann Intern Med 2002; 136(8):575–581.

17. Ramachandran A, Snehalatha C, Vijay V, et al. Derivation and validation of diabetes risk score for urban Asian-Indians. Diabetes Res Clin Pract 2005; 70(1):63–70.

18. National Health and Medical Research Council of Australia. National Evidence Based Guidelines for the Management of Type 2 Diabetes Mellitus. Part 3. Case Detection and Diagnosis of Type 2 Diabetes. 2001.

19. Ko GT, Chan JC, Yeung VT, et al. Combined use of a fasting plasma glucose concentration and HbA1c or fructosamine predicts the likelihood of having diabetes in high-risk subjects. Diabetes Care 1998; 21(8):1221–1225.

20. American Diabetes Association Report of the Expert Committee on the diagnosis and classification of diabetes mellitus. Diabetes Care 1997; 20:1183–1197.

21. Alberti K, Zimmet P. Definition, diagnosis and classification of diabetes mellitus and its complications. Part 1. Diagnosis and classification of diabetes mellitus. Report of a WHO Consultation. Diabetic Med 1998; 15(7):539–553.

22. Shaw JE, de Courten M, Boyko EJ, Zimmet PZ. Impact of new diagnostic criteria for diabetes on different populations. Diabetes Care 1999; 22(5):762–766.

23. Shaw J, Zimmet P, Hodge A, et al. Impaired fasting glucose: How low should it go? Diabetes Care 2000; 23:34–39.

24. Engelgau MM, Thompson TJ, Smith PJ, et al. Screening for diabetes mellitus in adults. The utility of random capillary blood glucose measurements. Diabetes Care 1995; 18(4):463–466.
25. Qiao Q, Keinanen-Kiukaanniemi S, Rajala U, et al. Random capillary whole blood glucose test as a screening test for diabetes mellitus in a middle-aged population. Scand J Clin Lab Invest 1995; 55(1):3–8.
26. Shaw J, Hodge A, de Courten M, et al. Isolated post-challenge hyperglycemia confirmed as a risk factor for mortality. Diabetologia 1999; 42:1050–1054.
27. Stern MP, Valdez RA, Haffner SM, et al. Stability over time of modern diagnostic criteria for type 2 diabetes. Diabetes Care 1993; 16:978–983.
28. Harris M, Eastman R, Cowie C, et al. Comparison of diabetes diagnostic categories in the United States population according to 1997, American Diabetes Association, and 1980–1985 World Health Organization diagnostic criteria. Diabetes Care 1997; 20:1859–1862.
29. de Vegt F, Dekker JM, Stehouwer CD, et al. The 1997 American Diabetes Association criteria versus the 1985 World Health Organization criteria for the diagnosis of abnormal glucose tolerance: Poor agreement in the Hoorn Study. Diabetes Care 1998; 21(10):1686–1690.
30. Wahl P, Savage P, Psaty B, et al. Diabetes in older adults: Comparison of diabetes mellitus with 1985 WHO classification. Lancet 1998; 352:1012–1015.
31. Ko G, Woo J, Chan JCN, Cockram CS. Use of the 1997 American Diabetes Association diagnostic criteria for diabetes in a Hong Kong Chinese population. Diabetes Care 1998; 21:2094–2097.
32. Shaw J, Zimmet P, de Courten M, et al. Impaired fasting glucose or impaired glucose tolerance. What best predicts future diabetes in Mauritius? Diabetes Care 1999; 22:399–402.
33. Gimeno S, Ferreira S, Franco L, Iunes M, The Japanese-Brazilian Diabetes Study Group: Comparison of glucose tolerance categories according to World Health Organization and American Diabetes Association diagnostic criteria in a population-based study in Brazil. Diabetes Care 1998; 21:1889–1892.

4

Role of Inflammation in the Pathogenesis of Insulin Resistance

Graeme I. Lancaster

Cellular and Molecular Metabolism Laboratory, Baker Heart Research Institute, Prahran, Victoria, Australia

Andrea Hevener

David Geffen School of Medicine, Division of Endocrinology, Diabetes and Hypertension, University of California, Los Angeles, California, U.S.A.

Mark A. Febbraio

Cellular and Molecular Metabolism Laboratory, Baker Heart Research Institute, Prahran, Victoria, Australia

INTRODUCTION

The evidence linking inflammation and diabetes dates back more than a century to the finding that treatment with high-dose sodium salicylate decreased glycosuria in patients presumed to have type 2 diabetes (for review see Ref. 1). Additional studies in the late 1950s further established a possible role for inflammatory processes in the etiology of diabetes and insulin resistance (2,3). However, the concept that inflammation may be critical to the pathogenesis of diabetes was not appreciated until Hotamisligil and colleagues (4) made the seminal observation that pro-inflammatory cytokines such as TNFα were highly expressed within adipose tissue and could significantly contribute to insulin resistance. Specifically, it was shown that administration of a neutralizing anti-TNF receptor-IgG chimera to genetically obese *fa/fa* rats improved insulin sensitivity (4). In addition, genetically obese *ob/ob* mice with targeted mutations in both p55 and p75 TNF receptors, and hence unresponsive to the effects of TNF, display an improved insulin sensitivity relative to *ob/ob* mice expressing fully functional alleles encoding the p55 and p75 TNF receptors (5). These studies stimulated a paradigm shift in our understanding of the nature of metabolic disease and were a harbinger for a new field of research that has subsequently characterized many aspects of the relationship between inflammation and metabolic disease.

INFLAMMATORY SIGNALING AND INSULIN RESISTANCE: IKK/NF-κB AND JNK AS MEDIATORS OF INSULIN RESISTANCE

While TNFα was identified as a key to the nexus linking inflammation to insulin resistance almost 15 years ago, the identification of key upstream signal transduction cascades over the last 5 to 10 years has markedly enhanced our understanding of the molecular processes that govern this link. Two molecules have been identified that appear critical to many aspects of inflammatory signaling, namely the inhibitor of kappa beta kinase (IKK) and c-Jun NH_2-terminal kinase (JNK). The IKK complex consists of three subunits: IKKα and IKKβ are catalytic acting principally as serine kinases, and IKKγ (also known as NEMO) is regulatory and required for the assembly of the IKK complex (6). IKK is best known for its essential role in the activation of nuclear factor of κB (NF-κB), a family of transcription factors known to be critical for the induction of inflammatory responses and innate immunity (7). In the basal state NF-κB family members p65, c-REL, and RELB are physically associated with inhibitor of κB (IκB) proteins thus preventing their nuclear translocation and subsequent transcriptional activities. In contrast, p100/p52 and p105/p50 family members contain C-terminal halves similar to the IκB proteins thus preventing their nuclear translocation. The induction of NF-κB transcriptional activity is dependent on the IKK-mediated phosphorylation of critical serine residues within the IκB proteins (canonical activation mediated via IKKβ) and the IκB "like" regions of p100/p52 and p105/p50 proteins (noncanonical activation mediated via IKKα). Phosphorylation at these sites promotes the ubiquitin-dependent degradation of both the IκB proteins and of the IκB regions of p100/p52 and p105/p50. Subsequently, liberated NF-κB family members are able to translocate to the nucleus and upregulate target genes such as TNFα.

In light of the observation that the anti-inflammatory agents aspirin and salicylate are potent and specific inhibitors of IKKβ/NF-κB signaling (8), and the early evidence described above that salicylates improve glucose tolerance, Shoelson and colleagues (9) investigated the potential role of IKKβ in genetic- and diet-induced insulin resistance. Initially, it was shown that both aspirin and salicylate improve glucose tolerance and insulin signaling in Zucker fatty rats and *ob/ob* mice. To specifically address the role of IKKβ in obesity-induced insulin resistance, mice heterozygous for a targeted disruption of the IKKβ locus (global IKKβ$^{-/-}$ deficiency results in midgestational lethality) were either fed a high fat diet or crossed with *ob/ob* mice. These investigators were able to demonstrate improved glucose tolerance and insulin sensitivity in IKKβ$^{+/-}$ mice compared with IKKβ$^{+/+}$ mice in response to both high fat feeding and after intercrossing with *ob/ob* mice (9). Subsequent studies, both *in vitro* (10,11) and *in vivo* (12,13), have confirmed the important role that the activation of IKKβ/NF-κB plays in mediating obesity-induced insulin resistance in numerous cells and tissues. For example, a transgenic mouse with liver-specific overexpression of IKKβ rendered the animal insulin resistant (12). In contrast, liver-specific IKKβ knockout animals are protected against diet-induced insulin resistance (12). Intriguingly, however, this pathway does not play a role in the etiology of insulin resistance in all tissue types since muscle-specific transgenic expression of activated IKKβ causes profound muscle wasting that resembles clinical cachexia, but intriguingly does not result in insulin resistance (14).

In addition to the IKK/NF-κB pathway, another important mediator of inflammatory and immune responses is JNK. Three genes encode the JNK proteins; *JNK1* and *JNK2* are ubiquitously expressed, whereas *JNK3* has a limited expression pattern. JNKs are members of the mitogen-activated protein kinase (MAPK) family and are essential for cells to respond to changes in environment, for example, alterations in the availability of nutrients to growth factors, cytokines, UV radiation, heat exposure, and cellular redox changes (15). One of the most critical and best-characterized roles of JNK is in regulating the transcriptional activity of the AP1 family of proteins, including c-Jun, JunB, JunD, and ATF4, via the phosphorylation of critical serine/threonine residues (16).

It has been demonstrated by numerous investigators that obesity and type 2 diabetes are associated with chronic elevations in various inflammatory molecules, e.g., cytokines, acute phase proteins, and free fatty acids (1). Given that many of these molecules are potent activators of JNK, Hotamisligil and colleagues (16) investigated the potential role of JNK in obesity and insulin resistance. JNK1- (JNK1$^{-/-}$) (but not JNK2) deficient mice displayed reduced body weight and adiposity compared to littermate controls following a high-fat diet. Furthermore, both high- fat–fed JNK1$^{-/-}$ mice, and JNK1$^{-/-}$ mice crossed with ob/ob (JNK1$^{-/-}$ x Lep$^{ob/ob}$) mice displayed markedly improved insulin sensitivity compared with JNK1$^{+/+}$ and JNK1$^{+/+}$ x Lep$^{ob/ob}$ control mice, respectively (16).

As discussed, both IKK and JNK are serine kinases that up-regulate pro-inflammatory gene expression via the activation of NF-κB and AP-1 transcription factors, respectively. In mediating insulin resistance, it is likely that IKK and JNK operate via two predominant mechanisms: (1) phosphorylation of critical phosphoacceptor residues in key insulin signaling molecules, and (2) transcriptional up-regulation of pro-inflammatory genes (1). Effective insulin signaling is critically dependent upon tyrosine phosphorylation of the insulin receptor and a family of adaptor proteins, the insulin receptor substrates (IRS). In contrast, serine phosphorylation of specific serine residues within IRS molecules inhibits insulin signaling, i.e., Ser^{307}/Ser^{312} of mouse/human IRS1. Critically, both IKKβ and JNK physically associate with IRS1 and phosphorylate Ser^{307} resulting in the inhibition of insulin signaling (17–20). Interestingly, an analogous phosphoacceptor site to Ser^{307} of IRS1 has recently been identified in IRS2 (21) and this site, Thr^{348}, is a substrate for JNK1. Therefore, the phosphorylation of key inhibitory residues within IRS1/2 by IKK and JNK appears to be a critical means by which these molecules induce insulin resistance in insulin-sensitive tissues.

IKK and JNK control the activation of two diverse families of transcription factors, NF-κB and AP-1, respectively. Key target genes upregulated by these transcription factors include several pro-inflammatory cytokines, e.g., TNFα, IL-1β, and IL-6. As discussed, TNFα appears to play an important role in mediating obesity-induced insulin resistance. Therefore, in addition to their kinase-dependent roles in mediating insulin resistance, the activation of IKK and JNK further promote insulin resistance via the induction of TNFα expression.

CYTOKINE AND LIPID REGULATION OF INFLAMMATION AND INSULIN ACTION

Cytokine Regulation of Inflammation and Insulin Action

The adipocyte is no longer viewed as a passive energy store but rather a dynamic endocrine organ that secretes hundreds of proteins. Thus, the adipocyte secretes a wide variety of hormones and cytokines (termed "adipokines") including, but not limited to leptin, adiponectin, TNFα, interleukin-6 and resistin. In this way, adipose tissue uses adipokines as a communication tool to signal changes in its mass and energy status to other organs that control fuel usage, such as the brain, skeletal muscle, and liver. It is generally accepted that cytokines such as leptin and adiponectin can enhance insulin sensitivity (22). The mechanism/s of action of both leptin and adiponectin are not fully elucidated, however both are potent activators of AMP-activated protein kinase (AMPK) (23,24), a kinase known to enhance fat oxidation and increase glucose uptake (25).

Of the pro-inflammatory cytokines, TNFα has been most strongly implicated in the pathogenesis of insulin resistance. Apart from the seminal work of Hotamisligil and colleagues in rodent models (4,5,26,27), TNFα expression is correlated with reduced insulin-stimulated glucose disposal in humans (28–31). Moreover, direct evidence supporting the role of TNFα in mediating insulin resistance comes from studies in humans demonstrating that acute infusion of TNFα inhibits insulin-stimulated glucose disposal (32). The mechanism of action of TNFα is well characterized. It is known that TNFα signals through a transmembrane family of TNF receptors ultimately resulting in the activation of both IκB kinase and JNK (33). The activation of IκB kinase not only can activate IKK leading to serine phosphorylation of IRS-1, but can also activate NFκB leading to the transcription and production of TNFα itself, allowing for the protein to be released from the cell to act on its receptor in an autocrine and paracrine manner (34). In addition, recent evidence suggests that TNFα can also contribute to insulin resistance by activating protein phosphatase 2C, thereby inhibiting AMPK and preventing fat oxidation and glucose uptake (35).

Like TNFα, systemic IL-6 concentrations are elevated in obesity and patients with type 2 diabetes (36–38). It is generally thought that elevations in the plasma and/or tissue concentrations of IL-6 have a negative effect on metabolism (22). Unlike the very careful analysis of TNFα-induced insulin resistance, the role of IL-6 in the etiology of obesity-induced insulin resistance is not resolved and whether IL-6 has positive or negative effects on metabolism is the subject of continuing controversy (39–42). Recent studies support the notion that IL-6, acting through its receptor (the gp130Rβ/IL6Rα homodimer) can activate pathways that have both anti-obesogenic and insulin-sensitizing effects (for review see Ref. 43). For example, IL-6 has been shown to activate AMPK in both skeletal muscle and adipose tissue (44–47) and therefore the acute insulin-sensitizing effects of IL-6 are most likely related to activation of AMPK.

Despite the fact that acute IL-6 treatment can enhance glucose uptake and fat oxidation in skeletal muscle there are, nonetheless, a number of studies both *in vitro* (48–51) and in rodents *in vivo* (52–54) that demonstrate that IL-6 is capable of inducing insulin resistance. Most, if not all, *in vivo* studies seem to suggest that IL-6 induces insulin resistance via adverse effects on the liver. Subjecting lean mice to chronically elevated IL-6 for 5 days causes hepatic insulin resistance (51), while treating either *ob/ob* (leptin deficient) mice (53) or liver-inducible kappa kinase (LIKK) transgenic mice that display hepatic insulin resistance (12) with IL-6 neutralizing antibodies attenuates hepatic insulin resistance. The IL-6-induced insulin resistance appears due to increased expression of SOCS-3 (51), thought to directly inhibit the insulin receptor (55). However, the negative effect of SOCS3 on insulin action has recently been brought into question. Liver-specific STAT3 knockout mice that express low levels of hepatic SOCS3 protein paradoxically are unable to suppress hepatic glucose production after intracerebral ventricular insulin infusion (56). Moreover, the prevention of IL-6 signaling either by neutralizing antibodies or by genetic deletion of IL-6 markedly reduced insulin-induced phosphorylation of hepatic STAT3 (56). These results suggest that the local production of IL-6 is important for the phosphorylation of hepatic STAT3 induced by the brain insulin action. In a more recent study, liver-specific SOCS3 knockout mice exhibited obesity and systemic insulin resistance with age (57), and insulin signaling was reduced in skeletal muscle (57) suggesting that deletion of the SOCS3 gene in the liver modulates insulin sensitivity in other organs. Possibly the most convincing evidence that IL-6 is anti-obesogenic is the observation that IL-6 knockout mice develop mature onset obesity and glucose intolerance (58), although even this is open to interpretation, as another study using the same IL-6 knockout mice found no such phenotype (59). The role of IL-6 in obesity and insulin action is clearly unresolved and requires further work.

Resistin (or FIZZ3) is an adipocyte-derived secretory factor that identified as a novel transcript produced exclusively by adipocytes (60). Despite the significant interest generated by the discovery of resistin in 2001, very little is known about the intracellular signaling pathways by which resistin induces its metabolic effects. A consistent finding *in vivo* is that resistin suppresses liver and muscle AMPK signaling (61–63), an effect also observed in L6 muscle cells (64). The mechanisms mediating this inhibition of AMPK signaling are still unclear and it is unknown whether the effects observed in vivo are due to direct effects on AMPK signaling or may be mediated through indirect pathways. One possibility is that a resistin-induced increase in SOCS3 (65) inhibit cytokine signaling known to activate AMPK and/or via direct inhibition of IRS1/2 signaling. Future studies are required to directly establish the mechanisms by which resistin suppresses AMPK signaling.

Lipid Regulation of Inflammation and Insulin Action

It is well known that obesity is the major promoter of insulin resistance in humans. There is emerging evidence to suggest that insulin resistance, at least in skeletal muscle and liver, is caused by dysregulated signaling processes secondary to the accumulation of lipid at these sites (66–68). Although the increase in muscle lipid content is manifest as the relatively inert lipid species, triacylglycerol (TAG), it is associated with accumulation of long-chain fatty acyl CoA (LCFA-CoA) species, diacylglyerols (DAG) and ceramides. DAG are important second messengers of intracellular signaling and are an intermediate of TAG and phospholipids. An association between insulin resistance and DAG accumulation has been repeatedly demonstrated in rodents. Although the underlying mechanisms are unresolved, they are thought to involve the activation of the DAG-sensitive protein kinase C (PKC) isoforms θ and ε (69,70). Despite current thinking that DAG primarily mediates lipid-induced insulin resistance (71), evidence is accumulating that ceramides are also a major lipid species that lead to insulin resistance. Ceramides are second-signal effector molecules shown to block insulin action via downregulation of the activation of Akt (72). In addition, ceramide has been shown to initiate inflammatory signaling pathways leading to the activation of both JNK and NFκB/IκK (73) which, as discussed, are key mediators in the development of insulin resistance (9,16). Recently, Summers and colleagues (74) have shown that mice deficient in the enzyme Des1, or wild-type mice treated with the drug myriocin, both of which prevent ceramide synthesis, are protected from high-fat diet induced obesity. These recent data (74) provide clear evidence that ceramide accumulation leads to dysregulated insulin signal transduction and insulin resistance.

Recently, Matsuzaka et al. (75) reported that mice lacking a long-chain fatty acid elongase, elongation of long-chain fatty acids family member- (Elovl6), do not develop insulin resistance even when fed a diet rich in saturated fats. Elovl6-deficient mice have increased levels of palmitate (C16:0) and palmitoleate (C16:1) but reduced levels of stearate (C18:0) and oleate (C18:1). When compared to wild-type mice, the Elovl6-deficient mice showed no difference in hepatosteatosis or in obesity induced by a high-fat diet but had improved insulin signaling, indicating that lipid levels can be dissociated from the insulin signaling pathway. The authors did not observe increased levels of ceramide or activation of JNK or IKK in the livers of Elovl6-deficient mice fed the high fat diet, but their livers did have smaller amounts of diacylglycerol and lower expression of PKCε compared with the wild-type mice. These results are considered important because they suggest that not all long-chain fatty acids cause the same metabolic consequences (76).

Finally, recent studies have implicated a conserved family of proteins, the "Toll-like" receptors (TLRs), involved in innate immunity in the interrelationship between lipid oversupply, inflammation, and insulin resistance TLRs recognize highly conserved molecular structures associated with infectious microorganisms, e.g., lipopolysaccharide, flagellin, double stranded RNA, peptidoglycan and lipoteichoic acid, and are crucial in promoting the generation of effective adaptive immune responses (77). Recent evidence has demonstrated that TLRs also recognize endogenous molecules, e.g., heat shock proteins, heparan sulphate, β-defensin 2 and the type III repeat extra domain A of fibronectin (77). Following recognition of their specific ligands, TLRs activate highly conserved signaling pathways. Briefly, except in the case of TLR3, the adaptor protein myeloid differentiation factor 88 (MyD88) is recruited to the cytosolic region of the TLR. This association promotes the recruitment of the serine-threonine kinases IL-1R-associated kinase 1 (IRAK1) and IRAK4 that phosphorylate and activate TNF receptor-associated factor 6 (TRAF6) resulting in the activation of IKK and subsequently the up-regulation of NF-κB-dependent genes (77). It is well known that some family members, particularly TLR4, are activated by saturated fatty acids (78,79). Moreover, Flier and colleagues (80) recently demonstrated that mice lacking TLR4 are protected from the ability of systemic lipid infusion to both suppress insulin signaling in muscle and induce systemic insulin resistance. Taken together, these data suggest that TLR4 is a molecular link between lipids, inflammation, and innate immunity.

ROLE OF IMMUNE CELLS IN REGULATING INFLAMMATION AND INSULIN RESISTANCE

Since the primary insulin-responsive tissues, including adipose tissue, are comprised of a variety of cell types all serving specific biological functions, it is important to discern which resident cell type within a given tissue of interest is responsible for producing proinflammatory cytokines. Adipocytes, for example, express receptors for a variety of proinflammatory molecules and produce macrophage migration factors during periods of metabolic stress, supporting the notion that other resident cell types, e.g., macrophages, could be involved in altering adipose tissue metabolism. F4/80-positive cells, i.e., macrophages, within the stromal vascular compartment comprise ~10% to 40% of the cells within adipose tissue (81) and produce IL-1β, TNF-α, IL-6, resistin, and prostaglandin (PG)-E2 (81–86). Furthermore, it was shown that macrophage-secreted factors and adipose tissue macrophage number are highly correlated with adiposity and insulin resistance in humans and rodents (81–83,87). These data provided the critical evidence that inspired a body of work focused on unraveling the physiological link between immune cell activation, inflammation, and insulin resistance.

The Impact of Macrophage Infiltration on Inflammation and Glucose Metabolism

One of the most extensively studied circulating factors involved in monocyte chemotaxis is monocyte chemoattractant protein (MCP)-1, which is known to be overexpressed in plasma and peripheral tissues from obese and insulin-resistant humans and rodents (86–88).To address the impact of alterations in monocyte recruitment to peripheral tissues on inflammation and insulin action, MCP-1 was selectively overexpressed or inhibited (89,90). As would be predicted, mice with adipose tissue-selective overexpression of MCP-1 exhibited increased adipose tissue macrophage content, elevated inflammatory markers, increased adiposity, impaired glucose tolerance and insulin resistance. Conversely, in the context of high-fat feeding, MCP-1 deletion led to diminished adipose tissue macrophage recruitment, reduced tissue inflammation and adiposity and improved insulin sensitivity (89). Findings from high fat-fed mice were extended to diabetic *db/db* mice, in which inhibition of MCP-1 led to a significant improvement in glucose metabolism and markedly reduced hepatic triglyceride content (89). In complementary studies, inhibition of macrophage infiltration into adipose tissue was further explored in MCP-1 receptor (CCR2) knockout mice, as this receptor regulates cellular chemotaxis and local macrophage-dependent inflammatory processes that have been previously linked with atherogenesis (87,88,91). Loss of CCR2 function by genetic ablation or antagonist treatment *in vivo* led to reduced macrophage content and inflammation as well as improved insulin action (92). It should be noted, however, that deletion of CCL2 and CCR2 do not yield consistent results in all mouse strains. Thus, studies by others (93,94) indicate that CCL2 and its receptor are not essential for high fat diet-induced macrophage recruitment to adipose tissue, possibly due to redundant or condition-specific chemokines.

Macrophage Phenotype and Insulin Sensitivity

While quantitative changes in adipose tissue macrophage content, in the context of high-fat feeding, genetic obesity and type 2 diabetes, are now well established, evidence is emerging that phenotypic differences between basal tissue resident macrophages and those recruited from the bone marrow during metabolic or inflammatory challenge are very important. A phenotypic evaluation of tissue resident macrophages was recently performed by Lumeng et al (95). In comparing resident adipose tissue macrophages (ATMs) from lean versus high-fat–fed mice, it was shown that macrophages from lean animals overexpress the anti-inflammatory cytokine, IL-10. Conversely, ATMs from high fat-fed mice display the "classically activated" M1 phenotype with increased expression of inflammatory genes including TNFα and iNOS (95). It is important to note that similar observations were recently made in human adipose tissue when lean vs. obese subjects were compared (96). Interestingly, the phenotypic response of human ATMs to stimulation (IFNγ, LPS, TNFα) was quite different than that of blood monocytes selectively differentiated to classic M1 or M2 macrophages *in vitro* (96). These data clearly implicate macrophage inflammation as playing a regulatory role in the etiology of obesity-induced insulin resistance. Genetic studies have highlighted a mechanistic link between macrophage inflammation and obesity-induced insulin resistance (13). Specifically, mice lacking IKKβ in myeloid cells (generated by crossing myeloid specific Lysozyme-Cre mice to floxed Ikbkb mice; IkbkbΔ mye) had greater insulin sensitivity compared with control mice (ikbkb floxed mice; IkbkbF/F) as determined from glucose and insulin tolerance testing (13). Furthermore, euglycemic-hyperinsulinemic clamps showed greater insulin-stimulated glucose disposal and enhanced suppression of hepatic glucose production in IkbkbΔ mye compared to IkbkbF/F mice, indicating improved muscle and hepatic insulin sensitivity (13). More recently, Karin and colleagues (97) have shown that deleting JNK1 from macrophages protects against insulin resistance. Conversely, these authors also showed that transplanting wild-type macrophages into global JNK1-/- mice rescues their negative metabolic pheneotype. Together, these data highlight the importance of myeloid cell inflammation in the etiology of systemic insulin resistance.

It is now well known that the peroxisome proliferator-activated receptor-γ (PPAR γ), a member of the nuclear receptor superfamily of ligand-dependent transcription factors, not only plays an essential role in fat cell development and metabolic homeostasis (98,99) but also is a negative regulator of macrophage activation (100). Accordingly, in parallel studies, work from our group (101) and others (102) showed that mice with a macrophage-specific deletion of PPAR γ led to NFκB target gene activation and a polarization of macrophages to an M1 inflammatory phenotype. Remarkably, macrophage-specific PPAR γ deletion *in vivo* caused hyperinsulinemia, impaired glucose tolerance, increased adipose mass, skeletal muscle inflammation, and skeletal muscle and hepatic insulin resistance even under normal chow fed conditions (101). While the exact tissue-specific role of the macrophage in the pathogenesis of whole body insulin resistance remains ill-defined, the finding that macrophage-specific deletion of PPARγ leads to skeletal muscle insulin resistance, even in lean animals with no detectable change in adipose tissue inflammation, suggests that the macrophage may serve as an initiator cell type in certain insulin-resistant states. Also of note is the observation that macrophage-specific deletion of PPARγ results not only in the activation of both IKK and JNK leading to impaired insulin signal transduction, but also to increased lipid accumulation in these tissues.

As discussed earlier, lipid-induced activation of inflammatory signaling may involve the activation of TLR4 (80). However, evidence exists that members of the scavenger receptor family, including fatty acid transporters, also may be important in mediating lipid-induced macrophage activation (103). In a recent study, Furuhashi et al. (104) demonstrated that inhibition of the fatty acid binding protein FABP4, also known as AP2, decreased both macrophage cholesterol efflux and expression of pro-inflammatory cytokines such as TNFα. In addition, inhibition of AP2 prevented both diabetes and athereosclerosis (104). These data are in line with previous studies demonstrating that macrophage-specific deletion of another fatty acid transporter, namely FAT/CD36, prevented atherosclerosis in a mouse model, Apo E-null mice, prone to this disease (105). These data suggest that one mechanism by which macrophages are activated is via the uptake and deposition of fatty acid within the cell.

PROXIMAL MEDIATORS OF OBESITY-INDUCED CELLULAR INFLAMMATION: ROLE OF THE ER

It was recently demonstrated that obesity is associated with the induction of a complex cellular homeostatic response known as the ER stress response, or the unfolded protein response (UPR) (106). ER stress is initiated in response to stimuli that impair the ability of the endoplasmic reticulum to correctly fold newly synthesized proteins and hence promotes the accumulation of unfolded or misfolded proteins within the ER lumen (107). Detection of unfolded proteins within the ER lumen and the subsequent initiation of the UPR is mediated by three molecules: inositol-requiring enzyme 1 (IRE1), PKR-like endoplasmic reticulum kinase (PERK) and activating transcription factor 6 (ATF6) (107). Both high-fat–fed mice and genetically obese *ob/ob* mice display an increase in eIF2α S51 phosphorylation, PERK T980 phosphorylation and IRE1α phosphorylation, all markers of ER stress, within adipose tissue and liver (106,108). Furthermore, deletion of one allele of the X-box-binding protein-1 (XBP1), a transcription factor essential in the UPR, exacerbated high-fat diet induced insulin resistance (106). Importantly, the induction of ER stress recruits and activates both JNK and IKK in an IRE1-dependent manner (109–111). Thus, it has been hypothesized that obesity-induced ER stress may be a crucial mediator of obesity-induced cellular inflammation and insulin resistance, and this area is the focus of intense research.

CONCLUSIONS AND CLINICAL IMPLICATIONS

It has become apparent over the last decade that the etiology of obesity-induced insulin resistance is complex. It appears that the major deleterious mediator molecules are long-chain saturated fatty acids and pro-inflammatory cytokines, principally TNF-α. These circulating molecules act on a multitude of transmembrane receptors located in metabolically active tissues such as skeletal muscle, liver and adipose tissue (Fig. 1). It is also clear that cells such as myeloid cells and organelles such as the endoplasmic reticulum play a role in the etiology of insulin resistance. Chronic, low-grade inflammation is a common theme in the complex interactions between environmental agents and genetically programmed signaling pathways that ultimately results in defective insulin signaling. We are heading back to where we were more than a century ago to identify key inflammatory molecules as drug targets for the treatment of obesity-induced insulin resistance.

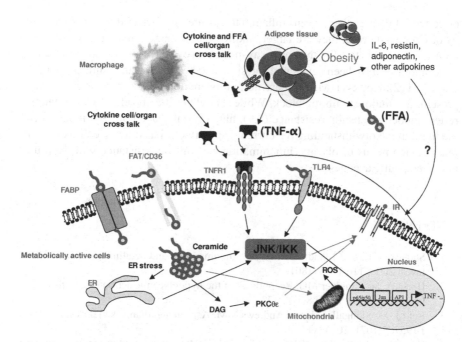

Figure 1 Schematic summarizing obesity-induced mediators of insulin resistance. Obesity (overfeeding and lack of physical activity) leads to enlarged, inflamed fat cells that initially recruit and activate myeloid cells such as macrophages. Macrophages and/or adipocytes can release a number of cytokines/adipokines than can affect multiple tissues by signaling through known and unknown receptors. Adipocytes can also release long-chain saturated fatty acids (LCSFA). Both LCSFA and TNF-α, can act on receptors in metabolically active tissue such as the liver and skeletal muscle. LCSFA can activate Toll like receptors (TLR4) and TNF can activate TNFR1 to signal to JNK and IKK, which can either directly dysregulate insulin signaling or can transcriptionally upregulate pro-inflammatory genes in the nucleus via the downstream transcription factor as NFκB, AP1, and c-Jun. Fatty acids can also enter and accumulate in the cell via transmembrane fatty acid transporters (FABP, FAT/CD36) to accumulate deleterious lipid species (ceramide and DAG) within the liver and skeletal muscle. Ceramide can activate JNK and IKK while DAG can signal to PKC isoforms to dysregulate insulin signaling. Intracellular fatty acid accumulation and lack of physical activity (skeletal muscle) can inhibit mitochondrial function and or capacity to result in ROS formation and activation of serine/threonine kinases. Finally both cytokines and fatty acids can lead to ER stress that can also result in JNK and IKK activity.

Despite the recent advances in identifying the molecular pathways that regulate obesity-induced inflammation and insulin resistance, translation to clinically effective therapy has yet to be realized. Since, as discussed in this chapter, TNF-α contributes to insulin resistance in rodents, one might expect that treating patients with type 2 diabetes with TNF receptor or TNF-α blockade drugs would be an effective therapeutic strategy. However, while Infliximab$^{®}$ or Embrel$^{®}$ are effective in treating other chronic inflammatory illnesses such as rheumatoid arthritis or Crohn's disease, they are largely ineffective in treating insulin resistance in humans. It appears that the JNK pathway may be an effective therapeutic target and JNK inhibitors have been developed and shown to be effective in animal models of obesity (112). However, MAP kinase inhibitors are notoriously nonspecific (113), presenting a major stumbling block. While salicylates may be effective in treating rodent models of insulin resistance (8,9), human trials have not been reported in the literature. Notwithstanding the current gap between basic science into clinical practice, the nexus of obesity, inflammation and insulin resistance will open up new therapeutic avenues.

REFERENCES

1. Shoelson SE, Lee J, and Goldfine AB. Inflammation and insulin resistance. J Clin Invest 2006; 116:1793–1801.
2. Hecht A, and Goldner MG. Reappraisal of the hypoglycemic action of acetylsalicylate. Metabolism 1959; 8:418–428.
3. Reid J, Macdougall A. I, and Andrews MM. Aspirin and diabetes mellitus. Br Med J 1957; 2:1071–1074.
4. Hotamisligil GS, Shargill NS, and Spiegelman BM. Adipose expression of tumor necrosis factor-alpha: Direct role in obesity-linked insulin resistance. Science 1993; 259:87–91.
5. Uysal KT, Wiesbrock SM, Marino MW, and Hotamisligil GS. Protection from obesity-induced insulin resistance in mice lacking TNF-alpha function. Nature 1997; 389:610–614.
6. Karin M, and Greten FR. NF-kappaB: Linking inflammation and immunity to cancer development and progression. Nat Rev Immunol 2005; 5:749–759.
7. Karin, M. Cao Y, Greten FR, and Li ZW. NF-kappaB in cancer: From innocent bystander to major culprit. Nat Rev Cancer 2002; 2:301–310.
8. Yin MJ, Yamamoto Y, and Gaynor RB. The anti-inflammatory agents aspirin and salicylate inhibit the activity of I(kappa)B kinase-beta. Nature 1998; 396:77–80.
9. Yuan M, Konstantopoulos N, Lee J, et al. Reversal of obesity- and diet-induced insulin resistance with salicylates or targeted disruption of Ikkbeta. Science 2001; 293:1673–1677.
10. Sinha S, Perdomo G, Brown NF, and O'Doherty RM. Fatty acid-induced insulin resistance in L6 myotubes is prevented by inhibition of activation and nuclear localization of nuclear factor kappa B. J Biol Chem 2004; 279:41294–41301.
11. Kim JK, Kim YJ, Fillmore JJ, et al. Prevention of fat-induced insulin resistance by salicylate. J Clin Invest 2001; 108:437–446.
12. Cai D, Yuan M, Frantz DF, et al. Local and systemic insulin resistance resulting from hepatic activation of IKK-beta and NF-kappaB. Nat Med 2005; 11:183–190.
13. Arkan MC, Hevener AL, Greten FR, et al. IKK-beta links inflammation to obesity-induced insulin resistance. Nat Med 2005; 11:191–198.
14. Cai D, Frantz JD, Tawa NE Jr, et al. IKKbeta/NF-kappaB activation causes severe muscle wasting in mice. Cell 2004; 119:285–298.

15. Davis RJ. Signal transduction by the JNK group of MAP kinases. Cell 2000; 103:239–252.
16. Hirosumi J, Tuncman G, Chang L, et al. A central role for JNK in obesity and insulin resistance. Nature 2002; 420:333–336.
17. Aguirre V, Uchida T, Yenush L, Davis R, and White MF. The c-Jun NH(2)-terminal kinase promotes insulin resistance during association with insulin receptor substrate-1 and phosphorylation of Ser(307). J Biol Chem 2000; 275:9047–9054.
18. Lee JY, Ye J, Gao Z, et al. Reciprocal modulation of Toll-like receptor-4 signaling pathways involving MyD88 and phosphatidylinositol 3-kinase/AKT by saturated and polyunsaturated fatty acids. J Biol Chem 2003 a; 278:37041–37051.
19. Gao Z, Hwang D, Bataille F, et al. Serine phosphorylation of insulin receptor substrate 1 by inhibitor kappa B kinase complex. J Biol Chem 2002; 277:48115–48121.
20. Nakamori Y, Emoto M, Fukuda N, et al. Myosin motor Myo1c and its receptor NEMO/IKK-gamma promote TNF-alpha-induced serine307 phosphorylation of IRS-1. J Cell Biol 2006; 173:665–671.
21. Solinas G, Naugler W, Galimi F, Lee MS, and Karin, M. Saturated fatty acids inhibit induction of insulin gene transcription by JNK-mediated phosphorylation of insulin-receptor substrates. Proc Natl Acad Sci U S A 2006; 103:16454–16459.
22. Lazar M. How obesity causes diabetes: Not a tall tale. Science 2005; 307:373–375.
23. Minokoshi Y, Kim YB, Peroni OD, et al. Leptin stimulates fatty-acid oxidation by activating AMP-activated protein kinase. Nature 2002; 415:339–343.
24. Yamauchi T, Kamon J, Waki H, et al. The fat-derived hormone adiponectin reverses insulin resistance associated with both lipoatrophy and obesity. Nat Med 2001; 7:941–946.
25. Kahn BB, Alquier T, Carling D, and Hardie DG AMP-activated protein kinase: Ancient energy gauge provides clues to modern understanding of metabolism. Cell Metabolism 2005; 1:15–25.
26. Hotamisligil GS, Murray DL, Choy LN, and Spiegelman BM. Tumor necrosis factor alpha inhibits signaling from the insulin receptor. Proc Natl Acad Sci USA 1994; 91:4854–4858.
27. Hotamisligil GS, Peraldi P, Budavari A, Ellis R., White MF, and Spiegelman BM. IRS-1-mediated inhibition of insulin receptor tyrosine kinase activity in TNF-alpha- and obesity-induced insulin resistance. Science 1996; 271:665–668.
28. Katsuki A, Sumida Y, Murashima S, et al. Serum levels of tumor necrosis factor-alpha are increased in obese patients with noninsulin-dependent diabetes mellitus. J Clin Endocrinol Metab 1998; 83:859–862.
29. Zinman B, Hanley AJG, Harris SB, Kwan J, and Fantus IG. Circulating tumor necrosis factor-alpha concentrations in a native Canadian population with high rates of Type 2 diabetes mellitus. J Clin Endocrinol Metab 1999; 84:272–278
30. Saghizadeh M, Ong JM, Garvey WT, Henry RR, and Kern PA The Expression of TNFalpha by Human Muscle. Relationship to Insulin Resistance. J. Clin. Invest 1996; 97:1111–1116.
31. Kern PA, Ranganathan S, Li C, Wood L. and Ranganathan L. Adipose tissue tumor necrosis factor and interleukin-6 expression in human obesity and insulin resistance. Am J Physiol 2001; 280:E745–E751.
32. Plomgaard P, Bouzakri K, Krogh-Madsen R, Mittendorfer B, Zierath JR, and Pedersen BK. Tumor necrosis factor-alpha induces skeletal muscle insulin resistance in healthy human subjects via inhibition of Akt substrate 160 phosphorylation. Diabetes 2006; 54:2939–2945.

33. Liu ZG, Hsu H, Goeddel DV, and Karin M. Dissection of TNF receptor 1 effector functions: JNK activation is not linked to apoptosis while NF-kappaB activation prevents cell death. Cell 1996; 87:565–576.
34. Wellen KE, and Hotamisligil GS. Inflammation, stress, and diabetes. J Clin Invest 2005; 115:1111–1119.
35. Steinberg GR, Michell BJ, van Denderen B, et al. Tumor necrosis factor-α induced skeletal muscle insulin resistance involves the suppression of AMP-kinase signaling. Cell Metab 2006; 4:465–474
36. Vozarova B, Weyer C, Hanson K, Tataranni PA, Bogardus C, and Pratley RE. Circulating interleukin-6 in relation to adiposity, insulin action, and insulin secretion. Obes Res 2001; 9:414–417.
37. Bastard JP, Maachi M, Van Nhieu JT, et al. Elevated levels of interleukin 6 are reduced in serum and subcutaneous adipose tissue of obese women after weight loss. J Clin Endocrinol Metab 2000; 85:3338–3342.
38. Carey AL, Bruce CR, Sacchetti M, et al. Interleukin-6 and tumor necrosis factor-alpha are not elevated in patients with type 2 diabetes: Evidence that plasma IL-6 is related to fat mass and not insulin responsiveness. Diabetologia 2004; 47:1029–1037.
39. Carey AL, and Febbraio MA. Interleukin-6 and insulin sensitivity: Friend or foe? Diabetologia 2004; 47:1135–1142.
40. Kristiansen OP, and Mandrup-Poulsen T. Interleukin-6 and diabetes: The good, the bad, or the indifferent? Diabetes 2005; 54 (Suppl 2):S114–S124.
41. Pedersen BK, and Febbraio MA Point: Interleukin-6 does have a beneficial role in insulin sensitivity and glucose homeostasis. J Appl Physiol 2007; 102:814–819.
42. Mooney RA. Counterpoint: Interleukin-6 does not have a beneficial role in insulin sensitivity and glucose homeostasis. J Appl Physiol 2007; 102:816–818.
43. Febbraio MA. gp130 receptor ligands as potential therapeutic targets for obesity. J Clin Invest 2007; 117:841–849.
44. Kelly M, Keller C, Avilucea PR, et al. AMPK activity is diminished in tissues of IL-6 knockout mice: The effect of exercise. Biochem Biophys Res Commun 2004; 320:449–454.
45. Al-Khalili L, Bouzakri K, Glund S, et al. Signaling specificity of interleukin-6 action on glucose and lipid metabolism in skeletal muscle. Mol Endocrinol 2006; 20:3364–3375.
46. Carey AL, Steinberg GR, Macaula SL, et al. IL-6 increases insulin stimulated glucose disposal in humans and glucose uptake and fatty acid oxidation in vitro via AMPK. Diabetes 2006; 55:2688–2697.
47. Glund S, Deshmukh A, Long YC, et al. Interleukin-6 directly increases glucose metabolism in resting human skeletal muscle. Diabetes 2007; 56:1630–1637.
48. Rotter V, Nagaev I, and Smith U. Interleukin-6 (IL-6) induces insulin resistance in 3T3-L1 adipocytes and is, like IL-8 and TNFalpha, overexpressed in human fat cells from insulin-resistant subjects. J Biol Chem 2003; 278:45777–45785.
49. Lagathu C, Bastard JP, Auclair M, et al. Chronic interleukin-6 (IL-6) treatment increased IL-6 secretion and induced insulin resistance in adipocyte: Prevention by rosiglitazone. Biochem Biophys Res Commun 2003; 311:372–379.
50. Senn JJ, Klover PJ, Nowak IA, and Mooney, RA Interleukin-6 induces cellular insulin resistance in hepatocytes. Diabetes 2002; 51:3391–3399.

51. Senn JJ, Klover PJ, Nowak IA, et al. Suppressor of Cytokine Signaling-3 (SOCS-3), a potential mediator of interleukin-6-dependent insulin resistance in hepatocytes. J Biol Chem 2003; 278:13740–13746.

52. Klover PJ, Zimmers TA, Koniaris LG, and Mooney, RA. Chronic exposure to Interleukin-6 causes hepatic insulin resistance in mice. Diabetes 2003; 52:2784–2789.

53. Klover PJ, Clementi AH, and Mooney RA. Interleukin-6 depletion selectively improves hepatic insulin action in obesity. Endocrinology. 2005; 146:3417–3427.

54. Kim HJ, Higashimori T, Park SY, et al. Differential effects of interleukin-6 and -10 on skeletal muscle and liver insulin action in vivo. Diabetes 2004; 53:1060–1067.

55. Ueki K, Kondo T, and Kahn CR. Suppressor of cytokine signaling 1 (SOCS-1) and SOCS-3 cause insulin resistance through inhibition of tyrosine phosphorylation of insulin receptor substrate proteins by discrete mechanisms. Mol Cell Biol 2004; 24:5434–5446.

56. Inoue H, Ogawa W, Asakawa A, et al. Role of hepatic STAT3 in brain-insulin action on hepatic glucose production. Cell Metab 2006; 3:267–275.

57. Torisu T, Sato N, Yoshiga D, et al. The dual function of hepatic SOCS3 in insulin resistance in vivo. Genes Cells 2007; 12:143–154.

58. Wallenius V, Wallenius K, Ahren B, et al. Interleukin-6-deficient mice develop mature-onset obesity. Nat Med 2002; 8:75–79.

59. Di Gregorio GB, Hensley L, Lu T, Ranganathan G, and Kern PA. Lipid and carbohydrate metabolism in mice with a targeted mutation in the IL-6 gene: Absence of development of age-related obesity. Am J Physiol Endocrinol Metab 2004; 287:E182–E187.

60. Steppan CM, Bailey ST, Bhat S, et al. The hormone resistin links obesity to diabetes. Nature 2001; 409:307–312.

61. Qi Y, Nie Z, Lee YS, et al. Loss of resistin improves glucose homeostasis in leptin deficiency. Diabetes 2006; 55:3083–3090.

62. Banerjee RR, Rangwala SM, Shapiro JS, et al. Regulation of Fasted Blood Glucose by Resistin. Science 2004; 303:1195–1198.

63. Satoh H, Nguyen MT, Miles PD, Imamura T, Usui I, and Olefsky JM Adenovirus-mediated chronic "hyper-resistinemia" leads to in vivo insulin resistance in normal rats. J Clin Invest 2004; 114:224–231.

64. Palanivel R. and Sweeney G. Regulation of fatty acid uptake and metabolism in L6 skeletal muscle cells by resistin. FEBS Lett 2005; 579:5049–5054.

65. Steppan CM, Wang J, Whiteman EL, Birnbaum MJ, and Lazar MA. Activation of SOCS-3 by resistin. Mol Cell Biol 2005; 25:1569–1575.

66. Pan DA, Lillioja S, Kriketos AD, et al. Skeletal muscle triglyceride levels are inversely related to insulin action. Diabetes 1997; 46:983–988.

67. Itani SI, Ruderman NB, Schmieder F, and Boden G. Lipid-induced insulin resistance in human muscle is associated with changes in diacylglyceol, protein kinase C, and IκB-α. Diabetes 2002; 51:2005–2011.

68. Adams JM, II, Pratipanawatr T, Berria R, et al.. Ceramide content is increased in skeletal muscle from obese insulin-resistant humans. Diabetes 2004; 53:25–31.

69. Schmitz-Peiffer C. Protein kinase C and lipid-induced insulin resistance in skeletal muscle. Ann NY Acad Sci 2002; 967:6–157.

70. Kim JK, Fillmore JJ, Sunshine MJ, et al, PKC-theta knockout mice are protected from fat-induced insulin resistance. J Clin Invest 2004; 114:823–827.

71. Qatanani M, and Lazar MA. Mechanisms of obesity-associated insulin resistance: Many choices on the menu. Genes Dev 2007; 21:1443–1455.

72. Summers SA, Garza LA, Zhou H, and Birnbaum MJ. Regulation of insulin-stimulated glucose transporter GLUT4 translocation and Akt kinase activity by ceramide. Mol Cell Biol 1998; 18:5457–5464.

73. Ruvolo PP. Intracellular signal transduction pathways activated by ceramide and its metabolites. Pharmacol Res 2003; 47:383–392.

74. Holland WL, Brozinick JT, Wang LP, et al. Inhibition of ceramide synthesis ameliorates glucocorticoid-, saturated-fat-, and obesity-induced insulin resistance. Cell Metab 2007; 5:167–179.

75. Matsuzaka T, Shimano H, Yahagi N, et al. Crucial role of a long-chain fatty acid elongase, Elovl6, in obesity-induced insulin resistance. Nat Med 2007; 13:1193–1202.

76. Bruce CR, and Febbraio MA. It's what you do with the fat that matters! Nat Med 2007; 13:1137–1138.

77. Akira S. Toll-like receptor signaling. J Biol Chem 2003; 278:38105–38108.

78. Lee JY, Ye J, Gao Z, et al. Reciprocal modulation of Toll-like receptor-4 signaling pathways involving MyD88 and phosphatidylinositol 3-kinase/AKT by saturated and polyunsaturated fatty acids, J Biol Chem 2003; 278:37041–37051.

79. Suganami T, Mieda T, Itoh M, Shimoda Y, Kamei Y, and Ogawa Y. Attenuation of obesity-induced adipose tissue inflammation in C3 H/HeJ mice carrying a Toll-like receptor 4 mutation. Biochem Biophys Res Commun. 2007; 354:45–49.

80. Shi H, Kokoeva MV, Inouye K, Tzameli I, Yin H, and Flier JS. TLR4 links innate immunity and fatty acid-induced insulin resistance. J Clin Invest 2006; 116:3015–3025.

81. Weisberg SP, McCann D, Rosenbaum DM, Leibel RL, and Ferrante AW. Obesity is associated with macrophage accumulation in adipose tissue. J Clin Invest 2003; 112:1796–1808.

82. Xu H, Barnes GT, Yang Q, et al. Chronic inflammation in fat plays a crucial role in the development of obesity-related insulin resistance. J Clin Invest 2003; 112:1821–1830.

83. Fain JN, Cheema PS, Bahouth SW, Lloyd Hiler M. Resistin release by human adipose tissue explants in primary culture. Biochem Biophys Res Commun 2003; 300:674–678.

84. Rajala MW, Lin Y, Ranalletta M, et al. Cell type-specific expression and coregulation of murine resistin and resistin-like molecule-α in adipose tissue. Mol Endocrinol 2002; 116:1920–1930.

85. Marshall LA, Bolognese B, and Roshak A. Characterization of phospholipase A2 release by elicited-peritoneal macrophage and its relationship to eicosanoid production. J Lipid Mediat Cell Signal 1994; 10:295–313.

86. Sartipy P, and Loskotoff DJ. Monocyte chemoattractant protein 1 in obesity and insulin resistance. Proc Natl Acad Sci USA 2003; 100:7265–7270.

87. Di Gregorio GB, Yao-Porengasser A, Rasouli N, et al. Expression of CD68 and macrophage chemoattractant protein-1 genes in human adipose and muscle tissues. Diabetes 2005; 54:2305–2313.

88. Christiansen T, Richelsen B, Bruun JM. Monocyte chemoattractant protein-1 is produced in isolated adipocytes, associated with adiposity and reduced after weight loss in morbid obese subjects. Int J Obes Relat Metab Disord 2005; 29: 146–150.

89. Kanda H, Tateya S, Tamori Y, et al. MCP-1 contributes to macrophage infiltration into adipose tissue, insulin resistance, and hepatic steatosis in obesity. J Clin Invest 2006; 116:1494–1505.

90. Kamei N, Tobe K, Suzucki R, et al. Overexpression of monocyte chemoattractant protein-1 in adipose tissue causes macrophage recruitment and insulin resistance. J Biol Chem 2006; 281:26602–26614.

91. Tsou C-L, Peters W, Si Y, et al. Critical roles for CCR2 and MCP-3 in monocyte mobilization from bone marrow and recruitment to inflammatory sites. J Clin Invest 2007; 117:902–909.

92. Weisberg SP, Hunter D, Huber R, et al. CCR2 modulates inflammatory and metabolic effects of high fat feeding. J Clin Invest 2006; 116:115–124.

93. Chen A, Mumick S, Zhang C, et al. Diet induction of monocyte chemoattractant protein-1 and its impact on obesity. Obesity Res 2005; 13:1311–1320.

94. Inouye KE, Shi H, Howard JK, et al. Absence of CC chemokine ligand 2 does not limit obesity-associated infiltration of macrophages. Diabetes 2007; 56:2242–2250.

95. Lumeng CN, Bodzin JL, and Saltiel AR. Obesity induces a phenotypic switch in adipose tissue macrophage polarization. J Clin Invest 2007; 117:175–184.

96. Zeyda M, Farmer D, Todoric J, et al. Human adipose tissue macrophages are of an anti-inflammatory phenotype but capable of excessive pro-inflammatory mediator production. Int J Obesity 2007; 31:1420–1428.

97. Solinas G, Vilcu C, Neels JG, et al. JNK1 in Hematopoietically Derived Cells Contributes to Diet-Induced Inflammation and Insulin Resistance without Affecting Obesity. Cell Metab 2007; 6:386–397.

98. Spiegelman BM. PPARγ: Adipogenic regulator and thiazolidinedione receptor. Diabetes 1998; 47:507–514.

99. Picard F, and Auwerx J. PPAR (gamma) and glucose homeostasis. Annu Rev Nutr 2002; 22:167–197.

100. Ricote M, Li AC, Willson TM, Kelly CJ, and Glass CK. The peroxisome proliferator-activated receptor-γ is a negative regulator of macrophage activation. Nature 1998; 391:79–82.

101. Hevener AL, Olefsky J, Reichart D, et al.. Macrophage PPAR γ is required for normal skeletal muscle and hepatic insulin sensitivity and full antidiabetic effects of TZDs. J Clin Invest 2007; 117:1658–1669.

102. Odegaard JI, Ricardo-Gonzalez RR, Goforth MH, et al. Macrophage-specific PPARgamma controls alternative activation and improves insulin resistance. Nature 2007; 447:1116–1120.

103. Karin M, Lawrence T, and Nizet V. Innate immunity gone awry: Linking microbial infections to chronic inflammation and cancer. Cell 2006; 124:823–835.

104. Furuhashi M, Tuncman G, Görgün CZ, et al. Treatment of diabetes and atherosclerosis by inhibiting fatty-acid-binding protein aP2. Nature 2007; 447:959–965.

105. Febbraio M, Guy E, and Silverstein RL. Stem cell transplantation reveals that absence of macrophage CD36 is protective against atherosclerosis. Arterioscler Thromb Vasc Biol 2004; 24:2333–2338.

106. Ozcan U, Cao Q, Yilmaz E, et al. Endoplasmic reticulum stress links obesity, insulin action, and type 2 diabetes. Science 2004; 306:457–461.

107. Marciniak S. J, and Ron D. Endoplasmic reticulum stress signaling in disease. Physiol Rev 2006; 86:1133–1149.

108. Ozcan U, Yilmaz E, Ozcan L, et al. Chemical chaperones reduce ER stress and restore glucose homeostasis in a mouse model of type 2 diabetes. Science 2006; 313:1137–1140.

109. Yang Q, Kim Y. S, Lin Y, et al. Tumour necrosis factor receptor 1 mediates endoplasmic reticulum stress-induced activation of the MAP kinase JNK. EMBO Rep 2006; 7:622–627.

110. Urano F, Wang X, Bertolotti A, et al. Coupling of stress in the ER to activation of JNK protein kinases by transmembrane protein kinase IRE1. Science 2000; 287:664–666.

111. Hu P, Han Z, Couvillon AD, Kaufman RJ, and Exton JH Autocrine tumor necrosis factor alpha links endoplasmic reticulum stress to the membrane death receptor pathway through IRE1alpha-mediated NF-kappaB activation and down-regulation of TRAF2 expression. Mol Cell Biol 2006; 26:3071–3084.

112. Kaneto H, Nakatani Y, Miyatsuka T, et al.. Possible novel therapy for diabetes with cell-permeable JNK-inhibitory peptide. Nat Med 2004; 10:1128–1132.

113. Bain J, Plater L, Elliott M, et al. The selectivity of protein kinase inhibitors: A further update. Biochem J 2007; 408:297–315.

5

How Do We Screen for and Predict Autoimmune Diabetes?

Peter Achenbach

Diabetes Research Institute, Munich, Germany

Ezio Bonifacio

CRTD, Dresden University of Technology, Dresden, Germany

Polly J. Bingley

Diabetes and Metabolism, Department of Clinical Science at North Bristol, University of Bristol, Bristol, U.K.

In recent years, the characteristics of the stages of pre-type 1 diabetes have been studied in different cohorts of individuals at risk, leading to the identification of disease-associated biomarkers that can now be applied to risk assessment and disease prediction. These studies have also demonstrated that progression to disease is not uniform and that, in order to optimize risk assessment, demographic, genetic, immune, and metabolic predictive markers should be combined. This chapter will summarize current knowledge on type 1 diabetes-associated risk markers and their potential use for screening purposes, and will suggest how prediction strategies could be translated into clinical application, if and when an effective form of intervention to prevent type 1 diabetes is identified.

WHY SHOULD WE SCREEN FOR TYPE 1 DIABETES?

Assessment of type 1 diabetes (T1D) risk and prediction of disease development remain primarily research tools, useful for identifying subjects suitable for recruitment into intervention trials which aim to prevent the clinical onset of T1D (1). In this chapter we have used the term "screening" as a form of shorthand, but it is important to realize that it will only be possible fully to evaluate screening according to standard criteria once one of these trials has been successful (2). Current strategies enable family members to be stratified into the majority who have levels of risk equivalent to those of the background population, and a small proportion at high risk for progression to disease (3–5). Recruitment into future trials can therefore be based on careful selection of participants who are best suited for the individual therapeutic approaches.

A number of different screening tools are available, but both their value and acceptable financial and other costs will depend on the purpose of risk assessment. Many of these cannot yet be quantified, but two major objectives of screening arise from the types of intervention trial currently envisaged.

Primary prevention trials aim to prevent the development of T1D by intervening at the earliest stage of pathogenesis before islet autoimmunity is initiated. Primary prevention is therefore applicable to islet autoantibody-negative young children who are at high genetic risk of T1D. In contrast, *secondary prevention trials* apply intervention to non-diabetic individuals who have already developed islet autoimmunity, with the aim of preventing progression to clinical disease. Islet autoantibody-positive relatives of people with T1D are currently the cohort of choice for recruitment into secondary prevention trials.

The Autoimmune Background of Type 1 Diabetes Determines Screening

Screening strategies should be based on the natural history of T1D development. For accurate risk assessment, it is useful to consider the characteristics at different stages of pathogenesis and the factors that contribute to the autoimmune process (Fig. 1).

Genes determine susceptibility to T1D and can influence the appearance and progression of islet autoimmunity (6). All the major T1D susceptibility genes identified to date have, in common, a functional relationship to the immune system, including involvement in antigen presentation (7), antigen expression (8), immune regulation (9,10), or signal transduction in immune cells (11). Whereas, some genes contribute to immune dysregulation and breakdown of immune tolerance to islet autoantigens, others can be protective; hence, a combination of genes shapes T1D susceptibility in the majority of cases (6,12). For the purposes of prediction, it is important to appreciate that different combinations of genes contributing to an individual's genetic susceptibility play a role in determining patterns of islet autoimmunity, associated diabetes risk, and/or speed of progression to disease. However, only a limited number of T1D-associated genes, mainly those in the human leukocyte antigen (HLA) class II region on chromosome 6, are currently used for screening purposes.

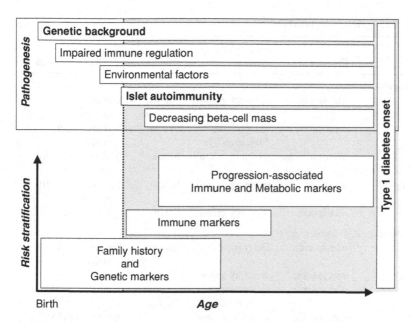

Figure 1 Pathogenesis and risk stratification of type 1 diabetes: Genetic background and impaired immune regulation are preconditions on which environmental factors can trigger islet autoimmunity, leading to β-cell destruction and decreasing β-cell mass, and finally to diabetes onset. Diabetes risk can be stratified by using markers related to the stage of pathogenesis.

Autoantigens

The autoimmune response in T1D is specifically directed against molecular targets that are predominantly expressed in β-cells. Autoantibody and T-cell responses to a wide range of molecules have been associated with T1D (Table 1) (13). While some of these antigens have been confirmed as major targets of the autoimmune process by many investigators (major T1D autoantigens), a number of others have been proposed but their relevance for the disease remains uncertain (minor or candidate T1D autoantigens). Interestingly, many of these autoantigens are related to cells of neuroendocrine origin with highly developed and regulated secretory mechanisms, and all of the major T1D autoantigens are related to the secretory apparatus (Table 1). The best-studied, major autoantigens in T1D are (pro)insulin (14,15), the 65-kDa isoform of glutamic acid decarboxylase (GAD65) (16), and the protein tyrosine phosphatase related molecules IA-2 (ICA512) and IA-2β (phogrin) (17–20). (Pro)insulin is present within β-cell secretory granules, and IA-2 and IA-2β are transmembrane proteins in these granules (20,21), whereas GAD65 is a membrane associated protein of β-cell synaptic-like microvesicles (22). Most recently, another transmembrane protein

Table 1 Autoantigens Reported in T1D

Antigen	Expression	Subcellular location	Antibodies	T cells	References
Major T1D autoantigens					
Insulin	islet specific	secretory granule	human, mouse	human, mouse	(14)
GAD65	neuroendocrine	synaptic-like microvesicle	human	human, mouse	(16)
IA-2 (ICA512)	neuroendocrine	secretory granule	human	human, mouse	(17,18)
IA-2β (phogrin)	neuroendocrine	secretory granule	human	human, mouse	(19,20)
ZnT8	islet specific	secretory granule	human		(24)
Minor or candidate T1D autoantigens					
Proinsulin	islet specific	Golgi apparatus	human	human, mouse	(15)
PreproIAPP	islet specific	secretory granule		human	(113)
IGRP	islet specific	endoplasmatic reticulum		mouse	(114)
HIP/PAP	islet specific	secretory granule		mouse	(115)
Reg II	islet specific	secretory granule		mouse	(116)
Reg Iα	islet specific	secretory granule	human		(117)
GAD67	neuroendocrine	cytosol	human	human, mouse	(118)
ICA69	neuroendocrine	Golgi apparatus	human	human, mouse	(119)
Carboxypeptidase H	neuroendocrine	secretory granule	human, mouse	mouse	(120)
Glima 38	neuroendocrine	secretory granule	human		(121)
Glycolipid GM2-1	neuroendocrine	secretory granule	human		(122)
Ganglioside GT3	neuroendocrine	cell membrane	human		(123)
Sulphatide	neuroendocrine	secretory granule	human		(124)
S100β	neuroendocrine	cytosol		human, mouse	(125)
Peripherin	neuroendocrine	cytosol	mouse	mouse	(126)
GLUT2	widely	cell membrane	human		(127)
DNA topoisomerase II	widely	nucleus	human		(128)
SOX13 (ICA12)	widely	nucleus	human		(129)
Jun-B	widely	nucleus	human	human	(130)
Imogen 38	widely	mitochondria		human	(131)
HSP60	widely	mitochondria	human, mouse	human, mouse	(132)
HSP70	widely	mitochondria, cytosol, ER	human	human	(133)
HSP90	widely	cytosol	human		(134)
AADC	widely	cytosol	human		(135)

of β-cell secretory granules, zinc transporter ZnT8 (23), has been identified as an additional major autoantigen in human T1D (24).

Islet Autoantibodies

Circulating autoantibodies to islet cell antigens are present in sera from new-onset T1D patients as well as prior to the clinical onset of disease, signaling an active and disease-specific–B-lymphocyte response (25). Because islet autoantibodies can precede the development of clinical onset diabetes by many years, they are used to identify individuals with higher risk for developing T1D (4,26–33). They can be very reproducibly detected and are currently the best-validated and most widely used predictive markers for T1D, particularly autoantibodies directed against the biochemically defined target antigens insulin (IAA), GAD65 (GADA), and IA-2 (IA-2A).

Much of our current understanding of islet autoantibodies and their role in prediction has derived from prospective studies in individuals with an increased genetic susceptibility, such as relatives of patients with T1D. The prevalence of islet autoantibodies in relatives is 5% to 10%, depending upon which antibodies are measured (4,31,34,35). The largest screening in relatives has been undertaken as part of the Diabetes Prevention Trial Type 1 (DPT-1) in North America (4). In a DPT-1 substudy, samples from 17,207 of the 71,148 first-degree relatives tested for islet cell antibodies (ICA), GADA, and IA-2A were also tested for IAA by microassay. At least one of the four autoantibodies (above the 99th centile) was found in 8.2% of relatives tested and more than one autoantibody in 2.3%. Although closely associated with future disease, not all subjects with islet autoantibodies will develop T1D. Substantial efforts have therefore been made to identify disease-specific characteristics of autoantibodies and other markers that will help distinguish which islet autoantibody-positive relatives will and will not develop T1D, and, if so, when is this likely to occur (5,36–39).

Autoreactive T Cells

T-cell responses to various β-cell antigens have been reported in T1D (13,40). T1D risk screening does not however currently involve routine measurement of T-cell reactivity because, compared to autoantibodies, human T-cell responses to islet antigens are considerably more difficult to detect reproducibly in the peripheral blood of patients with T1D or prior to clinical onset of disease. For years, it has been a challenge to show convincingly disease-specific T-cell responses in human T1D, and to distinguish quantitatively between specific T-cell responses of patients and control subjects (41,42), though the recent introduction of new methods, such as ELISpot-assay and tetramer-analysis into diabetes research has resulted in progress in this area (43–47). These measures may become more generally available and may begin to play a part in screening in the near future, particularly in monitoring the effect of immunointervention.

HOW SHOULD WE SCREEN?

In general, screening is hierarchical, starting from an a priori selection via genetics (including family history), followed by the detection of ongoing autoimmunity using islet autoantibody markers, and subsequent stratification of autoantibody-positive individuals on the basis of their islet autoantibody profile and an assessment of their ability to control glucose loads (Fig. 1). Where one stops, depends on the type of intervention trial (primary or secondary) and the target level of risk required for participation in the trial. *A proposed algorithm:*

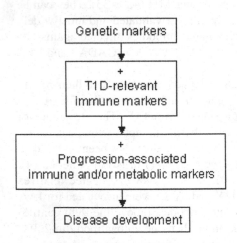

Screening for Primary Prevention Trials: Assessing Genetic Risk—Family History, Genes, and Both

As mentioned above, primary prevention trials target individuals who have not yet developed detectable markers of humoral autoimmunity. Screening must therefore make use of the "earlier" or "lower hierarchy" markers and must answer the primary question of "who is likely to develop T1D-relevant islet autoimmunity?" From the time of birth, family history and diabetes susceptibility genes can be used to identify individuals with an increased probability of developing islet autoimmunity and T1D (Fig. 2).

Risk Stratification by Family History

A *first-degree family history* of T1D is a major risk factor for islet autoimmunity and diabetes (6,48), and about 10% to 13% of newly-diagnosed children are from families with at least one affected first-degree relative (6,49). Overall, around 3% to 8% of relatives will develop islet autoimmunity and T1D, whereas, the risk in individuals without a T1D family history is around 10-fold lower (Fig. 2) (6). The risk of developing islet autoimmunity further varies depending on *which relative* is affected (Fig. 2). In the DPT-1 study, siblings of someone with T1D developed islet

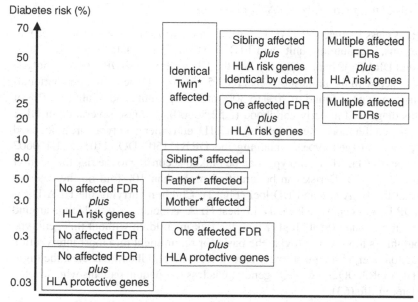

Risk stratification by T1D family history and HLA genotyping

Figure 2 T1D risk stratification by combining information on family history of T1D and HLA genotyping: Useful for primary risk assessment in islet autoantibody-negative individuals. *Risk is inversely related to the age at T1D onset in the affected relative. *Abbreviations*: FDR, first-degree relative; HLA risk genes, HLA DR3/DR4-DQ8.

autoantibodies more frequently than offspring or parents (50), and data from the German BABYDIAB study show that children with a healthy mother but a father with T1D are at higher risk of islet autoimmunity than the children of mothers with T1D (51). As a general rule, the risk of a child from an affected family is

If no first-degree relative with T1D $\ll$ if mother with T1D $<$ if father with T1D $<$ if sibling with T1D $<$ if identical twin with T1D.

Age at diagnosis of the affected family member and current age of the non-diabetic relative are important factors providing additional information on the inherited risk. For both of these, risk is inversely related to age, i.e., the probability that a person with a first-degree T1D family history will develop islet autoimmunity and diabetes decreases with increasing age of diagnosis in the affected relative with diabetes and falls with longer duration of autoimmunity-free survival (52,53).

Furthermore, risk depends upon *how many relatives* have T1D (Fig. 2). In the German BABYDIAB cohort, a child's risk for multiple islet autoantibodies was markedly higher (approximately 25%) if both parents or a parent and a sibling had T1D compared with a single affected family member (54).

Risk Stratification by HLA Genotyping

The HLA class II alleles *(IDDM1)* contribute most to T1D susceptibility (6,55). In Caucasians, islet autoimmunity and T1D are strongly associated with HLA DR3-DQ2 and DR4-DQ8 haplotypes (6), and the HLA DR3-DQ2/DR4-DQ8 genotype is associated with the highest diabetes risk (52,56–60). Depending upon nationality, this genotype is found in 20% to 30% of T1D patients and in almost 50% of patients diagnosed in early childhood (6,52,58–60). Because several other HLA genotypes confer moderate or high risk for T1D, and other genotypes are associated with protection (genotypes containing the DRB1*1501-DQA1*01/DQB1*0602 haplotype) (6,61), HLA genotypes can be ranked according to the risk they confer (57–59,62), and T1D risk can be stratified more than 100-fold on the basis of typing at the HLA-DR and DQ loci (Fig. 2). Children carrying the HLA DR3-DQ2/DR4-DQ8 genotype have the highest HLA-associated risk, which is around 4% and more than 10-fold higher than the risk in children without this genotype (6), but this is too low to provide the basis for recruitment into most intervention trials. Moreover, although strongly associated with childhood diabetes, the high-risk–HLA DR3-DQ2/DR4-DQ8 genotype is less frequent in patients who develop T1D later in life (63).

HLA genotyping helps to predict who will develop islet autoimmunity. In children without islet autoimmunity, HLA haplotypes can be used to identify those who are more likely to develop islet autoantibodies. Results from the German BABYDIAB study, the Finnish Type 1 Diabetes Prediction and Prevention (DIPP) study, and the Diabetes Autoimmunity Study in the Young (DAISY) consistently show that children carrying high-risk HLA genotypes are more likely to develop islet autoantibodies in infancy, and to do so at an earlier age, than those with intermediate risk, low risk, or protective HLA genotypes (64–66). Among BABYDIAB offspring who had at least one first-degree relative with T1D, the risk of developing islet autoantibodies by the age of 2 years was 20% in those with the high-risk DR3-DQ2/DR4-DQ8 or DR4-DQ8/DR4-DQ8 genotypes, compared with 2.7% in offspring without these genotypes, and overall 50% of islet autoantibody-positive offspring had at least one of these genotypes (65).

HLA genotyping helps to predict the characteristics of islet autoimmunity. Islet autoantibodies differ in their association with HLA haplotypes. HLA genotyping in antibody-negative children at risk may therefore help to predict the primary antigen(s) involved in a potential autoimmune process, and therefore direct targeted antibody screening. GADA are more frequent in individuals with HLA-DR3-DQ2 (67,68), whereas IAA and IA-2A are more common with HLA-DR4-DQ8 (64–67). Individuals without either of these haplotypes are more frequently islet autoantibody-negative (65–67,69).

HLA typing can also help to identify islet autoantibody responses that have T1D-relevant characteristics such as persistence, breadth, and maturity (see below). For example, the DAISY study found that the development of persistent islet autoantibodies was associated with the HLA-DR3-DQ2/DR4-DQ8 genotype in both relatives of patients with T1D and in children from the general population, whereas transient islet autoantibodies were not correlated with known genetic risk factors (66,70). The German BABYDIAB study showed that the genetic risk factors found in children who developed multiple islet autoantibodies were absent in children who developed single islet autoantibodies (54,59). Similarly, the Australian BabyDiab study found that HLA-DR4-DQ8 and DR3-DQ2 were more prevalent in children who developed persistent multiple islet autoantibodies than in children who were transient or single antibody positive (71), and the Karlsburg schoolchildren study found children with multiple islet autoantibodies, but not those with a single islet autoantibody, had HLA allele frequencies that were similar to those found in T1D (72). Finally, high-affinity IAA are associated with HLA-DR4-DQ8 containing genotypes (36); whereas, high-affinity GADA are associated with HLA-DR3-DQ2 (37), and most IA-2A positive offspring with the HLA-DR3-DQ2/DR4-DQ8 or DR4-DQ8/DR4-DQ8 genotypes immediately develop a broad antibody reactivity to multiple epitopes expressed in both IA-2 and IA-2β molecules (73). Altogether, this supports the view that HLA susceptibility genes may affect the magnitude and breadth of the autoimmune response.

HLA-genetic risk can be stratified by other genes and environment. HLA-associated risk is modified by several factors that include geographical region (background prevalence of genotypes and T1D incidence) (48,74,75), other genes (59,76,77) and, importantly, whether children have a T1D family history (48). Furthermore, HLA genes may interact with non-HLA genes or with the environment in a genotype-specific manner, so that the risk conferred by HLA is modified for some genotypes, but not others. This is the case for the risk conferred by a second T1D-susceptibility locus mapped to a variable number of tandem repeat (VNTR) in the insulin gene *(INS)* promoter region *(IDDM2)* (6). It has been suggested that the associated risk is conferred by differences in the level of expression of the insulin protein in the thymus leading to defective central tolerance to the insulin molecule (8,78,79). In accordance with this, IAA are less frequent in patients or relatives who have the T1D protective *INS* VNTR class I/III or III/III genotypes (59,68). Although genotype variation at *INS* significantly affects T1D susceptibility in all HLA risk categories, there is significant heterogeneity in the distribution of *INS* genotypes in patients carrying different HLA genotypes (76,80). In individuals with the high-risk HLA genotypes DR3-DQ2/DR4-DQ8 and DR4-DQ8/DR4-DQ8, risk can be further stratified by screening for predisposing *INS* VNTR class I/I genotype (59). Combining HLA and *INS* typing will therefore improve T1D risk stratification, but not in a manner strictly predicted from the multiplicative model.

Combined HLA Genotyping and T1D Family History can Identify Neonates at Highest Risk

Thousandfold differences in risk can be determined by combining the extent of an individual's family history with his or her HLA genotype (Fig. 2). Neonates carrying DR3-DQ2/DR4-DQ8 or DR4-DQ8/DR4-DQ8 can be further stratified by selection of those with multiple family history of diabetes (54), or who are HLA identical to the proband (81), to identify subgroups with more than 50% risk of developing islet autoantibodies. In the German BABYDIAB cohort, 55% of neonates who had a multiplex first-degree family history of T1D together with the DR3-DQ2/DR4-DQ8 or DR4-DQ8/DR4-DQ8 genotypes developed multiple islet autoantibodies (IAA, followed by GADA and IA-2A) in the first years of life, and the majority of those who developed these antibodies progressed to diabetes in childhood (54). In the DAISY cohort, siblings of children with T1D with the HLA-DR3-DQ2/DR4-DQ8 genotype and identical by descent for both HLA haplotypes with their diabetic sibling had a 65% risk of developing islet autoantibodies by age 7 and a 50% risk of developing diabetes by age 10 (81). Thus, it is possible to identify children with a 50% or higher risk of developing multiple antibodies in childhood, an early and specific marker for development of diabetes. Although these levels of risk are impressive, only a very small proportion of the future cases of T1D fall into these categories. These methods of screening will therefore only be applicable to very selective intervention trials, such as Pre-POINT (*P*rimary *O*ral/intranasal *IN*sulin *T*rial) (www.diabetes-point.org).

Screening for Secondary Prevention Trials: Islet Autoantibodies and Their Characteristics

Individuals with evidence of islet autoimmunity have entered a new stage in T1D pathogenesis, and may be suitable for inclusion into secondary prevention trials. Selection of participants for such trials therefore requires screening for *immune markers* (Fig. 1), which in T1D is currently synonymous with measurement of islet autoantibodies in peripheral blood. Prospective studies from birth such as the German BABYDIAB study (82), the Finnish DIPP project (83), the DAISY study from Colorado (84), the Australian BABYDIAB study (85), and the Prospective Assessment of Newborns for Diabetes Autoimmunity (PANDA) study from Florida (86) have contributed most of today's knowledge on the appearance and progression of islet autoimmunity in childhood. It has been demonstrated that IAA are almost always the first autoantibodies to appear in young children who subsequently progress to T1D (32,69,87), and that the typical natural history of T1D in children is the appearance of IAA, followed by relatively early/rapid spreading to other islet autoantibodies and eventually the development of diabetes (69,70,88). *We therefore recommend that in children, adolescents, and young adults (up to the age of around 25 years) screening includes all T1D-associated major autoantibodies, i.e., IAA, GADA, IA-2A, and ZnT8 autoantibodies.*

Screening in older relatives should take into consideration the frequencies of the individual antibodies in adult late-onset T1D. The prevalence of IAA decreases dramatically with increasing age (89), and IAA are therefore not particularly useful screening markers in the over 25 years age groups. The prevalence of GADA on the other hand, is relatively stable with age (90). IA-2A are slightly more prevalent in younger cases, whereas, the prevalence of ZnT8A is directly correlated with the age of T1D onset (24,34). *We therefore suggest that adults (older than 25 years) should be screened for GADA, IA-2A, and ZnT8A, with additional sequential testing for IAA for further risk stratification.*

Following its appearance, it is necessary to *confirm* the antibody marker and to monitor its *persistence* on follow-up. Only persistent islet autoantibodies signal an active autoimmune process relevant to diabetes development. Single positive test results or transient autoantibody appearance are not associated with progression to T1D (70,71). IAA are the major islet autoantibodies that are least likely to persist (69–71) and this is related to titer (70,71). Transient IAA are also associated with maternal transfer of insulin antibodies (91,92).

If autoantibodies are confirmed as stable, we need to look for *markers of progression* (Fig. 1). These may be immune and/or metabolic, may only develop during follow-up, and could potentially indicate relevant "events" in the underlying pathogenesis (93). It is therefore important to monitor autoantibodies at appropriate time intervals, especially in young individuals in whom changes are usually more frequent and rapid (93).

The development of *multiple islet autoantibodies* is a critical step in pathogenesis and, therefore, a highly relevant marker of risk of progression. It has been known for more than a decade that detection of two or more islet autoantibodies is associated with a significantly higher T1D risk than a single autoantibody (29,30,94). Whereas T1D risk is less than 20% within 10 years in relatives with just one islet autoantibody, it is approximately 35% within 5 years and 61% within 10 years in those with more than one autoantibody (5). Multiple islet autoantibody-positive subjects without a T1D family history also appear to have a high risk (33,95). However, the status "multiple autoantibody positivity" depends on which markers are tested. For example, recent data from the Munich family study show that around two-thirds of relatives found to be GADA positive, but IAA and IA-2A negative (i.e., previously defined as low risk) in fact had autoantibodies to the newly identified autoantigen ZnT8, moving them into the multiple antibody-positive category. This included all those who progressed to diabetes within this group of relatives (Ezio Bonifacio and Peter Achenbach, unpublished findings). It is therefore possible that further marker(s) will become available that can identify more advanced islet autoimmunity and higher risk among individuals who are currently categorized as "single autoantibody positive"

Who Will Progress in Islet Autoimmunity?

More recently, characteristics of islet autoantibodies themselves have been shown to identify relatives whose islet autoimmunity will progress. The major discriminating characteristics are related to the target specificity, the maturity and magnitude of the response, and the age at autoantibody appearance. Maturity and magnitude are reflected by antibody affinity, titer, and number of different IgG subclasses and target epitopes on individual and combined islet antigens.

Rule of thumb: "the more and the earlier, the higher the risk".

Target specificity matters. There appears to be a hierarchy of diabetes-relevance in the autoantibody response against different antigenic targets within and between islet autoantigens. For example, whereas risk is relatively low in relatives with GADA or IAA alone (approximately 20% within 10 years), the presence of IA-2A alone is associated with a similar risk (approximately 50% within 10 years) to multiple non-IA-2-autoantibodies (ICA, GADA and/or IAA) (5,34). Among IA-2A positive relatives, risk can be further stratified according to the presence or absence of autoantibodies to IA-2β (5,93). Also, IAA without proinsulin reactivity are associated with low risk, whereas proinsulin-reactive IAA are associated with very high risk of progression (36). For GADA, the N-terminal GAD-restricted antibodies are associated with low/no risk of progression, whereas individuals with antibodies directed towards the middle and/or C-terminal of the antigen progress to disease (37).

Maturity matters. Antibody affinity provides an indirect measure of maturity. In a typical antibody response, exposure to antigen in the presence of B-cell growth factors results in B lymphocyte expansion and IgM antibody production. Sustained or repeated antigen exposure leads to a switch from IgM to IgG production and selection of clones that produce antibodies of high affinity to the antigen (96,97). In T1D, high affinity autoantibodies are associated with progression of islet autoimmunity and are therefore "diabetes-relevant", whereas, low affinity antibodies are unrelated to diabetes development (36,37). The German BABYDIAB study has identified affinity as a marker for T1D-relevant IAA and GADA (36,37). IAA affinity varied considerably between IAA-positive children, and those who developed high-affinity IAA ($K_d > 10^9$ L/mol) had persistent IAA, developed multiple islet autoantibodies, and had a 50% risk of developing T1D within 6 years. In contrast, children with lower affinity IAA rarely progressed to multiple islet autoantibodies and did not develop T1D. High-affinity IAA differed from lower affinity IAA in insulin binding characteristics suggesting distinct epitope recognition and, in contrast to the lower affinity IAA, the associated epitope was also expressed on the proinsulin molecule (36). Similar findings were recently obtained for GADA, in that, single high-affinity GADA-positive children progressed to multiple islet autoantibodies and T1D more frequently than children with low-affinity GADA (37).

Magnitude matters. The magnitude of an autoantibody response is reflected by persistence, titer, affinity, and the breadth or range of autoantigen targets. Diabetes development has been associated with high-titer ICA (98), IAA (5,89), or IA-2A (5). High titer also determines other characteristics, such as breadth of the response in terms of IgG subclass usage and epitope reactivity. As expected, high titer responses are usually synonymous with multiple IgG subclass antibodies to multiple epitopes, though these features can also be independent indicators of disease risk in low-titer autoantibody-positive subjects (5). In a recent analysis of autoantibody-positive relatives followed for up to 15 years, the highest risks for T1D were associated with high-titer IAA and IA-2A responses, with the appearance of antibody subclasses IgG2, IgG3, and/or IgG4 of IAA and IA-2A, and antibodies to the IA-2-related molecule IA-2β (5). Using various combinations of these islet autoantibody characteristics, it was possible to stratify 5-year diabetes risk from less than 10% to approximately 90%.

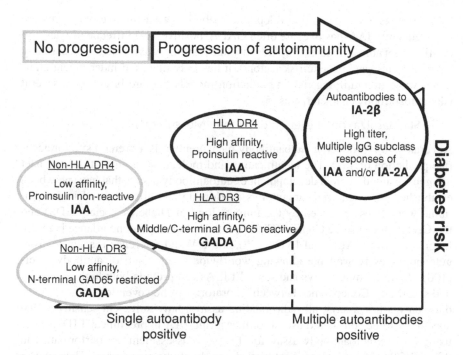

Figure 3 Type 1 diabetes risk stratification by islet autoantibody characteristics: Increase in T1D risk is associated with progression of islet autoimmunity from single to multiple autoantibodies. Immunization profiles in single IAA- or GADA-positive individuals that can signal progression to multiple autoantibodies are associated with mature high-affinity antibody responses against specific epitopes on the insulin/proinsulin and GAD65 molecules in the presence of HLA-DR4 and HLA-DR3, respectively. Further progression of autoimmunity in multiple autoantibody-positive individuals is signaled by broad intensive antibody responses of IAA and IA-2A, and the appearance of autoantibodies to IA-2β, and is associated with high risk of rapid diabetes development.

A schematic representation of our findings with respect to autoantibodies in the natural history and prediction of T1D is presented in Figure 3.

Age matters. Risk of developing T1D can be stratified on the basis of how early islet autoantibodies develop (88). The earlier in life the first autoantibody appears, the higher the risk of progression of islet autoimmunity and, in particular, the earlier multiple autoantibodies appear, the higher the risk of rapid progression to diabetes. In the German BABYDIAB cohort, 50% of children who already had multiple islet autoantibodies within the first year of life progressed to diabetes within 2 years of follow-up. This was significantly more rapid than progression in children who developed multiple islet autoantibodies at the age of 2 years (17%) or at the age of 5 years (7%) (88). In line with this, the magnitude of the autoantibody response in early childhood appears to be greater than that in later life. Children who develop islet autoantibodies before the age of 2 years, frequently have high-affinity IAA and progress to multiple islet autoantibodies

(36), whereas, children who develop autoantibodies after the age of 2 years are less frequently IAA-positive, are often GADA-positive, and infrequently develop multiple islet autoantibodies (88). Because age is strongly associated with antibody characteristics (and genetic risk factors), it has only marginal independent additional value in stratifying risk in prediction models that are based upon several islet autoantibody characteristics (5).

Standardization of Islet Autoantibody Measurement

Accurate and reproducible autoantibody measurement is a prerequisite for accurate prediction of T1D. The identification and molecular cloning of defined islet antigens resulted in rapid development of autoantibody assays that have now been established in specialized laboratories worldwide and are validated in international workshops organized by the Immunology of Diabetes Society (IDS) and the Centers for Disease Control (CDC) (99). There is high concordance between laboratories for GADA and IA-2A (99), and a WHO reference reagent for islet autoantibodies is available allowing worldwide comparison of antibody levels (100). Radio-binding assays and some ELISAs can provide both high sensitivity and specificity. Concordance between laboratories is, however, lower for IAA. To date, only a few assays, all radio-binding assays, have sufficient sensitivity and specificity to be considered useful for measuring IAA in preclinical T1D. Before using an islet autoantibody assay for T1D risk assessment, its performance in the IDS/CDC-based international workshops should be ascertained. These workshops are also useful in the validation of new assays and new autoantibodies. The Diabetes Autoantibody Standardization Program provides an established platform for rapid evaluation of new T1D markers by the wider research community. Examples are IAA affinity (101) or autoantibodies to IA-2β and ZnT8 (9th International Congress of the Immunology of Diabetes Society and American Diabetes Association Research Symposium, Miami, 2007). Future evaluation might include epitope and Ig subclass measurement, or determination of GADA affinity. In a complementary program, under the auspices of NIDDK, efforts are underway to align the best performing GADA and IA-2A assays by developing common assay protocols that will initially be used in the large type 1 diabetes research consortia such as TEDDY. The overall objective is to provide a basis for standard protocols for assessment of T1D risk.

Metabolic Markers of Progression to T1D

Metabolic markers are not primary screening tools in T1D risk assessment but can further refine risk assessment in autoantibody-positive individuals. First-phase insulin response (FPIR) in the intravenous glucose tolerance test is often impaired prior to diabetes onset and there have been attempts to determine the rate of progression to diabetes by combining islet autoantibody measurement and FPIR. Autoantibody-positive relatives with a low FPIR have a faster rate of progression (or are closer) to diabetes than those with normal FPIR (3,102,103). In DPT-1, T1D risk in ICA positive, IAA positive relatives with FPIR below the first centile was around 60% within 5 years (102). In the European Nicotinamide Diabetes Intervention Trial (ENDIT), the overall 5-year risk in ICA-positive relatives with low FPIR was approximately 55% (3), but among relatives positive for five autoantibodies (ICA, GADA, IA-2A, IAA, and IA-2βA), the risk associated with a low FPIR increased to >90%, and impaired oral glucose tolerance identified those with fastest progression to disease (>50% progression within one year) (104). Recent studies have also suggested that combining measures of insulin resistance and FPIR in islet autoantibody positive relatives may further contribute to risk assessment (105–107). Although risk assessment is clearly improved by the addition of metabolic measurements, and the intravenous glucose tolerance test and oral glucose tolerance test can stage the preclinical phase of T1D, these tests are difficult to standardize. Low FPIR was associated with T1D-related autoantibody characteristics such as high-titer ICA, the presence of IAA, and multiple islet autoantibodies in 52 children aged between 1 and 5 years in the DIPP study (108), and in older relatives participating in ENDIT (3), indicating that some of the increased risk conferred by low FPIR can be attributed to autoantibody characteristics. In accord with this, accurate T1D risk stratification was achieved on the basis of autoantibody characteristics that included titer, subclasses, and/or epitopes alone (5), suggesting that FPIR may not need to be included in the inclusion criteria for recruitment for future trials.

Many of the studies cited have demonstrated complex interactions between the determinants of risk of T1D, suggesting the need for integrated risk assessment models based on genetic, immune, and metabolic markers. Over the last decade, the data arising from large prospective studies such as DPT-1 and ENDIT have provided unprecedented opportunities to develop such models (3,109), but even larger populations are needed for multivariate analyses combining all the available markers.

FUTURE DIRECTIONS

Identification of novel autoantigens: It is likely that further islet autoantigens remain to be identified, and that these may enhance assessment of T1D risk. The recent identification of ZnT8 as a major target of islet autoantibodies in T1D is testimony to this, particularly the finding that antibodies to ZnT8 help identify relatives previously designated as single antibody-positive (for IAA, GADA, or IA-2A) who progress to T1D (Ezio Bonifacio and Peter Achenbach, unpublished).

Islet autoantibody profiling assays: With at least four autoantigen clusters and multiple epitope targets, efforts must be directed to developing islet autoantibody profiling and signature assays using array technology. Such assays would facilitate the tracking of changes in prediabetes that may help predict disease progression, and could also be of value in monitoring immune efficacy of intervention treatments.

Markers for adult autoimmune diabetes: Whereas children and adolescents usually develop T1D accompanied by multiple islet autoantibodies, adults are often only positive for GADA alone (110). As discussed, positivity for a single autoantibody has relatively low predictive value. Additional markers in this age group are therefore urgently required.

Transfer of findings in relatives to general population: Relatives of people with T1D have a 10- to 15-fold higher risk of developing T1D than people without a family history of T1D. Thus, a priori, the positive predictive value of islet autoantibodies for T1D progression will be higher in relatives than in nonrelatives. This difference becomes minimal with multiple islet autoantibodies and broad responses, because these are highly specific for T1D. Nevertheless, few studies have documented risk in the general population (95,111,112). Assuming that efficacious preventive therapies will be found, it will be important to establish T1D risk in islet autoantibody-positive individuals from the general population in order to decrease the overall incidence of T1D.

REFERENCES

1. Achenbach P, Bonifacio E, Ziegler AG. Predicting type 1 diabetes. Curr Diab Rep 2005; 5:98–103.
2. Staeva-Vieira T, Peakman M, von Herrath M. Translational mini-review series on type 1 diabetes: Immune-based therapeutic approaches for type 1 diabetes. Clin Exp Immunol 2007; 148:17–31.
3. Bingley PJ, Gale EA. Progression to type 1 diabetes in islet cell antibody-positive relatives in the European Nicotinamide Diabetes Intervention Trial: The role of additional immune, genetic and metabolic markers of risk. Diabetologia 2006; 49:881–890.
4. Krischer JP, Cuthbertson DD, Yu L, et al. Screening strategies for the identification of multiple antibody-positive relatives of individuals with type 1 diabetes. J Clin Endocrinol Metab 2003; 88:103–108.
5. Achenbach P, Warncke K, Reiter J, et al. Stratification of type 1 diabetes risk on the basis of islet autoantibody characteristics. Diabetes 2004; 53:384–392.
6. Redondo MJ, Eisenbarth GS. Genetic control of autoimmunity in Type I diabetes and associated disorders. Diabetologia 2002; 45:605–622.
7. Todd JA, Bell JI, McDevitt HO. HLA-DQ beta gene contributes to susceptibility and resistance to insulin-dependent diabetes mellitus. Nature 1987; 329:599–604.
8. Vafiadis P, Bennett ST, Todd JA, et al. Insulin expression in human thymus is modulated by INS VNTR alleles at the IDDM2 locus. Nat Genet 1997; 15:289–292.
9. Gambelunghe G, Ghaderi M, Cosentino A, et al. Association of MHC Class I chain-related A (MIC-A) gene polymorphism with Type I diabetes. Diabetologia 2000; 43:507–514.
10. Nistico L, Buzzetti R, Pritchard LE, et al. The CTLA-4 gene region of chromosome 2q33 is linked to, and associated with, type 1 diabetes. Belgian Diabetes Registry. Hum Mol Genet 1996; 5:1075–1080.
11. Bottini N, Musumeci L, Alonso A, et al. A functional variant of lymphoid tyrosine phosphatase is associated with type I diabetes. Nat Genet 2004; 36:337–338.
12. Todd JA, Farrall M. Panning for gold: Genome-wide scanning for linkage in type 1 diabetes. Hum Mol Genet 1996; (5 Spec No):1443–1448.

13. Lieberman SM, DiLorenzo TP. A comprehensive guide to antibody and T-cell responses in type 1 diabetes. Tissue Antigens 2003; 62:359–377.
14. Palmer JP, Asplin CM, Clemons P, et al. Insulin antibodies in insulin-dependent diabetics before insulin treatment. Science 1983; 222:1337–1339.
15. Kuglin B, Gries FA, Kolb H. Evidence of IgG autoantibodies against human proinsulin in patients with IDDM before insulin treatment. Diabetes 1988; 37:130–132.
16. Baekkeskov S, Aanstoot HJ, Christgau S, et al. Identification of the 64 K autoantigen in insulin-dependent diabetes as the GABA-synthesizing enzyme glutamic acid decarboxylase. Nature 1990; 347:151–156.
17. Lan MS, Lu J, Goto Y, Notkins AL. Molecular cloning and identification of a receptor-type protein tyrosine phosphatase, IA-2, from human insulinoma. DNA Cell Biol 1994; 13:505–514.
18. Rabin DU, Pleasic SM, Shapiro JA, et al. Islet cell antigen 512 is a diabetes-specific islet autoantigen related to protein tyrosine phosphatases. J Immunol 1994; 152:3183–3188.
19. Lu J, Li Q, Xie H, et al. Identification of a second transmembrane protein tyrosine phosphatase, IA-2beta, as an autoantigen in insulin-dependent diabetes mellitus: Precursor of the 37-kDa tryptic fragment. Proc Natl Acad Sci U S A 1996; 93:2307–2311.
20. Wasmeier C, Hutton JC. Molecular cloning of phogrin, a protein-tyrosine phosphatase homologue localized to insulin secretory granule membranes. J Biol Chem 1996; 271:18161–18170.
21. Solimena M, Dirkx R, Jr., Hermel JM, et al. ICA 512, an autoantigen of type I diabetes, is an intrinsic membrane protein of neurosecretory granules. Embo J 1996; 15:2102–2114.
22. Reetz A, Solimena M, Matteoli M, et al. GABA and pancreatic beta-cells: Colocalization of glutamic acid decarboxylase (GAD) and GABA with synaptic-like microvesicles suggests their role in GABA storage and secretion. Embo J 1991; 10:1275–1284.
23. Chimienti F, Devergnas S, Favier A, Seve M. Identification and cloning of a beta-cell-specific zinc transporter, ZnT-8, localized into insulin secretory granules. Diabetes 2004; 53:2330–2337.
24. Wenzlau JM, Juhl K, Yu L, et al. The cation efflux transporter ZnT8 (Slc30A8) is a major autoantigen in human type 1 diabetes. Proc Natl Acad Sci U S A 2007; 104:17040–17045.
25. Atkinson MA, Eisenbarth GS. Type 1 diabetes: New perspectives on disease pathogenesis and treatment. Lancet 2001; 358:221–229.
26. Bingley PJ, Bonifacio E, Ziegler AG, et al. Proposed guidelines on screening for risk of type 1 diabetes. Diabetes Care 2001; 24:398.
27. Srikanta S, Ganda OP, Rabizadeh A, et al. First-degree relatives of patients with type I diabetes mellitus. Islet-cell antibodies and abnormal insulin secretion. N Engl J Med 1985; 313:461–464.
28. Gorsuch AN, Spencer KM, Lister J, et al. Evidence for a long prediabetic period in type I (insulin-dependent) diabetes mellitus. Lancet 1981; 2:1363–1365.
29. Bingley PJ, Christie MR, Bonifacio E, et al. Combined analysis of autoantibodies improves prediction of IDDM in islet cell antibody-positive relatives. Diabetes 1994; 43:1304–1310.

30. Verge CF, Gianani R, Kawasaki E, et al. Prediction of type I diabetes in first-degree relatives using a combination of insulin, GAD, and ICA512bdc/IA-2 autoantibodies. Diabetes 1996; 45:926–933.

31. Kulmala P, Savola K, Petersen JS, et al. Prediction of insulin-dependent diabetes mellitus in siblings of children with diabetes. A population-based study. The Childhood Diabetes in Finland Study Group. J Clin Invest 1998; 101:327–336.

32. Ziegler AG, Hummel M, Schenker M, Bonifacio E. Autoantibody appearance and risk for development of childhood diabetes in offspring of parents with type 1 diabetes: The 2-year analysis of the German BABYDIAB Study. Diabetes 1999; 48:460–468.

33. LaGasse JM, Brantley MS, Leech NJ, et al. Successful prospective prediction of type 1 diabetes in schoolchildren through multiple defined autoantibodies: An 8-year follow-up of the Washington State Diabetes Prediction Study. Diabetes Care 2002; 25:505–511.

34. Decochez K, De Leeuw IH, Keymeulen B, et al. IA-2 autoantibodies predict impending Type I diabetes in siblings of patients. Diabetologia 2002; 45:1658–1666.

35. Bingley PJ, Williams AJ, Gale EA. Optimized autoantibody-based risk assessment in family members. Implications for future intervention trials. Diabetes Care 1999; 22:1796–1801.

36. Achenbach P, Koczwara K, Knopff A, et al. Mature high-affinity immune responses to (pro)insulin anticipate the autoimmune cascade that leads to type 1 diabetes. J Clin Invest 2004; 114:589–597.

37. Mayr A, Schlosser M, Grober N, et al. GAD autoantibody affinity and epitope specificity identify distinct immunization profiles in children at risk for type 1 diabetes. Diabetes 2007; 56:1527–1533.

38. Fourlanos S, Narendran P, Byrnes GB, et al. Insulin resistance is a risk factor for progression to type 1 diabetes. Diabetologia 2004; 47:1661–1667.

39. Chase HP, Cooper S, Osberg I, et al. Elevated C-reactive protein levels in the development of type 1 diabetes. Diabetes 2004; 53:2569–2573.

40. Tree TI, Peakman M. Autoreactive T cells in human type 1 diabetes. Endocrinol Metab Clin North Am 2004; 33:113–133, ix–x.

41. Roep BO. T-cell responses to autoantigens in IDDM. The search for the Holy Grail. Diabetes 1996; 45:1147–1156.

42. Roep BO, Atkinson MA, van Endert PM, et al. Autoreactive T cell responses in insulin-dependent (Type 1) diabetes mellitus. Report of the first international workshop for standardization of T cell assays. J Autoimmun 1999; 13:267–282.

43. Schloot NC, Meierhoff G, Karlsson Faresjo M, et al. Comparison of cytokine ELISpot assay formats for the detection of islet antigen autoreactive T cells. Report of the third immunology of diabetes society T-cell workshop. J Autoimmun 2003; 21:365–376.

44. Arif S, Tree TI, Astill TP, et al. Autoreactive T cell responses show proinflammatory polarization in diabetes but a regulatory phenotype in health. J Clin Invest 2004; 113:451–463.

45. Durinovic-Bello I, Rosinger S, Olson JA, et al. DRB1*0401-restricted human T cell clone specific for the major proinsulin73-90 epitope expresses a down-regulatory T helper 2 phenotype. Proc Natl Acad Sci U S A 2006; 103:11683–11688.

46. Oling V, Marttila J, Ilonen J, et al. GAD65- and proinsulin-specific CD4+ T-cells detected by MHC class II tetramers in peripheral blood of type 1 diabetes patients and at-risk subjects. J Autoimmun 2005; 25:235–243.

47. Reijonen H, Novak EJ, Kochik S, et al. Detection of GAD65-specific T-cells by major histocompatibility complex class II tetramers in type 1 diabetic patients and at-risk subjects. Diabetes 2002; 51:1375–1382.

48. Familial risk of type I diabetes in European children. The Eurodiab Ace Study Group and The Eurodiab Ace Substudy 2 Study Group. Diabetologia 1998; 41:1151–1156.

49. Dahlquist G, Blom L, Holmgren G, et al. The epidemiology of diabetes in Swedish children 0-14 years–A six-year prospective study. Diabetologia 1985; 28:802–808.

50. Yu L, Cuthbertson DD, Eisenbarth GS, Krischer JP. Diabetes Prevention Trial 1: Prevalence of GAD and ICA512 (IA-2) autoantibodies by relationship to proband. Ann N Y Acad Sci 2002; 958:254–258.

51. Bonifacio E, Pflüger M, Marienfelds, Winkler C, Hummel M, Ziegler AG. Maternal type 1 diabetes reduces the risk of islet autoantibodies: relationships with birthweight and maternal HbA(1C). Diabetologia 2008; Epub ahead of print (doi: 10.1007/s00125-008-1022-z).

52. Gillespie KM, Gale EA, Bingley PJ. High familial risk and genetic susceptibility in early onset childhood diabetes. Diabetes 2002; 51:210–214.

53. Redondo MJ, Yu L, Hawa M, et al. Heterogeneity of type I diabetes: Analysis of monozygotic twins in Great Britain and the United States. Diabetologia 2001; 44:354–362.

54. Bonifacio E, Hummel M, Walter M, et al. IDDM1 and Multiple Family History of Type 1 Diabetes Combine to Identify Neonates at High Risk for Type 1 Diabetes. Diabetes Care 2004; 27:2695–2700.

55. Todd JA. Genetic analysis of type 1 diabetes using whole genome approaches. Proc Natl Acad Sci U S A 1995; 92:8560–8565.

56. Hermann R, Bartsocas CS, Soltesz G, et al. Genetic screening for individuals at high risk for type 1 diabetes in the general population using HLA Class II alleles as disease markers. A comparison between three European populations with variable rates of disease incidence. Diabetes Metab Res Rev 2004; 20:322–329.

57. Van der Auwera BJ, Schuit FC, Weets I, et al. Relative and absolute HLA-DQA1-DQB1 linked risk for developing type I diabetes before 40 years of age in the Belgian population: Implications for future prevention studies. Hum Immunol 2002; 63:40–50.

58. Lambert AP, Gillespie KM, Thomson G, et al. Absolute risk of childhood-onset type 1 diabetes defined by human leukocyte antigen class II genotype: A population-based study in the United Kingdom. J Clin Endocrinol Metab 2004; 89:4037–4043.

59. Walter M, Albert E, Conrad M, et al. IDDM2/insulin VNTR modifies risk conferred by IDDM1/HLA for development of Type 1 diabetes and associated autoimmunity. Diabetologia 2003; 46:712–720.

60. Nejentsev S, Sjoroos M, Soukka T, et al. Population-based genetic screening for the estimation of Type 1 diabetes mellitus risk in Finland: Selective genotyping of markers in the HLA-DQB1, HLA-DQA1 and HLA-DRB1 loci. Diabet Med 1999; 16:985–992.

61. She JX. Susceptibility to type I diabetes: HLA-DQ and DR revisited. Immunol Today 1996; 17:323–329.

62. Buzzetti R, Galgani A, Petrone A, et al. Genetic prediction of type 1 diabetes in a population with low frequency of HLA risk genotypes and low incidence of the disease (the DIABFIN study). Diabetes Metab Res Rev 2004; 20:137–143.

63. Sabbah E, Savola K, Ebeling T, et al. Genetic, autoimmune, and clinical characteristics of childhood- and adult-onset type 1 diabetes. Diabetes Care 2000; 23:1326–1332.

64. Kimpimaki T, Kupila A, Hamalainen AM, et al. The first signs of beta-cell autoimmunity appear in infancy in genetically susceptible children from the general population: The Finnish Type 1 Diabetes Prediction and Prevention Study. J Clin Endocrinol Metab 2001; 86:4782–4788.

65. Schenker M, Hummel M, Ferber K, et al. Early expression and high prevalence of islet autoantibodies for DR3/4 heterozygous and DR4/4 homozygous offspring of parents with Type I diabetes: The German BABYDIAB study. Diabetologia 1999; 42:671–677.

66. Yu J, Yu L, Bugawan TL, et al. Transient antiislet autoantibodies: Infrequent occurrence and lack of association with "genetic" risk factors. J Clin Endocrinol Metab 2000; 85:2421–2428.

67. Kulmala P, Savola K, Reijonen H, et al. Genetic markers, humoral autoimmunity, and prediction of type 1 diabetes in siblings of affected children. Childhood Diabetes in Finland Study Group. Diabetes 2000; 49:48–58.

68. Graham J, Hagopian WA, Kockum I, et al. Genetic effects on age-dependent onset and islet cell autoantibody markers in type 1 diabetes. Diabetes 2002; 51:1346–1355.

69. Kimpimaki T, Kulmala P, Savola K, et al. Natural history of beta-cell autoimmunity in young children with increased genetic susceptibility to type 1 diabetes recruited from the general population. J Clin Endocrinol Metab 2002; 87:4572–4579.

70. Barker JM, Barriga KJ, Yu L, et al. Prediction of autoantibody positivity and progression to type 1 diabetes: Diabetes Autoimmunity Study in the Young (DAISY). J Clin Endocrinol Metab 2004; 89:3896–3902.

71. Colman PG, Steele C, Couper JJ, et al. Islet autoimmunity in infants with a Type I diabetic relative is common but is frequently restricted to one autoantibody. Diabetologia 2000; 43:203–209.

72. Schlosser M, Wassmuth R, Strebelow M, et al. Multiple and high-titer single autoantibodies in schoolchildren reflecting the genetic predisposition for type 1 diabetes. Ann N Y Acad Sci 2003; 1005:98–108.

73. Naserke HE, Ziegler AG, Lampasona V, Bonifacio E. Early development and spreading of autoantibodies to epitopes of IA-2 and their association with progression to type 1 diabetes. J Immunol 1998; 161:6963–6969.

74. Kukko M, Virtanen SM, Toivonen A, et al. Geographical variation in risk HLA-DQB1 genotypes for type 1 diabetes and signs of beta-cell autoimmunity in a high-incidence country. Diabetes Care 2004; 27:676–681.

75. Kondrashova A, Viskari H, Kulmala P, et al. Signs of beta-cell autoimmunity in nondiabetic schoolchildren: A comparison between Russian Karelia with a low incidence of type 1 diabetes and Finland with a high incidence rate. Diabetes Care 2007; 30:95–100.

76. Laine AP, Hermann R, Knip M, et al. The human leukocyte antigen genotype has a modest effect on the insulin gene polymorphism-associated susceptibility to type 1 diabetes in the Finnish population. Tissue Antigens 2004; 63:72–74.

77. Steck AK, Bugawan TL, Valdes AM, et al. Association of Non-HLA Genes With Type 1 Diabetes Autoimmunity. Diabetes 2005; 54:2482–2486.

78. Mathis D, Benoist C. Back to central tolerance. Immunity 2004; 20:509–516.

79. Pugliese A, Zeller M, Fernandez A, Jr., et al. The insulin gene is transcribed in the human thymus and transcription levels correlated with allelic variation at the INS VNTR-IDDM2 susceptibility locus for type 1 diabetes. Nat Genet 1997; 15:293–297.

80. Motzo C, Contu D, Cordell HJ, et al. Heterogeneity in the magnitude of the insulin gene effect on HLA risk in type 1 diabetes. Diabetes 2004; 53:3286–3291.

81. Aly TA, Ide A, Jahromi MM, et al. Extreme genetic risk for type 1 A diabetes. Proc Natl Acad Sci USA 2006; 103:14074–14079.

82. Ziegler AG, Hillebrand B, Rabl W, et al. On the appearance of islet associated autoimmunity in offspring of diabetic mothers: A prospective study from birth. Diabetologia 1993; 36:402–408.

83. Kupila A, Muona P, Simell T, et al. Feasibility of genetic and immunological prediction of type I diabetes in a population-based birth cohort. Diabetologia 2001; 44:290–297.

84. Rewers M, Bugawan TL, Norris JM, et al. Newborn screening for HLA markers associated with IDDM: Diabetes autoimmunity study in the young (DAISY). Diabetologia 1996; 39:807–812.

85. Honeyman MC, Coulson BS, Stone NL, et al. Association between rotavirus infection and pancreatic islet autoimmunity in children at risk of developing type 1 diabetes. Diabetes 2000; 49:1319–1324.

86. Bennett Johnson S, Baughcum AE, Carmichael SK, et al.Maternal anxiety associated with newborn genetic screening for type 1 diabetes. Diabetes Care 2004; 27:392–397.

87. Yu L, Robles DT, Abiru N, et al. Early expression of antiinsulin autoantibodies of humans and the NOD mouse: Evidence for early determination of subsequent diabetes. Proc Natl Acad Sci U S A 2000; 97:1701–1706.

88. Hummel M, Bonifacio E, Schmid S, et al. Brief communication: Early appearance of islet autoantibodies predicts childhood type 1 diabetes in offspring of diabetic parents. Ann Intern Med 2004; 140:882–886.

89. Vardi P, Ziegler AG, Mathews JH, et al. Concentration of insulin autoantibodies at onset of type I diabetes. Inverse log-linear correlation with age. Diabetes Care 1988; 11:736–739.

90. Achenbach P, Ziegler AG. Diabetes-related antibodies in euglycemic subjects. Best Pract Res Clin Endocrinol Metab 2005; 19:101–117.

91. Naserke HE, Bonifacio E, Ziegler AG. Prevalence, characteristics and diabetes risk associated with transient maternally acquired islet antibodies and persistent islet antibodies in offspring of parents with type 1 diabetes. J Clin Endocrinol Metab 2001; 86:4826–4833.

92. Hamalainen AM, Ronkainen MS, Akerblom HK, Knip M. Postnatal elimination of transplacentally acquired disease-associated antibodies in infants born to families with type 1 diabetes. The Finnish TRIGR Study Group. Trial to Reduce IDDM in the Genetically at Risk. J Clin Endocrinol Metab 2000; 85:4249–4253.

93. Achenbach P, Warncke K, Reiter J, et al. Type 1 diabetes risk assessment: Improvement by follow-up measurements in young islet autoantibody-positive relatives. Diabetologia 2006; 49:2969–2976.

94. Ziegler AG, Ziegler R, Vardi P, et al. Life-table analysis of progression to diabetes of anti-insulin autoantibody-positive relatives of individuals with type I diabetes. Diabetes 1989; 38:1320–1325.

95. Strebelow M, Schlosser M, Ziegler B, et al. Karlsburg Type I diabetes risk study of a general population: Frequencies and interactions of the four major Type I diabetes-associated autoantibodies studied in 9419 schoolchildren. Diabetologia 1999; 42:661–670.

96. Burnet FM. The new approach to immunology. N Engl J Med 1961; 264:24–34.

97. Wabl M, Cascalho M, Steinberg C. Hypermutation in antibody affinity maturation. Curr Opin Immunol 1999; 11:186–189.

98. Bonifacio E, Bingley PJ, Shattock M, et al. Quantification of islet-cell antibodies and prediction of insulin-dependent diabetes. Lancet 1990; 335:147–149.

99. Bingley PJ, Bonifacio E, Mueller PW. Diabetes antibody standardization program: First assay proficiency evaluation. Diabetes 2003; 52:1128–1136.

100. Mire-Sluis AR, Gaines Das R, Lernmark A. The World Health Organization International Collaborative Study for islet cell antibodies. Diabetologia 2000; 43:1282–1292.

101. Achenbach P, Schlosser M, Williams AJ, et al. Combined testing of antibody titer and affinity improves insulin autoantibody measurement: Diabetes Antibody Standardization Program. Clin Immunol 2007; 122:85–90.

102. Effects of insulin in relatives of patients with type 1 diabetes mellitus. N Engl J Med 2002; 346:1685–1691.

103. Chase HP, Cuthbertson DD, Dolan LM, et al. First-phase insulin release during the intravenous glucose tolerance test as a risk factor for type 1 diabetes. J Pediatr 2001; 138:244–249.

104. Achenbach P, Bonifacio E, Gale EA, Bingley PJ. Antibodies to IA-2beta improve diabetes risk assessment in high risk relatives. Diabetologia 2008; 51:488–492.

105. Xu P, Cuthbertson D, Greenbaum C, Palmer JP, Krischer JP, Diabetes Prevention Trial–Type 1 Study Group. Role of insulin resistance in predicting progression to type 1 diabetes. Diabetes Care 2007; 30:2314–2320.

106. Bingley PJ, Mahon JL, Gale EAM, The European Nicotinamide Diabetes Intervention Trial (ENDIT) Group. Insulin resistance and progression to type 1 diabetes in the European Nicotinamide Diabetes Intervention Trial (ENDIT). Diabetes Care 2008; 31:146–150.

107. Fourlanos S, Narendran P, Byrnes GB, Colman PG, Harrison LC. Insulin resistance is a risk factor for progression to type 1 diabetes. Diabetologia 2004; 47:1661–1667.

108. Keskinen P, Korhonen S, Kupila A, et al. First-phase insulin response in young healthy children at genetic and immunological risk for Type I diabetes. Diabetologia 2002; 45:1639–1648.

109. Sosenko JM, Krischer JP, Palmer JP, et al. A Risk Score for Type 1 Diabetes Derived from Autoantibody Positive Participants in The Diabetes Prevention Trial- Type 1. Diabetes Care 2008; 31:528–533.

110. Fourlanos S, Dotta F, Greenbaum CJ, et al. Latent autoimmune diabetes in adults (LADA) should be less latent. Diabetologia 2005; 48:2206–2212.

111. Bingley PJ, Bonifacio E, Williams AJ, et al. Prediction of IDDM in the general population: Strategies based on combinations of autoantibody markers. Diabetes 1997; 46:1701–1710.
112. Maclaren NK, Lan MS, Schatz D, et al. Multiple autoantibodies as predictors of type 1 diabetes in a general population. Diabetologia 2003; 46:873–874.
113. Panagiotopoulos C, Qin H, Tan R, et al. Identification of a beta-cell-specific HLA class I restricted epitope in type 1 diabetes. Diabetes 2003; 52:2647–2651.
114. Lieberman SM, Evans AM, Han B, et al. Identification of the beta cell antigen targeted by a prevalent population of pathogenic CD8+ T cells in autoimmune diabetes. Proc Natl Acad Sci U S A 2003; 100:8384–8388.
115. Gurr W, Yavari R, Wen L, et al. A Reg family protein is overexpressed in islets from a patient with new-onset type 1 diabetes and acts as T-cell autoantigen in NOD mice. Diabetes 2002; 51:339–346.
116. Gurr W, Shaw M, Li Y, Sherwin R. RegII is a beta-cell protein and autoantigen in diabetes of NOD mice. Diabetes 2007; 56:34–40.
117. Shervani NJ, Takasawa S, Uchigata Y, et al. Autoantibodies to REG, a beta-cell regeneration factor, in diabetic patients. Eur J Clin Invest 2004; 34:752–758.
118. Honeyman MC, Cram DS, Harrison LC. Glutamic acid decarboxylase 67-reactive T cells: A marker of insulin-dependent diabetes. J Exp Med 1993; 177:535–450.
119. Pietropaolo M, Castano L, Babu S, et al. Islet cell autoantigen 69 kD (ICA69). Molecular cloning and characterization of a novel diabetes-associated autoantigen. J Clin Invest 1993; 92:359–371.
120. Castano L, Russo E, Zhou L, et al. Identification and cloning of a granule autoantigen (carboxypeptidase-H) associated with type I diabetes. J Clin Endocrinol Metab 1991; 73:1197–1201.
121. Aanstoot HJ, Kang SM, Kim J, et al. Identification and characterization of glima 38, a glycosylated islet cell membrane antigen, which together with GAD65 and IA2 marks the early phases of autoimmune response in type 1 diabetes. J Clin Invest 1996; 97:2772–2783.
122. Dotta F, Gianani R, Previti M, et al. Autoimmunity to the GM2–1 islet ganglioside before and at the onset of type I diabetes. Diabetes 1996; 45:1193–1196.
123. Gillard BK, Thomas JW, Nell LJ, Marcus DM. Antibodies against ganglioside GT3 in the sera of patients with type I diabetes mellitus. J Immunol 1989; 142:3826–3832.
124. Buschard K, Josefsen K, Horn T, Fredman P. Sulphatide and sulphatide antibodies in insulin-dependent diabetes mellitus. Lancet 1993; 342:840.
125. Winer S, Tsui H, Lau A, et al. Autoimmune islet destruction in spontaneous type 1 diabetes is not β-cell exclusive. Nat Med 2003; 9:198–205.
126. Boitard C, Villa MC, Becourt C, et al. Peripherin: An islet antigen that is cross-reactive with nonobese diabetic mouse class II gene products. Proc Natl Acad Sci U S A 1992; 89:172–176.
127. Inman LR, McAllister CT, Chen L, et al. Autoantibodies to the GLUT-2 glucose transporter of beta cells in insulin-dependent diabetes mellitus of recent onset. Proc Natl Acad Sci U S A 1993; 90:1281–1284.
128. Chang YH, Hwang J, Shang HF, Tsai ST. Characterization of human DNA topoisomerase II as an autoantigen recognized by patients with IDDM. Diabetes 1996; 45:408–414.

129. Kasimiotis H, Myers MA, Argentaro A, et al. Sex-determining region Y-related protein SOX13 is a diabetes autoantigen expressed in pancreatic islets. Diabetes 2000; 49:555–561.

130. Honeyman MC, Cram DS, Harrison LC. Transcription factor jun-B is target of autoreactive T-cells in IDDM. Diabetes 1993; 42:626–630.

131. Arden SD, Roep BO, Neophytou PI, et al. Imogen 38: A novel 38-kD islet mitochondrial autoantigen recognized by T cells from a newly diagnosed type 1 diabetic patient. J Clin Invest 1996; 97:551–561.

132. Birk OS, Elias D, Weiss AS, et al. NOD mouse diabetes: The ubiquitous mouse hsp60 is a beta-cell target antigen of autoimmune T cells. J Autoimmun 1996; 9:159–166.

133. Abulafia-Lapid R, Gillis D, Yosef O, et al. T cells and autoantibodies to human HSP70 in type 1 diabetes in children. J Autoimmun 2003; 20:313–321.

134. Qin HY, Mahon JL, Atkinson MA, et al. Type 1 diabetes alters anti-hsp90 autoantibody isotype. J Autoimmun 2003; 20:237–245.

135. Rorsman F, Husebye ES, Winqvist O, et al. Aromatic-L-amino-acid decarboxylase, a pyridoxal phosphate-dependent enzyme, is a beta-cell autoantigen. Proc Natl Acad Sci U S A 1995; 92:8626–8629.

6

What are the Prospects for Preventing Autoimmune Diabetes?

Carla J. Greenbaum

Diabetes Program, Benaroya Research Institute, Seattle, Washington, U.S.A.

Leonard C. Harrison

The Walter and Eliza Hall Institute of Medical Research, Parkville, Victoria, Australia

INTRODUCTION

The first major breakthrough in understanding type 1 diabetes (T1D) was in 1889 when Von Mering & Minkowski at the University of Strasbourg showed that removing the pancreas of dogs caused diabetes (1). It took 33 years for this knowledge to translate into the isolation of insulin for therapy, thereby changing a fatal disease into a less fatal, chronic disease. It was another 28 years before Bornstein, using a crude insulin bioassay, clearly delineated insulin-dependent (type 1) diabetes and non-insulin-dependent (type 2) diabetes as insulin deficient and non-insulin-deficient, respectively (2). This was soon confirmed with the development of the insulin radioimmunoassay by Berson and Yalow (3). The concept that T1D might be an immune-mediated disease was spurred by the histologic description of immune cells in the islets (insulitis) by Gepts in 1965 (4), and subsequently cemented by a larger analysis of pancreas samples by Foulis in the 1980s (5). Meanwhile, in 1974, Nerup et al. (6) and others (7) reported the association of T1D with specific HLA types and Bottazzo et al. (8) and Irving et al. (9), the association with islet cell antibodies (ICA) detected by indirect immunofluorescence. By the 1980s, autoantibodies to insulin had been identified particularly in younger patients by Palmer et al. (8,10) and ICA as well as impaired insulin secretion (first phase–insulin response to IV glucose–FPIR) shown by Eisenbarth et al (11–13) to identify at-risk individuals prior to clinical disease. This was the basis, together with further definition of HLA specificities (14), for prediction algorithms for clinical T1D in relatives and subsequently in the general population (15). The immunoserological basis of risk prediction depended on the discovery of specific autoantigens, in addition to insulin, namely glutamic acid decarboxylase molecular weight isoform 65,000 (GAD-65) (16), insulinoma-like antigen-2 (IA-2) (17) and, more recently, zinc transporter 8 (18), and the development of biochemical assays for antibodies to these antigens (19) that have been subjected to quality control in international workshops (20,21). As described in chapter 5, identification of those at risk for T1D using serological and other markers has been a great success story, crossing the first hurdle in prevention, the requirement to identify those who could benefit. Combined with advances in understanding preclinical natural history and immunotherapeutics, clinical trials aimed at primary prevention before initiation of the autoimmune process and secondary prevention during the autoimmune process are now a reality. To date, however, most trials represent tertiary prevention aimed at retarding further β-cell destruction in people with clinical T1D (Fig. 1). Primary, secondary, and tertiary prevention trials have been previously reviewed (22–25) and guidelines suggested (26). In this chapter, we describe current and planned clinical trials for T1D prevention, while identifying issues that continue to challenge translational investigators.

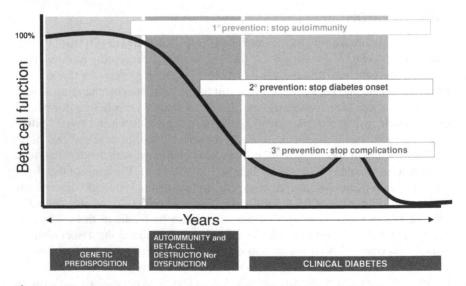

Figure 1 Potential for prevention at stages of the natural history of diabetes.

CURRENT AND PLANNED CLINICAL TRIALS

Intervention to prevent T1D could involve prevention of the immune-mediated–β-cell destructive process through blocking of its initiation or effector phases, direct enhancement of β-cell growth, and survival or metabolic interventions to reduce β-cell demand. Most likely, success will come from a combination of these approaches.

Prevention of Immune-Mediated β-Cell Destruction

The cyclosporine trial demonstrated that immunosuppression may retard loss of β-cell function in the short-term and was thus an important sentinel (27–29). Yet, the worsening of renal function in that study (30–32), together with increasing evidence of metabolic (hyperlipidemia), infectious, and long-term cancer risk in individuals treated with life-long–potent immunosuppression for other purposes [e.g., transplantation (33)], led to a consensus that the preferred approach would be to induce disease-specific tolerance rather than chronically suppress the immune response.

Numerous reviews describe current approaches to block the initial or subsequent phases of autoimmune disease, targeted to a range of mechanisms. Current understanding of the immune response to a putative antigen describes interactions between antigen presenting cells and T cells, the latter through the T cell receptor. The characteristic of the immune response depends upon additional signaling by costimulatory molecules and intracellular pathways with effector cells propagating and regulatory cells dampening the response. The balance between these effector and regulatory functions influences whether the outcome is beneficial (ridding the individual of an external pathogen), or harmful (autoimmune disease). Induction of tolerance in the context of autoimmunity therefore implies a return to a stable state in which the immune response is self regulated. Tolerance may be induced by autoantigen administration. Other approaches include interruption of the T- or B-cell responses with antibodies to surface markers such as CD3 or CD20, respectively, or costimulation molecules or the IL-2 receptor, drugs that primarily affect intracellular processes resulting in alteration of immune cell signaling or potential depletion of autoreactive cells, including mycophenolate mofetil and rapamycin, cytokine blockade or alteration and direct administration of autologous, regulatory T cells. Clinical trials of these agents that are or soon will be underway are listed (Table 1).

In addition to these pharmaceutical approaches, the geographic variation in disease incidence, the increasing incidence particularly among the very young, and the broadening of HLA types in people presenting with T1D, have lead many to consider environmental interventions to block initiation of autoimmunity (see chap. 1 for further information). The role of the environment in diabetes development is also supported by observations in animal models. For example, there is an increased incidence of diabetes in NOD housed in a germ-free versus

Table 1 Current Immunotherapeutic Approaches to T1D Prevention[a]

	Drug	Dose	Sponsor/date	Subjects/Study design	Proposed Mechanism
Tertiary prevention	Mycophenilate Mofetil and Daclizumab	MMF po 600 mg/m2 for 2 yr; DZB IV 1 mg/kg every other wk × 2 wk	NIH: Diabetes Trial Net/2004	Phase II: Masked, placebo $N = 120$ Age = 8–45 yr	MMF blocks T-cell proliferation, DZB blocks IL-2 receptor on activated T cells
Tertiary prevention	Rituximab	375 mg/m2 for weekly IV infusion	NIH: Diabetes Trial Net/2005	Phase II: Masked, placebo $N = 66$ Age = 8–45 yr	Deletes B cells. In T1DM, these may be serving as antigen presenting cells
Tertiary prevention	IL-2 + Rapamycin (Sirolimus)	Rapamycin po target trough level 5–10 µg/mL for 3 mo IL-2, 4.5 × 106 IU SQ 3 times weekly for 28 days	NIH: Immune Tolerance Network: /2007	Phase 1 open label $N = 10$ adults 4 yr from dx with C-peptide	Induction of Treg cells IL-2 signals both effector and regulatory cells whereas rapamycin blocks only effecter T cell population
Tertiary prevention	Thymoglobulin	Four IV doses	NIH: Immune Tolerance Network: 2005/2007	Phase II: Masked, placebo $N = 66$ 2 mo from diagnosis Age = 12–35 yr	Pan T cell immunosuppression
Tertiary prevention	hOKT3γ1(ala-ala)	9034 µg/m2 over 14-day course	NIH	4–12 mo from diagnosis Masked, placebo Ages = 8–30 yr	Immunomodulation
Tertiary prevention	hOKT3γ1 (ala-ala)	Two 14-day courses a year apart with total dose per course of 9034 µg/m2	NIH: Immune Tolerance Network: 2005	Phase II: randomized, open label $N = 81$ Age = 8–30 yr 8 wk from diagnosis	Immunomodulation
Secondary prevention	hOKT3γ1(ala-ala)	9034 µg/m2 over 14-day course	NIH: Diabetes Trial Net /2008	Antibody positive relatives with abnormal glucose tolerance	Immunomodulation
Tertiary prevention	CTLA4-Ig (Abatacept)	10 mg/kg IV monthly for 2 yr	NIH: Diabetes Trial Net /2008	Phase II: Masked, placebo $N = 108$ 3 mo from diagnosis	Co-stimulatory blockade

Prevention	Intervention	Protocol	Sponsor/Year	Study design	Mechanism/Comment
Tertiary prevention	Dendritic cells with anti-sense olignucleotides targeting CD40, CD80, and CD86 mRNA	SQ injections of AS-ODN dendritic cells obtained through apheresis	NIH	Phase I open label N = 10	Costimulatory blockade Anergizing signal to T cells in pancreas–draining lymph nodes, interrupting anti-B-cell antigen spreading
Secondary prevention	Oral insulin	7.5 mg po q day ongoing	NIH: Diabetes Trial Net /2007	Relatives at risk for diabetes: masked, placebo	Antigen therapy: Oral tolerance
Tertiary prevention	GAD65-Alum	Three arm trial with placebo, two, or three injections of 20 µg	NIH: Diabetes Trial Net /2008	Phase II; masked, placebo N = 150 3 mo from diagnosis	Antigen therapy; tolerance induction
Primary prevention	Oral and nasal insulin (pre-point)	Three arm trial: oral insulin (2.5/7.5/22.5/67.5 mg), nasal insulin (0.28, 0.88, 2.5, 7.5 for 10 days and then twice weekly	JDRF/2008	Antibody negative children with genetic risk N = 40	Antigen therapy; tolerance induction
Secondary prevention	Nasal insulin (INIT II)	Three arm trial: nasal insulin (1.6 or 16 mg) or placebo, daily 7 days, then weekly for 1 yr	Diabetes Vaccine Development Center	Antibody positive relatives at risk for disease	Antigen therapy: Mucosal tolerance
Tertiary prevention	Anakinra (Anti-IL1 receptor)	100 mg sq	JDRF/Øresund Diabetes Academy and the Steno Diabetes Center 2008	Phase IIa: Masked, Placebo N = 80 Age = 18–35 yr ≤12 wk of diabetes symptoms	IL-1B directly impairs insulin secretion and inhibits β-cell survival
Tertiary prevention	Umbilical cord blood	Variable number of nucleated cells; single IV infusion	JDRF	Open label pilot study N = 23	Regulatory cells in cord blood Regeneration of B-cells from stem cells in cord blood

[a] Pharmaceutical sponsored trials not included.

conventional "dirty" environment (34) and the incidence can be altered by changing conditions of housing and feeding (35). It is felt that the mucosa plays a key role in maintenance of self-tolerance in TID. Under dirty conditions, bacterial colonization of the intestine leads to maturation of mucosal immune function (36), which may be a requirement for the generation of regulatory T cells in response to oral antigen, (37,38). This provides theoretical support for the "hygiene hypothesis" (38,39), which posits that the increasing incidence of autoimmune and allergic disorders in the developed world is related to "clean living" conditions.

Epidemiology data both support (40) and refute (41–43) an effect of early introduction of cow's milk as a risk factor for islet autoantibody development. This question should be answered by the ongoing primary prevention clinical trial called TRIGR in which, genetically-at-risk babies are randomly assigned to formula with and without cow's milk and followed for development of islet autoantibodies. Early introduction of gluten [BABYDIAB study (43)] and cereal [DAISY study (44)] were reported to be associated with islet autoimmunity. These observations led to the BabyDiet study testing whether development of autoantibodies differs in babies randomized to early (at the age of 6 months) or late (at the age of 12 months) introduction of gluten (45). The changing western diet with a shift from anti-inflammatory to proinflammatory fatty acids over the past half century (46) and an increase in prostaglandin synthase in children with diabetes (47), together with epidemiology data suggesting a protective effect of cod liver oil (48), led to the hypothesis that omega-3–fatty acids may protect against autoimmune disease. A pilot trial, the Nutritional Intervention to Prevent diabetes (NIP) study, to test this hypothesis began in 2007. Epidemiological data also indicate that vitamin D insufficiency is a risk factor for T1D, and basic science studies demonstrate multiple effects of vitamin D on immune and metabolic function pertinent to development of T1D (49,50). Recent pilot studies indicate that vitamin D can be safely administered even to the very young (51), and a primary prevention trial may be considered by NIH Diabetes TrialNet in the near future. Finally, it has been suggested that gut flora play an important role in maintenance of mucosal immunity (52,53). This idea has raised the possibility that administration of protobiotics may offer protection from autoimmunity, and a pilot study has demonstrated the safety of this approach (54).

Enhancement of β-Cell Growth and Survival

Aside from immunotherapy, consideration has been given to therapies that could support the β-cell directly by promoting growth (through augmentation of β-cell replication or differentiation of ductal or acinar cells), or by reducing B-cell death. The former assumes that there is a capacity for β-cell replication and differentiation after birth in humans, and to assert this there is as yet, no evidence. Absent such information in humans however, there is considerable in vitro and some in vivo data indicating that pharmacologic manipulation can increase the functional β-cell mass (55). For example, NOD mice treated at diabetes onset with epidermal growth factor (EGF) and gastrin resolve their hyperglycemia and have an increased β-cell mass (56). Similar data has been reported in strepto-zotocin treated rats (57). However, careful analysis of pancreas specimens from patients with Zollinger-Ellison syndrome secondary to gastrin-producing tumors demonstrated an increase in β-cell size and replication, only in islets adjacent to the tumors. There was no effect of excess gastrin on cells more than 1-cm away from the tumor, suggesting that there would be limited benefit to thera-peutic administration of gastrin in humans (58). In addition to EGF and gastrin, the incretin hormone, glucagon-like peptide 1 (GLP-1) has been shown in vitro and in vivo animal studies, to impact the β-cell both by effects on B-cell growth and replication and through inhibition of apoptosis (see chap. 7 for further infor-mation) (59). Despite widespread clinical use of GLP-1 mimetics in patients with T2 diabetes, and more recently in subjects receiving islet transplantation in which salutatory effects on glucose tolerance has been demonstrated, no effects of therapy have been clearly attributable to improvement in β-cell mass. Never-theless, the concept that administration of readily available pharmacologic agents could augment β-cell growth is so attractive that clinical trials in patients with T1DM with gastrin and EGF have occurred. (http://www.transitiontherapeutics. com/technology/diabetes.php). Of course, if the assumptions about the disease process were correct, such therapies would be expected to be most useful in com-bination with therapies to block the immune assault. Such a trial using Anti-CD3 and Exenatide (GLP-1 mimetic) is being developed under the auspices of Diabetes TrialNet.

Metabolic Intervention

An alternate but not exclusive approach to prevention involves intervening in the metabolic rather than immune process. Two concepts are key to this approach. One is that hyperglycemia itself contributes to ongoing β-cell destruction whether directly by an unspecified glucose toxicity on the immune system or β-cells, or indirectly by increasing the demand on the β-cell at a time when its function is compromised by an abnormal cytokine milieu or by direct T-cell attack. The other is that insulin resistance either intrinsic to the underlying immuno-inflammatory process or induced by hyperglycemia increases the need for insulin secretion to maintain normoglycemia. Since β-cell destruction and insulin resistance both appear to contribute to the rate of onset of disease (60–62) (see chap. 1 for further information), immediate and aggressive correction of hyperglycemia and insulin resistance may prevent disease progression. Insulin resistance has implications not only for alternative preventative approaches directed at improving insulin action in T1D, but for stratifying autoantibody-positive subjects in prevention trials. The benefits of aggressive control of glycemia were suggested by the Diabetes Control and Complications Trial (DCCT) in a study in which subjects in the intensive insulin therapy group maintained better β-cell function over time (63) and in a study in which the "Biostator" insulin delivery pump was used to control blood glucose from the time of diagnosis (64). A metabolic intervention trial within NIH Diabetes TrialNet using more modern closed loop–insulin delivery-glucose monitoring systems to aggressively control hyperglycemia will begin in 2008.

TRANSLATIONAL CHALLENGES

Investigators perceive that we have entered an era in which the way type 1 diabetes is treated will profoundly change. For people with diabetes, this refers to the introduction of closed loop insulin delivery systems, further improvements in islet transplantation, and the emergence of stem cell therapy. It is important to appreciate that all forms of cure for T1D that involve restoring endogenous β-cell function will involve prevention because the immune system has a memory and the disease is recurrent. Therefore, the requirement is for safe and effective forms of preventative therapies that can be used in combination with therapies to restore β-cell function. The thoughtful researcher must keep in mind the ongoing challenges in translating these concepts into reality.

Translational Issues: Concept to Clinical Trial

In our modern era, basic scientific information about disease mechanisms and molecules is used to design drugs against specific therapeutic targets, an approach which promises improved efficacy and safety. Yet, the maxim that we do not know what we do not know demands that we approach new therapies with caution. Novel tools and techniques may allow for identification of new therapeutic targets, yet the exquisitely complex systems developed over millennia which constitute physiological immune surveillance require us to assume redundancies in any particular process as well as unpredictable responses to perturbations of the system. Bringing new science to clinical trial therefore creates challenges for any translational investigator. For those aiming to prevent T1D, specific issues include the inaccessibility of the lesion in the pancreas in humans, lack of a large animal model of autoimmune β-cell destruction, significant differences in both innate and adaptive immunity between rodents and humans, and genetic and clinical heterogeneity in humans compared to inbred rodent models. This may lead to unpredictability regarding both efficacy and safety when translating results of rodent studies to human trials. Further, as discussed below, extrapolation from animal models regarding dose and timing of an intervention may lead to miscalculations in design of clinical trials and the possibility of discarding an effective therapy.

The fact that so many therapies alter the disease process in the NOD mouse while few are able to reverse or stabilize overt disease (65,66) has led to the assumption that a therapy that works late in the disease process of the NOD has crossed a higher bar and thus is more likely to be successful in humans. This was one of the strongest arguments for rapidly bringing anti-CD3 monoclonal antibody therapy to trial in individuals with recent-onset T1D; when administered to euglycemic NOD mice (with insulitis only) there was a limited, short-term effect, yet in NOD mice with overt hyperglycemia prolonged remission of the diabetes was seen (67). Indeed, early studies showed a significant short-term retention of β-cell function in individuals with recent-onset clinical diabetes, appearing to validate this assumption (68,69). More controversial is, whether this therapy will be useful in humans prior to clinical disease onset. Under the supposition that antibody-positive relatives with abnormal, but not yet diabetic, glucose tolerance are more akin to the recently-diabetic NOD mice; an NIH Diabetes TrialNet study testing whether anti-CD3 therapy can prevent the progression from abnormal to diabetic glucose tolerance is being planned and may provide further insight into the appropriate timing of this intervention.

The concept underlying antigen-specific immunotherapy is that autoantigen-specific immunoregulatory mechanisms are physiological and can be boosted or restored to prevent pathological autoimmunity. Strategies to achieve this include the delivery of autoantigen by a "tolerogenic" route (e.g., mucosal), cell type (e.g., resting dendritic cell), mode (e.g., with blockade of costimulation molecules), or form (e.g., as an "altered peptide ligand'). These can prevent or suppress experimental autoimmune diseases in rodents by several possible mechanisms including clonal deletion or anergy, or induction of regulatory T cells (70–72). While results from clinical trials of intranasal (73) and oral (74) insulin in individuals at risk of T1D are suggestive, the astute reader will also recognize that antigen administration is a double-edge sword that has also been used to induce cytotoxic immunity in the setting of cancer. It is likely that the presence or absence of activated effector cells, the nature of the antigen (e.g., presence of CD4 and CD8 T-cell epitopes), dose, timing, and route of administration determine the nature of the response. In contrast to anti-CD3, autoantigen-specific therapy has only been efficacious prior to overt disease in the NOD mouse (75,76). Consistent with this observation, oral insulin in newly-diagnosed subjects had no effect (77,78), whereas, a post hoc analysis indicated benefit in "at risk" subjects with high levels of insulin autoantibodies (74) (an observation being tested anew in the NIH Diabetes Trial-Net Oral Insulin Prevention Trial). In contrast to animal data suggesting efficacy would only be seen prior to disease onset, in an initial study administration of SC GAD-65 to subjects with T1D may have been associated with preservation of C-peptide secretion (79,80). On the other hand, administration of nasal insulin to antibody-positive, young genetically-at-risk children in the DIPP trial had no effect on diabetes development (81). Thus far, the available data serve to highlight that since we do not know whether progression from peri-insulitis to destructive insulitis to clinical disease characteristic of some mouse models (82,83) also occurs in humans, looking to rodents to decide timing of intervention is fraught with untested assumptions.

In addition to timing, antigen therapy may not yet have been effectively translated to humans because of difficulties in determining an effective dose. For example, despite compelling animal data, daily administration of 0.25 U/kg of ultralente insulin had no effect on the progression to clinical disease in high-risk relatives studied as part of the Diabetes Prevention Trial (84). In this study, the decision about the insulin dose used was largely based in concerns about possible hypoglycemia, and was significantly less than that shown to be efficacious in the rodent studies (75,85,86). Similarly, the DIPP trial used approximately 1 U/kg/d of nasal insulin. While this dose did not cause hypoglycemia, in antibody positive very young children, it was not effective in preventing or delaying onset of disease as noted above.

New animal models—transgenic, gene targeted, and "humanized" mice (87–97) help to understand mechanistic pathways, identify β-cell autoantigens that influence disease and facilitate direct testing of new immunotherapeutics. While they yield publishable information, this is not necessarily the knowledge relevant to human T1D. Manipulation of one or another component of a rodent's immune system is unlikely to fully mimic the human condition. Another novel approach is biosimulation in silico, which incorporates multiple aspects of the disease process to allow for virtual manipulation (98). While the utility of this approach is not yet proven, it may be less reductionist than "real" animal models and thus better predict outcomes in human studies.

Wrestling with these issues, some investigators have suggested that a therapy should have a plausible hypothesis and be shown to work in more than one animal model of diabetes before consideration is given to trials in people at risk for or with T1D. Others, presupposing similarities in human disease mechanisms, have proposed that more emphasis be given to testing therapies in T1D that have been shown to be beneficial in other human autoimmune diseases. Results from the current generation of clinical trials may provide insights as to which approach best translates into effective therapy for individuals with T1D.

Translational Issues: Clinical Trial Design

The notion that immune-mediated β-cell destruction should be amenable to treatment led to more than 35 clinical trials in individuals with recently-diagnosed diabetes between 1985 and 2001 (22). It is important to bring a critical eye to these reports, as only 14 of these have reported a negative outcome, yet no therapy is in clinical use today. Aside from the well-known difficulty in getting journals to accept reports of negative trials, other important factors related to study design have contributed to the uncertainty as to whether any intervention has worked and the relative merits of different interventions.

Outcome Measures

A fundamental issue with all trials is the question of endpoint. How will it be determined whether or not the therapy has worked? The Immunology of Diabetes Intervention Group grappled with this problem in the early 1980s suggesting that maintenance of good glucose control without insulin therapy should be a measurable and clinically relevant endpoint. Yet this idea fell out of favor for several reasons. First, careful evaluation of subjects not receiving study drug during the first year after diagnosis revealed that virtually all went through a "honeymoon" period and many attained good blood glucose control of insulin.

Thus, the natural history of the disease limited the value of insulin withdrawal as an endpoint. Second, with the widespread use of home blood glucose monitoring and newer methods of delivering insulin, the variability in patient and physician behavior appeared to account for insulin withdrawal at least as much changes in the underlying pathology. Third, there was accumulating though indirect evidence that insulin itself may be beneficial to β-cell survival and thus many clinicians, at least in the United States, kept their patients on minimal doses of insulin even when blood glucose control did not demand this. The suggestion to use insulin dose as an endpoint under the assumption that as insulin secretion was preserved, less exogenous insulin would be required, also came up against same problems as insulin withdrawal. Furthermore, it was compounded by the impact of insulin sensitivity on insulin requirements. Thus, with no change in β-cell function, an increase in insulin dose is necessary to maintain glucose control in children entering puberty, a time of increasing insulin resistance.

The decision to measure insulin secretion directly appeared to be a better solution, yet raised new issues. The first was how to determine the clinical relevance of residual insulin secretory function. As discussed below, this remains a difficult question. The β-cell responds to glucose, amino acids, and other secretagogues administered orally or IV, leading investigators to measure the insulin response to a meal to reflect a clinically relevant response. Therefore, insulin secretion was determined before and after consumption of a hearty breakfast with standard amounts of carbohydrate, fat, and protein. To standardize the time for consumption, the standard meal was eventually formulated into a measured liquid preparation consumed within several minutes. This mixed meal tolerance test (MMTT) demonstrated deficits in insulin secretion in those with T1D, but it required several hours to perform. Administration of IV glucagon was shown to elicit a robust C-peptide secretory response within a few minutes in healthy subjects but not in those with T1D. It was not until 2006, however, that these two tests were formally compared. The 2-hour MMTT elicited a slightly higher and more reproducible C-peptide response than IV glucagon, indicating it is a more sensitive and reliable measure of β-cell function (submitted for publication Carla J. Greenbaum, Benaroya Research Institute, Seattle, WA).

Several studies have used the area under the curve response to a 4-hour (as compared with 2-hour) MMTT (68,99). Recently, the benefit of anti-CD3 monoclonal antibody therapy in recent-onset T1D subjects was demonstrated by differences in both glucose clamp and glucagon induced–C-peptide secretion (69). Unfortunately, it is unknown if the clinical trial outcome would have been the same if either the 2-hour area under the curve (AUC) from the MMTT or peak C-peptide response from glucagon stimulation was used.

Variations in measurements directly impact the utility of the test. Thus, an endpoint that is poorly reproducible due to assay or biological variation requires either more subjects or a large effect to see a treatment difference. A series of studies examined the impact of antecedent glucose status and insulin dosing on the acute β-cell secretory response, leading to guidelines for standardization. Thus, subjects were required to have a glucose value between 70 and 200 mg/dL before testing. Tests were to be conducted before 10 AM. Subjects were instructed to take their usual long-acting insulin or continue their basal rate if using an insulin pump, but very short acting insulin and regular insulin was not permitted within several hours of the test. Under these conditions, both the glucagon stimulation test and the MMTT were shown to be highly reproducible within a 3 to 10 days period (submitted for publication Carla J. Greenbaum, Benaroya Research Institute, Seattle, WA).

Standardization allows for improvements in clinical trials in which differences in secretion are used to determine whether a therapy preserved β-cell function. This alone is, however, not sufficient because new therapies must demonstrate clinical benefit in relation to possible risks and we do not yet know what level of insulin secretion over what period of time conveys clinical benefit. This is analogous to our ability to measure the effect of a therapy on blood pressure, yet without knowing what level of blood pressure reduction results in reduction in morbidity and mortality.

The most compelling data for a clinical benefit associated with preservation of β-cell function comes from the DCCT, in which individuals with T1D were required to have MMTT-stimulated C-peptide ≤ 0.50 pmol/mL. In a post hoc analysis, 303/855 subjects within 1 to 5 years of diagnosis were found to have a stimulated C-peptide between 0.2 and 0.5 pmol/mL. Of these "responders", 138 had been assigned to the DCCT intensive therapy group. Of the 552 "nonresponders", 274 were in the intensive therapy group. Among the intensively treated subjects, responders had a lower HbA1c, a 50% reduced risk for retinopathy progression, and a 65% reduced risk for severe hypoglycemia (63). These data suggested that 0.2 pmol/mL was a clinically significant level of C-peptide. A subsequent analysis demonstrated that those who were able to sustain this level of C-peptide for a year or more had greater clinical benefit (100). Similar conclusions about clinical benefit in relation to C-peptide comes from smaller studies such as that of Sjoberg et al. (101). However, longitudinal studies are required to understand the relationship between plasma C-peptide concentrations across a range of values with clinical outcomes.

A second issue with using C-peptide secretion as a marker of residual β-cell function in intervention trials has been the increasing recognition that insulin secretion persists after diagnosis in a large number of subjects. Observations from the control arm of some (77,102,103) but not all (68) recent intervention trials show no change in fasting or glucagon- or MMTT-stimulated C-peptide between baseline and 1 year after diagnosis. While this may reflect the impact of intensive insulin therapy and better glucose control, it should be noted that eligibility evaluations for the DCCT found that 48% of adults and 33% of adolescents (aged between 13–18 years) 1 to 5 years after diagnosis had stimulated C-peptide levels > 0.2 pmol/L, with 8% of adults and 3% of adolescents above this value even 5 to 15 years after diagnosis (104). Evidence for sustained β-cell function had also been reported (and underappreciated) in smaller studies in previous eras. Several studies have reported that HLA type, autoantibody status, HbA1C, and most importantly age, all impact on the postdiagnosis decline in C-peptide (105). Yet, a recent cross-sectional population-based study revealed persistent β-cell function even among youth with T1D (Carla J. Greenbaum, Benaroya Research Institute, Seattle, WA unpublished observations: SEARCH study). It has been suggested that the rate of fall of C-peptide secretion postdiagnosis may be similar across age groups, but that younger subjects start with less C-peptide and thus reach undetectable β-cell function more rapidly. Unfortunately, little information about C-peptide secretion in normal healthy children is available.

Another key point in interpreting results from intervention studies involves understanding the analysis plan for the primary outcome. Thus, some studies directly compare C-peptide responses at 1 or 2 years between treatment and control groups, whereas others do the same, but adjust for baseline values. In contrast, some studies compare the proportion of individuals in treatment and control groups that have a given percent decline in C-peptide from baseline. Considering the wide variation in baseline C-peptide values, the conclusion from a particular study may greatly depend upon what analysis plan was employed. To further complicate interpretation of results and particularly our ability to compare across studies, the timing of the "baseline" C-peptide may have a great impact. For example, if the inclusion criteria require individuals to be within 6 to 8 weeks from diagnosis, few, if any subjects will likely be in the "honeymoon" period. A baseline value obtained before resolution of hyperglycemia and acidosis or stabilization of insulin dose may result in an "artificially" low "baseline" value. On the other hand, if enrollment is allowed to 3 or 6 months, the "baseline" value may be considerably higher and conclusions regarding outcome significantly different. These concepts are illustrated in Figure 2. Of course, if studies were large enough, then randomization and/or adjustment for time from diagnosis may help to resolve these issues, but this has not yet been the case.

While there is current consensus that some measure of β-cell function is the most appropriate primary outcome measure for clinical trials, this requires that a relatively large number of subjects be followed for several years. A key advance would be the development of other surrogate markers of either disease progression or therapeutic effect. Although autoantibodies can be used to accurately predict risk for diabetes, they have not yet been shown to reflect an effect of therapy (106). Efforts to standardize measures of cellular immune function akin to autoantibody standardization (107) have begun (108–114) and may influence future clinical trial design and outcome assessment.

Subject Selection

To diminish the risk of exposure to unproven therapies in individuals who do not yet have a clinical disease, new therapies with potentially untoward adverse effects are usually first tested in individuals with established clinical disease before consideration is given to testing in those at risk. Often overlooked in this paradigm is the potential benefit of new therapies in the two populations of subjects. Prevention or delay of clinical disease in those at risk for disease provides an unambiguous benefit, whereas, we can only surmise about the potential benefit of retarding

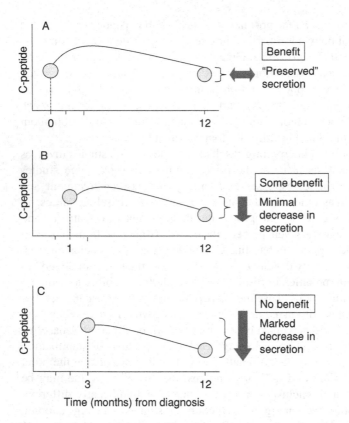

Figure 2 Impact of timing of baseline measure on interpretation of outcome in tertiary prevention trials. Theoretical illustration of a single subject's stimulated C-peptide over time postdiagnosis. (**A**) If baseline sample is obtained at the time of diagnosis and metabolic dysregulation, the stimulate C-peptide value will be relatively low. The difference between this baseline and C-peptide level at one year suggests that C-peptide has been preserved; if receiving therapy, one might conclude that the drug was beneficial to the subject. (**B**) However, if baseline sample is obtained when metabolic dysregulation is resolved, there will be a fall in C-peptide between baseline and 1 year, suggesting minimal preservation of C-peptide and lesser/no benefit. (**C**) If the baseline sample is obtained during the honeymoon period, when stimulated C-peptide is often high, the difference between baseline and 1-year value is large, suggesting a marked fall in C-peptide production and failure of therapy.

β-cell destruction in individuals treated after clinical diagnosis. This potential benefit could become tangible if, at the time of diagnosis, we could identify and thus target those destined to develop complications regardless of diabetes control. Preserving β-cell function could have a profound impact in these individuals and identifying them is a challenge for translational investigators.

The second problem with the sequential approach to trialing a candidate intervention therapy, described above, is scientific. If a therapy does not work in individuals with disease, is it really appropriate to stop testing it for prevention, particularly if the hypothesis and animal models suggest increased efficacy earlier in the disease process? In this regard, it may be more appropriate to consider interventions first in the population of antibody-positive relatives with abnormal glucose tolerance that, if left untreated, almost inevitably will progress to clinical diabetes within 5 years.

Another important unanswered question is whether it is critical for subjects with diabetes to be entered into a clinical trial as soon as feasible after clinical diagnosis. Certainly, subjects must have sufficient β-cell function at the time of enrollment to potentially benefit from intervention. Yet, since significant insulin secretion is found in a high percentage of individuals even several years from diagnosis, this requirement alone would allow enrollment of subjects outside of the immediate diagnosis period. The critically important and as yet unanswered question is whether there are immunologic processes occurring around the time of diagnosis that require intervention at that time to be effective. It is surprising that how little is understood about the transition from prediabetes to overt disease in humans. Recent analysis of data from the Diabetes Prevention Trial suggests little change in stimulated C-peptide just prior to diagnosis, implying but not proving that an abrupt destructive event does not occur (115). Without such knowledge, the only evidence in humans that early treatment could be important is from a post hoc analysis of the cyclosporine (116) and one of the anti-CD3 trials (69), suggesting increased benefit in those closer to diagnosis or with greater β-cell function.

Despite the limited data in humans, given that early treatment seems to make sense intuitively, why is there controversy about this issue in current clinical trial design? The most important reason is the difficulty in obtaining true informed consent for subjects in such a study. Having just been confronted with the news that they or their child has a life-long disease requiring a complete change in lifestyle, individuals may expect therapeutic benefit or even cure from a clinical trial. Although study personnel and consent forms explicitly deny this, families are often unable to truly comprehend that message. Another consideration relates to equipoise, the need to extend the potential of benefit of an intervention to the large number of individuals with persisting β-cell function outside of the immediate postdiagnosis period.

Translational investigators must also wrestle with the question of subject age for trial entry. Because primary and secondary prevention studies are not feasible without the inclusion of children, well-designed trials of therapies with limited potential for adverse effects are generally uncontroversial in this setting. On the other hand, because T1D presents throughout adulthood, most clinical investigators would agree that phase I (safety) tertiary intervention studies should be carried out in adults. However, it is not clear whether an effect in adults will be the same in children and therefore phase II and phase III studies (conducted with prespecified safety parameters and careful monitoring) should include children. It is also important to consider the upper age limit for inclusion in trials, because of the limited information available about the natural history of β-cell loss after diagnosis in different age groups. If, after accounting for variables such as HLA type, antibody status, and baseline C-peptide secretion, the rate of fall of β-cell function was similar among various ages, then it would be reasonable to include individuals who are in their 40s or even older. However, if this is not the case, and the number of subjects enrolled in a trial is too small to adequately stratify by age, then including a wide range of ages may limit the ability to detect an effect of therapy. Pooling data from the control arms of recent trials may provide sufficient data to better answer this question.

Translational Issues: Clinical Trial to Clinical Use

Moving from clinical trial to clinical use will require vigilance in several areas. First, endocrinologists will have to learn how to administer and monitor immunotherapy. Most currently practicing physicians and training programs have no experience with these forms of therapy. Thus, at some point, additional training and credentialing may be needed. Second, "postmarketing" surveillance and a willingness to openly evaluate benefits and risks will be needed particularly in comparison to advances in "mechanical" treatments for diabetes. For example, if a closed loop insulin delivery system is developed which allows for minimal intrusion on the day-to-day life of the person with diabetes and lessens the risk of complications, there will be limited tolerance for any risk associated with immune intervention therapies. It is important to acknowledge that very long-term eval-uation will be required to determine if preservation of β-cell function reduces vascular and other complications such as hypoglycemic unawareness.

Future Approaches

Future approaches to prevent immune-mediated diabetes will use new knowl-edge about the genetic and environmental factors underlying disease progress to formally stage subjects. Prevention of T1D will no doubt occur incrementally with different interventions suited to risk level (Fig. 3). Ideally, prevention should be directed to individuals at-risk, with early, sub-clinical disease, or better still, to those at genetic risk without any evidence of underlying disease. The case for intervening early in such asymptomatic individuals rests on the likelihood of greater efficacy before the disease process is underway, but it is constrained by the requirement for safety. Autoantigen-based immunotherapy in this popula-tion is likely to be an important therapeutic component due to its relative safety compared to conventional immunosuppressive agents and compelling data from rodent models. In asymptomatic individuals, the majority of whom are likely to be children unable to give autonomous informed consent, safety is the first consider-ation. In end-stage autoimmune disease, combinatorial approaches that not only enhance immune regulation but also suppress pathogenic immunity are likely to be required. Advances in manipulating gene expression safely in stem cells and conditioning the recipient immune system could open new avenues for stem cell

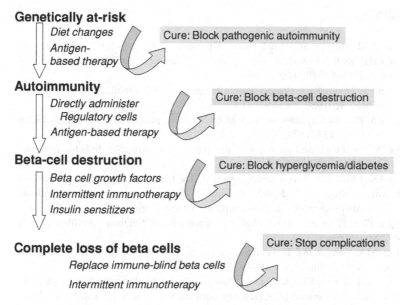

Figure 3   Vision of future therapeutic algorithms for type 1 diabetes prevention.

based–self-antigen vaccination. Prevention of T1D will facilitate the replacement or regeneration of β-cells in people with established diabetes or at risk of recurrent autoimmune β-cell destruction. Finally, lessons learned from the prevention of T1D should apply to other autoimmune diseases.

This vision requires answers to key questions on both sides of the bridge between basic and clinical research, including:

1. Will genetic markers allow for better selection of subjects for targeted therapies?
2. Can surrogate markers of disease progression or therapeutic effect be improved/discovered?
3. Is T1D a disease of remission and relapses?
4. Is there an abrupt immunologic or metabolic event that precipitates onset of clinical disease, or is the transition to overt diabetes solely the result of chronic progression of the underlying process?
5. How are data on timing and/or dose of an intervention optimally translated from animal studies to a clinical trial?
6. At the time of diagnosis, can subjects be identified who are most likely to develop complications despite excellent glucose control, as primary targets for intervention?
7. Are there differences in the natural history of disease after diagnosis in different age groups, or according to other potentially relevant variables such as HLA, insulin resistance?
8. What is the most efficient way to bring combination therapies to clinical trial?

REFERENCES

1. Dittrich HM. History of the discovery of pancreatic diabetes by von Mering and Minkowski 1889. A historical overview on the occasion of the 100th anniversary. Z Gesamte Inn Med 1989; 44:335–340.
2. Bornstein J, Trewhella P. Plasma insulin levels in diabetes mellitus in man. Aust J Exp Biol Med Sci 1950; 28:569–572.
3. Yalow RS, Berson SA. Immunoassay of endogenous plasma insulin in man. J Clin Invest 1960; 39:1157–1175.
4. Gepts W. Pathology and anatomy of the pancreas in juvenile diabetes mellitus. Diabetes 1965; 14:619–33.
5. Foulis AK, Liddle CN, Farquharson MA, et al. The histopathology of the pancreas in type 1 (insulin-dependent) diabetes mellitus: a 25-year review of deaths in patients under 20 years of age in the United Kingdom. Diabetologia 1986; 29:267–74.
6. Nerup J, Platz P, Andersen OO, et al. HL-A antigens and diabetes mellitus. Lancet 1974; 2:864–866.
7. Menser MA, Forrest JM, Honeyman MC, et al. Letter: Diabetes, HL-A antigens, and congenital rubella. Lancet 1974; 2:1508–1509.
8. Bottazzo GF, Florin-Christensen A, Doniach D. Islet-cell antibodies in diabetes mellitus with autoimmune polyendocrine deficiencies. Lancet 1974; 2:1279–1283.
9. MacCuish A, Barnes E, Irvine W, et al. Antibodies to islet cells in insulin-dependent diabetics with coexistent autoimmune disease. Lancet 1974 Dec 28; 2(7896):1529–1531.
10. Palmer J, Asplin C, Clemons P. Insulin autoantibodies in insulin-dependent diabetes before insulin treatment. Science 1983; 222:1337–1339.
11. Bleich D, Jackson RA, Soeldner JS, et al. Analysis of metabolic progression to type I diabetes in ICA+ relatives of patients with type I diabetes. Diabetes Care 1990; 13:111–118.
12. Ganda OP, Srikanta S, Brink SJ, et al. Differential sensitivity to beta-cell secretagogues in "early" type I diabetes mellitus. Diabetes 1984; 33:516–521.
13. Srikanta A, Ganda OP, Gleason RE, et al. Pre-Type I diabetes: Linear loss of beta-cell response to intravenous glucose. Diabetes 1984; 33:717–720.
14. Kim SJ, Holbeck SL, Nisperos B, et al. Identification of a polymorphic variant associated with HLA-DQW3 and characterized by specific restriction sites within the DQ beta-chain gene. Proc Natl Acad Sci U S A 1985; 82:8139–8143.
15. Eisenbarth GS. Type I diabetes mellitus. A chronic autoimmune disease. N Engl J Med 1986; 314:1360–1368.
16. Baekkeskov S, Aanstoot H, Christgau S, et al. Identification of the 64kD autoantigen in insulin-dependent diabetes as the GABA-synthesizing enzyme glutamic acid decarboxylase. Nature 1990; 347:151–156.
17. Lu J, Li Q, Xie H, et al. Identification of a second transmembrane protein tyrosine phosphatase, IA-2beta, as an autoantigen in insulin-dependent diabetes mellitus: Precursor of the 37-kDa tryptic fragment. Proc Natl Acad Sci U S A 1996; 93:2307–2311.
18. Wenzlau JM, Juhl K, Yu L, et al. The cation efflux transporter ZnT8 (Slc30A8) is a major autoantigen in human type 1 diabetes. Proc Natl Acad Sci U S A 2007; 104:17040–17045.

19. Grubin CE, Daniels T, Toivola B, et al. A novel radioligand binding assay to determine diagnostic accuracy of isoform-specific glutamic acid decarboxylase antibodies in childhood IDDM. Diabetologia 1994; 37:344–350.

20. Achenbach P, Schlosser M, Williams AJ, et al. Combined testing of antibody titer and affinity improves insulin autoantibody measurement: Diabetes Antibody Standardization Program. Clin Immunol 2007; 122:85–90.

21. Bingley PJ, Bonifacio E, Mueller PW. Diabetes Antibody Standardization Program: First assay proficiency evaluation. Diabetes 2003; 52:1128–1136.

22. Greenbaum CJ. Type 1 diabetes intervention trials: What have we learned? A critical review of selected intervention trials. Clin Immunol 2002; 104:97–104.

23. Pozzilli P. Immuno-intervention and preservation of beta-cell function in type 1 diabetes. Diabetes Metab Res Rev 2007; 23:255–256.

24. Skyler JS. Prediction and prevention of type 1 diabetes: Progress, problems, and prospects. Clin Pharmacol Ther 2007; 81:768–771.

25. Staeva-Vieira T, Peakman M, von Herrath M. Translational mini-review series on type 1 diabetes: Immune-based therapeutic approaches for type 1 diabetes. Clin Exp Immunol 2007; 148:17–31.

26. Greenbaum CJ, Harrison LC. Guidelines for intervention trials in subjects with newly diagnosed type 1 diabetes. Diabetes 2003; 52:1059–1065.

27. Assan R, Feutren G, Sirmai J, et al. Plasma C-peptide levels and clinical remissions in recent-onset type I diabetic patients treated with cyclosporin A and insulin. Diabetes 1990; 39:768–774.

28. Stiller CR, Laupacis A, Dupre J, et al. Cyclosporine for treatment of early type I diabetes: Preliminary results. N Engl J Med 1983; 308:1226–1227.

29. Stiller CR, Dupre J, Gent M, et al. Effects of cyclosporine immunosuppression in insulin-dependent diabetes mellitus of recent onset. Science 1984; 223:1362–1367.

30. Parving HH, Tarnow L, Nielsen FS, et al. Cyclosporine nephrotoxicity in type 1 diabetic patients. A 7-year follow-up study. Diabetes Care 1999; 22:478–483.

31. Ribstein J, Rodier M, Mimran A. Effect of cyclosporine on blood pressure and renal function of recent type 1 diabetes mellitus. J Hypertens Suppl 1989; 7:S198–S199.

32. Stiller CR, Dupre J, Gent M, et al. Effects of cyclosporine in recent-onset juvenile type 1 diabetes: Impact of age and duration of disease. J Pediatr 1987; 111:1069–1072.

33. Gutierrez-Dalmau A, Campistol JM. Immunosuppressive therapy and malignancy in organ transplant recipients: A systematic review. Drugs 2007; 67:1167–1198.

34. Pozzilli P, Signore A, Williams AJ, et al. NOD mouse colonies around the world–Recent facts and figures. Immunol Today 1993; 14:193–196.

35. Funda DP, Fundova P, Harrison LC. Microflora-dependency of selected diabetes-preventive diets: Germ-free and ex-germ-free monocolonized NOD mice as models for studying environmental factors in type 1 diabetes. In: 13th International Congress of Immunology, Rio de Janeiro, Brazil, 2007.

36. Macpherson AJ, Harris NL. Interactions between commensal intestinal bacteria and the immune system. Nat Rev Immunol 2004; 4:478–485.

37. Locke NR, Stankovic S, Funda DP, et al. TCR gamma–delta intraepithelial lymphocytes are required for self-tolerance. J Immunol 2006; 176:6553–6559.

38. Ke Y, Pearce K, Lake JP, et al. Gamma–delta T lymphocytes regulate the induction and maintenance of oral tolerance. J Immunol 1997; 158:3610–3618.
39. Strachan DP. Hay fever, hygiene, and household size. BMJ 1989; 299:1259–1260.
40. Virtanen SM, Saukkonen T, Savilahti E, et al. Diet, cow's milk protein antibodies and the risk of IDDM in Finnish children. Childhood Diabetes in Finland Study Group. Diabetologia 1994; 37:381–387.
41. Norris JM, Beaty B, Klingensmith G, et al. Lack of association between early exposure to cow's milk protein and beta-cell autoimmunity. Diabetes Autoimmunity Study in the Young (DAISY). JAMA 1996; 276:609–614.
42. Couper JJ, Steele C, Beresford S, et al. Lack of association between duration of breast-feeding or introduction of cow's milk and development of islet autoimmunity. Diabetes 1999; 48:2145–2149.
43. Ziegler AG, Schmid S, Huber D, et al. Early infant feeding and risk of developing type 1 diabetes-associated autoantibodies. JAMA 2003; 290:1721–1728.
44. Norris JM, Barriga K, Klingensmith G, et al. Timing of initial cereal exposure in infancy and risk of islet autoimmunity. JAMA 2003; 290:1713–1720.
45. Fuchtenbusch M, Ziegler AG, Hummel M. Elimination of dietary gluten and development of type 1 diabetes in high-risk subjects. Rev Diabet Stud 2004; 1:39–41.
46. Simopoulos AP. Essential fatty acids in health and chronic disease. Am J Clin Nutr 1999; 70:560S–569S.
47. Litherland SA, Xie XT, Hutson AD, et al. Aberrant prostaglandin synthase 2 expression defines an antigen-presenting cell defect for insulin-dependent diabetes mellitus. J Clin Invest 1999; 104:515–523.
48. Stene LC, Joner G. Use of cod liver oil during the first year of life is associated with lower risk of childhood-onset type 1 diabetes: A large, population-based, case-control study. Am J Clin Nutr 2003; 78:1128–1134.
49. Mathieu C, Badenhoop K. Vitamin D and type 1 diabetes mellitus: State of the art. Trends Endocrinol Metab 2005; 16:261–266.
50. Adorini L. Intervention in autoimmunity: The potential of vitamin D receptor agonists. Cell Immunol 2005; 233:115–124.
51. Wicklow BA, Taback SP. Feasibility of a type 1 diabetes primary prevention trial using 2000 IU vitamin D3 in infants from the general population with increased HLA-associated risk. Ann NY Acad Sci 2006; 1079:310–312.
52. Calcinaro F, Dionisi S, Marinaro M, et al. Oral probiotic administration induces interleukin-10 production and prevents spontaneous autoimmune diabetes in the non-obese diabetic mouse. Diabetologia 2005; 48:1565–1575.
53. Matsuzaki T, Nagata Y, Kado S, et al. Prevention of onset in an insulin-dependent diabetes mellitus model, NOD mice, by oral feeding of Lactobacillus casei. Apmis 1997; 105:643–649.
54. Ljungberg M, Korpela R, Ilonen J, et al. Probiotics for the prevention of beta-cell autoimmunity in children at genetic risk of type 1 diabetes—The PRODIA study. Ann N Y Acad Sci 2006; 1079:360–364.
55. Bonner-Weir S, Weir GC. New sources of pancreatic beta-cells. Nat Biotechnol 2005; 23:857–861.
56. Suarez-Pinzon WL, Yan Y, Power R, et al. Combination therapy with epidermal growth factor and gastrin increases beta-cell mass and reverses hyperglycemia in diabetic NOD mice. Diabetes 2005; 54:2596–2601.

57. Brand SJ, Tagerud S, Lambert P, et al. Pharmacological treatment of chronic diabetes by stimulating pancreatic beta-cell regeneration with systemic co-administration of EGF and gastrin. Pharmacol Toxicol 2002; 91:414–420.
58. Meier JJ, Butler AE, Galasso R, et al. Increased islet beta-cell replication adjacent to intrapancreatic gastrinomas in humans. Diabetologia 2006; 49:2689–2696.
59. Drucker DJ. Biologic actions and therapeutic potential of the proglucagon-derived peptides. Nat Clin Pract Endocrinol Metab 2005; 1:22–31.
60. Fourlanos S, Narendran P, Byrnes GB, et al. Insulin resistance is a risk factor for progression to type 1 diabetes. Diabetologia 2004; 47:1661–1667.
61. Greenbaum CJ. Insulin resistance in type 1 diabetes. Diabetes Metab Res Rev 2002; 18:192–200.
62. Xu P, Cuthbertson D, Greenbaum C, et al. Role of insulin resistance in predicting progression to type 1 diabetes. Diabetes Care 2007; 30:2314–2320.
63. Effect of intensive therapy on residual beta-cell function in patients with type 1 diabetes in the diabetes control and complications trial. A randomized, controlled trial. The Diabetes Control and Complications Trial Research Group. Ann Intern Med 1998; 128:517–523.
64. Shah S, Malone J, Simpson N. A randomized trial of intensive insulin therapy in newly diagnosed insulin-dependent diabetes mellitus. NEJM 1989; 320:550–554.
65. Roep BO. Are insights gained from NOD mice sufficient to guide clinical translation? Another inconvenient truth. Ann N Y Acad Sci 2007; 1103:1–10.
66. Shoda LK, Young DL, Ramanujan S, et al. A comprehensive review of interventions in the NOD mouse and implications for translation. Immunity 2005; 23:115–126.
67. Chatenoud L, Thervet E, Primo J, et al. Anti-CD3 antibody induces long-term remission of overt autoimmunity in nonobese diabetic mice. Proc Natl Acad Sci U S A 1994; 91:123–127.
68. Herold KC, Hagopian W, Auger JA, et al. Anti-CD3 monoclonal antibody in new-onset type 1 diabetes mellitus. N Engl J Med 2002; 346:1692–1698.
69. Keymeulen B, Vandemeulebroucke E, Ziegler AG, et al. Insulin needs after CD3-antibody therapy in new-onset type 1 diabetes. N Engl J Med 2005; 352:2598–2608.
70. Faria AM, Weiner HL. Oral tolerance: Mechanisms and therapeutic applications. Adv Immunol 1999; 73:153–264.
71. Faria AM, Weiner HL. Oral tolerance: Therapeutic implications for autoimmune diseases. Clin Dev Immunol 2006; 13:143–157.
72. Harrison LC, Hafler DA. Antigen-specific therapy for autoimmune disease. Curr Opin Immunol 2000; 12:704–711.
73. Harrison LC, Honeyman MC, Steele CE, et al. Pancreatic beta-cell function and immune responses to insulin after administration of intranasal insulin to humans at risk for type 1 diabetes. Diabetes Care 2004; 27:2348–2355.
74. Skyler JS, Krischer JP, Wolfsdorf J, et al. Effects of oral insulin in relatives of patients with type 1 diabetes: The Diabetes Prevention Trial–Type 1. Diabetes Care 2005; 28:1068–1076.
75. Atkinson M, Maclaren N, Luchetta R. Insulitis and diabetes in NOD mice reduced by prophylactic insulin therapy. Diabetes 1990; 39:933–937.
76. Zhang ZJ, Davidson L, Eisenbarth G, et al. Suppression of diabetes in nonobese diabetic mice by oral administration of porcine insulin. Proc Natl Acad Sci U S A 1991; 88:10252–10256.

77. Chaillous L, Lefevre H, Thivolet C, et al. Oral insulin administration and residual beta-cell function in recent- onset type 1 diabetes: a multicentre randomised controlled trial. Diabete Insuline Orale group. Lancet 2000; 356:545–549.
78. Pozzilli P, Pitocco D, Visalli N, et al. No effect of oral insulin on residual beta-cell function in recent-onset type I diabetes (the IMDIAB VII). IMDIAB Group. Diabetologia 2000; 43:1000–1004.
79. Ludvigsson J. Immune intervention at diagnosis—Should we treat children to preserve beta-cell function ? Pediatr Diabetes 2007; 6(Suppl 8):34–39.
80. Agardh CD, Cilio CM, Lethagen A, et al. Clinical evidence for the safety of GAD65 immunomodulation in adult-onset autoimmune diabetes. J Diabetes Complications 2005; 19:238–246.
81. Simell, O. Oral presentation at the Immunology of Diabetes Society. Meet, Nov 15, 2007.
82. Matos M, Park R, Mathis D, et al. Progression to islet destruction in a cyclophosphamide-induced transgenic model: A microarray overview. Diabetes 2004; 53:2310–2321.
83. Poirot L, Benoist C, Mathis D. Natural killer cells distinguish innocuous and destructive forms of pancreatic islet autoimmunity. Proc Natl Acad Sci U S A 2004; 101:8102–8107.
84. Diabetes Prevention Trial Study Group. Effects of insulin in relatives of patients with type 1 diabetes mellitus. N Engl J Med 2002; 346:1685–1691.
85. Gotfredsen CF, Buschard K, Frandsen EK. Reduction of diabetes incidence of BB Wistar rats by early prophylactic insulin treatment of diabetes-prone animals. Diabetologia 1985; 28:933–935.
86. Gottlieb PA, Handler ES, Appel MC, et al. Insulin treatment prevents diabetes mellitus but not thyroiditis in RT6-depleted diabetes resistant BB/Wor rats. Diabetologia 1991; 34:296–300.
87. Blankenhorn EP, Descipio C, Rodemich L, et al. Refinement of the IDDM4 diabetes susceptibility locus reveals TCRVbeta4 as a candidate gene. Ann N Y Acad Sci 2007; 1103:128–131.
88. Carson BD, Ziegler SF. Impaired T-cell receptor signaling in Foxp3+ CD4 T cells. Ann N Y Acad Sci 2007; 1103:167–178.
89. Gebe JA, Falk B, Unrath K, et al. Autoreactive T cells in a partially humanized murine model of T1D. Ann N Y Acad Sci 2007; 1103:69–76.
90. Hamilton-Williams EE, Martinez X, Lyman M, et al. The use of idd congenic mice to identify checkpoints of peripheral tolerance to islet antigen. Ann N Y Acad Sci 2007; 1103:118–127.
91. King M, Pearson T, Shultz LD, et al. Development of new-generation HU-PBMC-NOD/SCID mice to study human islet alloreactivity. Ann N Y Acad Sci 2007; 1103:90–93.
92. Luo B, Wu T, Pan Y, et al. Resistance to the induction of mixed chimerism in spontaneously diabetic NOD mice depends on the CD40/CD154 pathway and donor MHC disparity. Ann N Y Acad Sci 2007; 1103:94–102.
93. Pechhold K, Chakrabarty S, Harlan DM. Cytotoxic T-cell mediated diabetes in RIP-CD80 transgenic mice: Autoantigen peptide sensitivity and fine specificity. Ann N Y Acad Sci 2007; 1103:132–142.
94. Serreze DV, Marron MP, Dilorenzo TP. "Humanized" HLA-transgenic NOD mice to identify pancreatic beta-cell autoantigens of potential clinical relevance to type 1 diabetes. Ann N Y Acad Sci 2007; 1103:103–111.

95. Shultz LD, Pearson T, King M, et al. Humanized NOD/LtSz-scid IL2 receptor common gamma chain knockout mice in diabetes research. Ann N Y Acad Sci 2007; 1103:77–89.

96. Tracy S, Drescher KM. Coxsackievirus infections and NOD mice: Relevant models of protection from, and induction of, type 1 diabetes. Ann N Y Acad Sci 2007; 1103:143–151.

97. Unger WW, Pinkse GG, Mulder-van der Kracht S, et al. Human clonal CD8 autoreactivity to an IGRP islet epitope shared between mice and men. Ann N Y Acad Sci 2007; 1103:192–195.

98. Zheng Y, Kreuwel HT, Young DL, et al. The virtual NOD mouse: Applying predictive biosimulation to research in type 1 diabetes. Ann N Y Acad Sci 2007; 1103:45–62.

99. Skyler JS, Rabinovitch A. Cyclosporine in recent onset type I diabetes mellitus. Effects on islet beta-cell function. Miami Cyclosporine Diabetes Study Group. J Diabetes Complications 1992; 6:77–88.

100. Steffes MW, Sibley S, Jackson M, et al. Beta-cell function and the development of diabetes-related complications in the diabetes control and complications trial. Diabetes Care 2003; 26:832–836.

101. Sjoberg S, Gjotterberg M, Berglund L, et al. Residual C-peptide excretion is associated with a better long-term glycemic control and slower progress of retinopathy in type I (insulin- dependent) diabetes mellitus. J Diabet Complications 1991; 5: 18–22.

102. Schnell O, Eisfelder B, Standl E, et al. High-dose intravenous insulin infusion versus intensive insulin treatment in newly diagnosed IDDM. Diabetes 1997; 46:1607–1611.

103. Pozzilli P, Di Mario U. Autoimmune diabetes not requiring insulin at diagnosis (latent autoimmune diabetes of the adult): Definition, characterization, and potential prevention. Diabetes Care 2001; 24:1460–1467.

104. Palmer JP, Fleming GA, Greenbaum CJ, et al. C-peptide is the appropriate outcome measure for type 1 diabetes clinical trials to preserve beta-cell function: Report of an ADA workshop, 21–22 October 2001. Diabetes 2004; 53:250–264.

105. Sherry NA, Tsai EB, Herold KC. Natural history of beta-cell function in type 1 diabetes. Diabetes 2005; 54(Suppl 2):S32–S39.

106. Mandrup-Poulsen T, Molvig J, Andersen HU, et al. Lack of predictive value of islet cell antibodies, insulin antibodies, and HLA-DR phenotype for remission in cyclosporin-treated IDDM patients. The Canadian-European Randomized Control Trial Group. Diabetes 1990; 39:204–210.

107. Bingley PJ, Williams AJ. Validation of autoantibody assays in type 1 diabetes: workshop programme. Autoimmunity 2004; 37:257–260.

108. Pinkse GG, Boitard C, Tree TI, et al. HLA class I epitope discovery in type 1 diabetes: Independent and reproducible identification of proinsulin epitopes of CD8 T cells—Report of the IDS T-Cell Workshop Committee. Ann N Y Acad Sci 2006; 1079:19–23.

109. Tree TI, Roep BO, Peakman M. A mini meta-analysis of studies on CD4+CD25+ T cells in human type 1 diabetes: Report of the Immunology of Diabetes Society T-Cell Workshop. Ann N Y Acad Sci 2006; 1079:9–18.

110. Peakman M, Tree TI, Endl J, et al. Characterization of preparations of GAD65, proinsulin, and the islet tyrosine phosphatase IA-2 for use in detection of autoreactive T-cells in type 1 diabetes: Report of phase II of the Second International Immunology

of Diabetes Society Workshop for Standardization of T-cell assays in type 1 diabetes. Diabetes 2001; 50:1749–1754.

111. Roep BO, Atkinson MA, van Endert PM, et al. Autoreactive T-cell responses in insulin-dependent (Type 1) diabetes mellitus. Report of the first international workshop for standardization of T-cell assays. J Autoimmun 1999; 13:267–282.

112. Schloot NC, Meierhoff G, Karlsson FM, et al. Comparison of cytokine ELISpot assay formats for the detection of islet antigen autoreactive T cells. Report of the third immunology of diabetes society T-cell workshop. J Autoimmun 2003; 21:365–376.

113. Nagata M, Kotani R, Moriyama H, et al. Detection of autoreactive T cells in type 1 diabetes using coded autoantigens and an immunoglobulin-free cytokine ELISPOT assay: Report from the fourth immunology of diabetes society T-cell workshop. Ann N Y Acad Sci 2004; 1037:10–15.

114. Seyfert-Margolis V, Gisler TD, Asare AL, et al. Analysis of T-cell assays to measure autoimmune responses in subjects with type 1 diabetes: Results of a blinded controlled study. Diabetes 2006; 55:2588–2594.

115. Sosenko JM, Palmer JP, Greenbaum CJ, et al. Patterns of metabolic progression to type 1 diabetes in the Diabetes Prevention Trial-Type 1. Diabetes Care 2006; 29:643–649.

116. Martin S, Pawlowski B, Greulich B, et al. Natural course of remission in IDDM during 1st year after diagnosis. Diabetes Care 1992; 15:66–74.

7

The Incretin Effect: Regulation of Insulin Secretion and Glucose Tolerance by GI Hormones

David A. D'Alessio, Benedikt A. Aulinger, and Marzieh Salehi

Department of Medicine, Division of Endocrinology, Vontz Center for Molecular Studies, University of Cincinnati, Cincinnati, Ohio, U.S.A.

THE INTEGRATED INSULIN RESPONSE AND GLUCOSE TOLERANCE IN VIVO

The concentration of glucose in the blood is a highly regulated physiologic parameter. The adaptive significance of maintaining glucose levels within narrow bounds is probably related to minimization of fluid shifts, appropriate allocation of glucose to storage depots, and retention of calories. The system for glucose regulation is complex and very effective. For example, nondiabetic humans have the capacity to eat large carbohydrate meals, with only minor, 30% to 50%, changes in circulating glucose concentrations that are typically returned to basal levels within 1 to 2 hours. Signaling by the islet hormone insulin is the principle means of shifting glucose from the circulation into cells and the control of insulin secretion is at the core of normal glucose tolerance. The islet β-cell is regulated by the interaction of substrate, neural, and hormonal stimuli. An increase in ambient glucose is the best established stimulus for insulin release, and is essential for normal secretion *in vivo* since the response to other physiologic β-cell stimuli are substantially reduced at basal glucose levels. However, it is clear from the pattern of β-cell secretory rates after meals that other factors also have important roles in this process. Insulin secretion is most pronounced in the early part of meals, before a peak in blood glucose (1) suggesting that other factors, in addition to hyperglycemia, stimulate the β-cell after meals. For effective homeostasis it is important that insulin secretion should not change as a strictly linear function of plasma glycemia but rather preempt major changes in blood glucose. In other words, the β-cells should anticipate an increase in glycemia rather than simply chasing the rising glucose levels. This system has at its core inputs from the gastrointestinal (GI) tract that act as a feed forward mechanism to link nutrient absorption with insulin secretion in order to promote efficient nutrient assimilation (2–4). In addition, there are neural stimuli to the β-cell that play a role in physiologic insulin secretion (5). Signals carried by parasympathetic nerves contribute to anticipatory insulin secretion, termed cephalic insulin release, and also to the postprandial insulin response. Thus, the model that has emerged from a large body of research over the last three decades is that the insulin response to eating is controlled by a system that integrates circulating glucose levels, neural inputs, and stimulation by hormones released from the GI tract to allow glycemia to be restored rapidly, and without hypoglycemia.

THE INCRETIN EFFECT AND ROLE OF GI HORMONES IN GLUCOSE METABOLISM

It has long been known that the GI tract plays an important role in the disposition of carbohydrate meals. That this must be the case was deduced from a number of studies demonstrating that circulating insulin levels are significantly higher after glucose is ingested than when it is administered intravenously (IV) (Fig. 1). Based on these observations it was postulated that the GI tract released substances during carbohydrate absorption that could stimulate insulin secretion. These substances were called incretins, a term first used in the early 20th century to refer to stimuli of internal secretions. The augmentation of glucose-stimulated insulin secretion that occurs when carbohydrate is absorbed through the gut is called the incretin effect (2,4). Subsequently it has become clear that in healthy humans stimulation by incretins accounts for 30% to 70% of postprandial insulin secretion (6).

The glycemic excursion in healthy humans following the ingestion of liquid glucose is nearly identical across ranges of intake from 25 to 100 g. However, there is a progressive increase of insulin secretion and the incretin effect with the amount of carbohydrate ingested (6). This set of observations demonstrates two important points, namely that the postprandial β-cell response is not quantitatively dependent on the glycemic level, and that signals from the gut increase in proportion to nutrients presented for digestion. Based on these observations, the insulin response to meals fits a model whereby glucose activates β-cell secretion, while the incretin effect controls the gain on insulin output.

There are two known hormones that act as incretins, glucose-dependent insulinotropic polypeptide (GIP) and glucagon-like peptide 1 (GLP-1). These peptides are produced by specialized cells in the intestinal mucosa, and secreted in response to carbohydrate and lipid containing meals. There are specific GIP and GLP-1 receptors that are expressed on islet cells, as well as in other tissues,

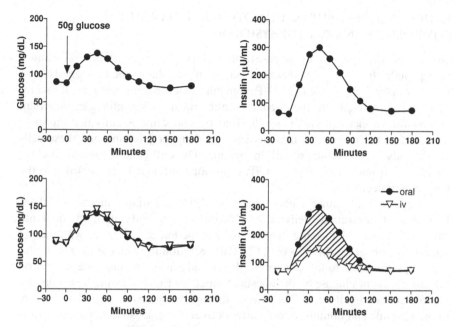

Figure 1 Schematic representation of the incretin effect. The left panel shows plasma glucose following ingestion of a glucose solution (upper) and plasma glucose during an intravenous infusion of glucose to match the glycemia during the oral glucose administration (bottom). The right panel shows the insulin response to oral glucose (upper) and the response to IV glucose relative to oral glucose (bottom). Despite nearly indentical levels of plasma glucose, insulin secretion is substantially higer with oral compared to IV glucose (the incretin effect-shaded area right bottom panel).

and deletion of these receptors in mouse models leads to glucose intolerance (3). These data and corroborating studies using GIP and GLP-1 receptor antagonists have demonstrated that enteroinsular signaling is a physiologic process that is necessary for normal glucose homeostasis.

The incretin effect has been demonstrated to be defective in several disease states. Patients with type 2 diabetes have only minimal augmentation by oral compared to IV glucose stimulus (7,8). Similarly, first-degree relatives of type 1 diabetic patients with normal fasting glucose but diabetic responses to an oral glucose tolerance test (OGTT) have a significant reduction of the incretin effect (9). But even nondiabetic individuals can have a reduction in the incretin effect, since this has been demonstrated in persons with impaired glucose tolerance (10) and in heart and liver transplant recipients taking immunosuppressive drugs known to affect the β-cell (11). While the mechanism of the abnormal incretin effect in these conditions is not clear, these subject groups have in common abnormal β-cell function, and one reasonable supposition is that a defective response of the islet to gut stimulus is an early and fundamental aspect of impaired insulin secretion.

GLUCOSE-DEPENDENT INSULINOTROPIC POLYPEPTIDE: PHYSIOLOGY AND PATHOPHYSIOLOGY

GIP (originally referred to as gastric inhibitory polypeptide) is a 42 amino-acid peptide that is highly conserved across mammalian species suggesting an important physiologic role (12). GIP augments glucose-stimulated insulin secretion, and is secreted into the circulation after meal consumption, an important criteria for an incretin. GIP is synthesized by endocrine K-cells that are most prevalent in the mucosa of the duodenum and upper jejunum, and these cells are the only known source of GIP in humans. The GIP gene is located on chromosome 17q and encodes preproGIP, a prohormone that is processed into the bioactive molecule.

Ingestion of either carbohydrate or lipid containing meals stimulates K-cells, and intravenous delivery of glucose, amino acids, or lipids does not cause GIP release, indicating that luminal interaction of substrates with the gut mucosa is critical for this process (12). GIP secretion in response to enteral glucose is proportional to the amount of glucose administered and is dependent on the absorption of glucose by the intestinal mucosa (13). Following ingestion of a glucose containing drink, GIP is released throughout the entire period of delivery to the intestine and diminishes only after delivery of glucose to the duodenum is complete (13). Consistent with this, glucose-stimulated GIP release is inhibited by factors that reduce carbohydrate digestion and uptake (2). The addition of fat to a glucose meal greatly accentuates the GIP response. Taken as a whole, the available data indicate that GIP secretion is regulated directly by the products of meal digestion in a dose-dependent manner, consistent with a role as a quantitative signal of nutrient absorption to the endocrine pancreas (14).

Following release into the circulation, GIP is rapidly metabolized by the enzyme dipeptidyl peptidase IV (DPP-IV), a ubiquitous protease located on capillary endothelium as well as in the circulation. DPP-IV cleaves specifically between residues 2 and 3 leaving $GIP_{(3-42)}$ (12,15). This conversion occurs rapidly, so that the circulating half-life of full-length GIP is only 5 to 7 minutes in mammals, and is inactivating since $GIP_{(3-42)}$ does not stimulate insulin secretion.

A single GIP receptor (GIPr) has been identified and is currently believed to mediate all of the physiologic effects of the peptide. The GIPr has seven-transmembrane domains and substantial homology with receptors in the secretin-VIP receptor family, particularly the glucagon and GLP-1 receptors. The GIPr is expressed in pancreatic islet cells, the upper gastrointestinal tract, adipocytes, adrenal cortex, pituitary, and a variety of brain regions (3). Binding by GIP to its receptor activates adenylyl cyclase and increases intracellular cAMP, but also acts through PI3 kinase and growth factor pathways.

GIP is insulinotropic only when ambient glucose concentrations are elevated, typically to greater than 5 to 6 mM (16). This action has been demonstrated uniformly in a wide range of experimental settings including cultured β-cells, animal models, and humans. In humans both porcine and synthetic human GIP stimulate insulin secretion when infused to concentrations mimicking those occurring after meals as long as some degree of hyperglycemia is present. The glucose dependence of GIP-stimulated insulin secretion is also a feature of the actions of GLP-1 and other GI peptides that activate the β-cell, and probably represents an adaptation to prevent hypoglycemia during normal postprandial metabolism.

The incretin role of GIP has been demonstrated by several experimental techniques such as immunoneutralization of circulating GIP and by administration of competitive antagonists of the GIP receptor, both of which cause glucose intolerance (17,18). Similarly, targeted gene deletion of the GIP receptor in a line of mice resulted in animals with normal fasting glucose levels and responses to intraperitoneal glucose loads (19). However, in response to oral glucose loading the GIP receptor knockout mice had significant glucose intolerance and impaired insulin secretory responses. Taken together these studies in rodents indicate that the incretin action of GIP is necessary for normal glucose tolerance.

Beyond a role as an incretin, GIP has several other actions that may be important for normal metabolic function. GIP stimulates the proliferation of β-cell lines, and seems to protect them from toxic exposures that increase apoptosis (20,21). In addition, the GIP receptor is expressed in adipose tissue and evidence exists to suggest that GIP promotes triglyceride accumulation in adipocytes. GIP receptor knock-out mice (GIPr -/-) are resistant to obesity when chronically fed a high-rat diet, and a cross of the GIPr -/- line with *ob/ob* mice mutes the striking obesity of the latter (19,22). Interestingly, the effects of GIP on β-cells and adipocytes may combine for distinct effects in different settings. Administration of a GIPr antagonist to normal mice causes glucose intolerance (17). However, the same agent improves glucose metabolism and insulin sensitivity in diabetic *ob/ob* mice (23).

Because GIP plays an important role in the normal physiology of insulin secretion after ingested nutrients it has been widely studied as a factor contributing to diabetes. The best evidence is that GIP is not deficient in diabetic patients, and in fact meal-stimulated levels may in fact be greater in these individuals. However, a number of studies have demonstrated that GIP has greatly reduced effectiveness to stimulate insulin secretion in persons with type 2 diabetes (24). The pathophysiology of reduced GIP action in diabetes is unclear. It has been suggested that the GIPr is downregulated by hyperglycemia or expressed in reduced amounts in the diabetic state (25). Alternatively the results of several recent studies have suggested that the reduction of GIP signaling is proportional to the reduction in overall β-cell function in diabetic patients (26). Regardless, it seems likely that one explanation for the impaired incretin effect in diabetes is a reduced effect of GIP.

GLUCAGON-LIKE PEPTIDE 1: PHYSIOLOGY AND PATHOPHYSIOLOGY

GLP-1 is cleaved from proglucagon in specific intestinal mucosal cells termed L-cells, and secreted primarily as an amidated 30 amino acid peptide GLP-1 (7-36)NH$_2$ (4). The distribution of the L-cells that produce GLP-1 is greatest in the distal small intestine and colon. Despite the fact that nutrients do not reach this region of the GI tract until 30 to 60 minutes after eating, GLP-1 is released in the early phases of meal absorption, similar to GIP. It has generally been presumed that the bulk of secreted GLP-1 is from the distal gut, rather than from the smaller numbers of cells in the jejunum. Therefore, a variety of mechanisms have been proposed to explain how nutrients in the upper GI tract activate L-cells in the distal intestine to release GLP-1. In rats meal-induced GLP-1 release appears to be mediated by neural signals (27). However, studies seeking to demonstrate a role for the parasympathetic nervous system in the secretion of GLP-1 in humans have been negative (5).

Upon reaching the bloodstream GLP-1, like GIP, is metabolized by DPP-IV, which cleaves the N-terminal dipeptide His-Ala leaving the circulating congener GLP-1(9-36)NH_2 (15,28). Because of this rapid metabolism bioactive GLP-1 has a plasma half-life of 1 to 2 minutes (29). There is currently no known physiologic role for GLP-1(9-36). Although *in vitro* studies have suggested that this peptide acts as a GLP-1 antagonist, this does not occur in humans at physiologic concentrations (30). Furthermore at concentrations achieved following meals, GLP-1(9-36) does not stimulate insulin secretion. While some studies have demonstrated effects of GLP-1(9-36) to lower blood glucose (31), others have not (30).

GLP-1 binds to a specific GLP-1 receptor (GLP-1 r) that was cloned from an islet cell library (32) and is expressed on β-cells. In addition, the GLP-1r is made by cells in the gastric and small intestinal mucosa, cardiac and endothelial cells, and neurons in the hypothalamus, hindbrain, and other brain regions, and vagal afferent nerves (33,34). In β-cells activation of the GLP-1r by ligand binding stimulates the generation of cAMP and the activation of protein kinase A (PKA) or guanine nucleotide exchange factors as proximal steps in the stimulation of insulin exocytosis (35). However, it is now clear that some aspects of GLP-1 mediated actions in the β-cell involve the PI 3-kinase pathway (36). Little is known about the intracellular signaling through the GLP-1r in cell types other than β-cells.

In β-cells the classic action of GLP-1 is to augment glucose-stimulated insulin secretion (35,36). Like GIP, GLP-1 stimulates insulin release in cultured β-cells, animals, and humans in a glucose-dependent manner. However, beyond acting as an acute insulin secretagogue, GLP-1 increases the biosynthesis of important β-cell products including insulin, glucokinase, and the GLUT 2 glucose transporter (37). More recently it has been shown that GLP-1 signaling plays a role in pancreatic islet growth and development. In cultured cells and rodent models, GLP-1 and its analogues directly stimulate β-cell growth and replication to promote an increase in islet mass (38,39). GLP-1 signaling also promotes the differentiation of pancreatic duct cells into insulin-producing cells (40). Moreover, it appears that GLP-1 inhibits β-cell apoptosis, another action that would promote expansion of β-cell mass (38). These findings point to important possibilities for GLP-1 in normal islet development and have therapeutic implications as well.

The important effects of GLP-1 signaling on β-cell function have been elegantly demonstrated in studies of mice with a targeted deletion of the GLP-1r gene. These mice have glucose intolerance and delayed and diminished insulin secretion (41). When the islets from GLP-1r -/- mice was examined there was a slight reduction in islet size with a relative increase in the proportion of α-cells

(42). In addition, the islets of these mice are more susceptible to the toxic effects of streptozotocin than control mice (43). Finally, absence of the GLP-1r blunts the compensatory growth following partial pancreatectomy (44). In sum, studies with GLP-1r -/- mice demonstrates broad effects of GLP-1 signaling on β-cell function.

GLP-1 has other important effects on islet hormones in addition to stimulating insulin secretion from β-cells. Importantly, GLP-1 lowers fasting and postprandial glucagon concentrations in humans, animals, and cultured islets (2–4,38). The degree of glucagon lowering induced by GLP-1 is sufficient to reduce fasting blood glucose concentrations in diabetic and nondiabetic subjects (45,46). In fact recent work suggests that GLP-1 is responsible for the majority of glucagon suppression following glucose meals (46).

In addition to these important effects on the islet hormones, the other established action of GLP-1 that limits blood glucose excursions is delayed gastric emptying (47). This effect is complex, involving both reduced antral motility and increased fundic capacity (48,49), and is likely mediated through the autonomic nervous system since the effect of GLP-1 is abolished by vagotomy (50). The effects of GLP-1 to delay gastric emptying can be profound at high doses, and has been associated with nausea.

GLP-1 is produced by a discrete set of neurons in the hindbrain and the GLP-1 receptor is expressed on cells in the hypothalamus. Administration of GLP-1 into the central nervous system (CNS) of rats acutely reduces food intake, and chronic administration reduces body weight (51). This raises the possibility that GLP-1 contributes to the regulation of satiety and/or energy balance. Since short-term intravenous administration of GLP-1 to humans suppresses consumption of a subsequent lunch (52) it appears that at least some of the satiety effects of GLP-1 are mediated by peripherally, rather than centrally, derived peptide. It is possible that effects of GLP-1 on food intake are mediated through the same visceral neural circuits that regulate gastric emptying. One hypothesis that has been advanced by several groups is that GLP-1 interacts with neural sensors located in the hepato-portal bed and mediates effects on the islet, stomach, and potentially other organs involved with glucose tolerance such as the islet and liver (30,53) via CNS mediation (54–57). Such a pathway would be available to signal satiety as well.

Expression of the GLP-1r in the heart has effects on cardiac performance and other metabolism. GLP-1 signaling seems to play a role in cardiac development since mice with a targeted gene deletion of the GLP-1r have enlarged hearts (58). In addition, GLP-1 improves cardiac output in humans and animals with cardiomyopathy (59,60) suggesting acute functional effects as well. It appears that GLP-1 promotes glucose metabolism in cardiac myocytes and this is correlated with improved myocardial function (59). Beyond affecting myocardial performance, there is recent evidence that GLP-1r signaling protects against ischemic damage (61,62). Taken together recent studies indicate that GLP-1 has direct effects on the heart, and that signaling through cardiac GLP-1r may have important effects on myocardial function and health. This promises to become a very active area of research because of the novelty of the mechanism and the substantial potential to have clinical impact.

APPLICATION OF THE INCRETINS TO THERAPEUTICS

Because of the wide spectrum of GLP-1 actions that combine to lower blood glucose there has been a concerted effort to develop diabetes treatments around this hormone. Lesser efforts have been made to specifically apply the GIP system for this purpose since it does not appear to have significant insulinotropic effects in diabetic individuals. The use of either incretin directly for chronic treatment of diabetes is impractical because of their rapid metabolism by DPP-IV, and the fact that small peptides are subject to digestion and so generally not available as oral preparations. However, two basic strategies have been employed to circumvent these limitations. The first is the development of metabolism-resistant, long-acting GLP-1 receptor agonists; the second is inhibition of DPP-IV by a number of orally available small molecules. Both approaches have yielded successful agents that are now in use in the clinic.

GLP-1 Receptor Agonists

There is currently one long-acting GLP-1 receptor agonist that has been approved for treatment and several others in advanced phases of development. Exendin-4 is a naturally occurring reptilian peptide of 39 amino acids with considerable homology to GLP-1 (63). Exendin-4 is a potent GLP-1 receptor agonist that shares many of the physiologic and pharmacologic effects of GLP-1, but is not metabolized by DPP-IV and so has a plasma half-life of 4 hours in humans following subcutaneous injection. Importantly exendin-4 causes glucose-dependent insulin secretion, delayed gastric emptying and lower glucagon levels. In a short-term study of diabetic subjects with a broad range of pre-existing glycemic control, subcutaneous injections of exenatide reduced both fasting and postprandial glucose levels and were effective over a 5-day course of treatment (64). In randomized controlled trials comparing subcutaneous exenatide with placebo added to sulfonylurea, metformin, metformin and sulfonylurea, or thiazolidenedione exenatide caused a dose-dependent decrease in hemoglobin A1c of 0.8% to 0.9% over 30-week time. Importantly exenatide also caused significant weight loss of ~2.5 kg in these trials, indicating that the effects of chronic activation of the GLP-1 receptor can affect energy balance in humans. Nausea has been the most common side effect of exenatide treatment, affecting nearly half of subjects taking it, but is rarely a cause for patients to stop the drug. Hypoglycemia associated with exenatide treatment in the absence of other diabetes drugs that cause low blood glucose is rare. Exenatide has been available for use in diabetic patients since mid-2005 and estimated use to date is between 500,000 and one million patients.

There are a number of other GLP-1 mimetics in development. The most advanced of these is liraglutide, a modified GLP-1 molecule that includes a C-16 fatty acyl derivative that promotes binding to albumin. Liraglutide is resistant to metabolism by DPP-IV, is absorbed gradually from the subcutaneous space after injection and reaches peak levels 9 to 12 hours after administration (65). Like exenatide the actions of liraglutide are predictable from what is known about the physiology of GLP-1. The trend for development of GLP-1 analogues is to create compounds with longer durations of action and that require a reduced number of injections.

DPP-IV Inhibitors

DPP-IV is especially critical for the inactivation of GLP-1. Several compounds are currently available that provide nearly complete, and long-lasting inhibition of DPP-IV, which increases the proportion of active GLP-1 from 10 to 20% of total circulating GLP-1 immunoreactivity to nearly 100% (63). A DPP-IV inhibitor named sitagliptin is now available for use, with a second one, vildagliptin, likely to be approved soon.

Sitagliptin is an orally available, highly specific inhibitor of DPP-IV, and in doses used for therapy can lower the measurable activity of the enzyme by up to 96% for 12 hours (66). Sitagliptin treatment causes a greater than twofold elevation of active GIP and GLP-1 and these are associated with increased insulin secretion, reduced glucagon levels and improvements in both fasting and post-prandial hyperglycemia. In a randomized, placebo-controlled study of sitagliptin monotherapy in type 2 diabetic patients, active treatment reduced hemoglobin A1c levels by an average of > 1% (67). Sitagliptin also caused significant improvements in chronic glucose control when added to the treatment of diabetic patients receiving pioglitazone or metformin (68,69). In these clinical trials sitagliptin was very well tolerated with no increase in side effects compared to placebo. In contrast to exenatide there was no increase in gastrointestinal side effects in treated subjects. However, treatment with sitagliptin does not affect body weight.

Vildagliptin is another DPP-IV inhibitor that has been studied extensively. The effectiveness of vildagliptin for inhibiting DPP-IV seems to be equivalent to sitagliptin. In a 4-week study of vildagliptin in moderate to well-controlled type 2 diabetic subjects, once daily administration reduced DPP-IV activity by 90% to 95% for up to 12 hours and by nearly 50% 24 hours after dosing (63,70,71). In this study fasting GLP-1 levels were double than those seen in placebo-treated subjects, and fasting, prandial, and average 24 hr glucose levels were significantly decreased, as was hemoglobin A1c. Vildagliptin increased β-cell function and reduced plasma glucagon. Body weight did not change over the course of the study and there was no difference in adverse events between the vildagliptin and placebo groups. In a larger trial, 107 diabetic subjects taking metformin were randomized to receive vildagliptin or placebo for 12 weeks (63,70,71). The addition of vildagliptin caused a significant reduction in HbA1c compared to placebo with rare occurrences of hypoglycemia and no increase in adverse events.

DPP-IV is expressed on lymphocytes; in the immunology literature the enzyme is referred to as CD26 (3). While there is some evidence of minor effects on *in vitro* lymphocyte function with DPP-IV inhibitors, there is no evidence from clinical studies of any adverse effects in humans. This area bears scrutiny as more patients are treated with these compounds.

Based on current clinical and pharmacologic studies it appears that the effects of GLP-1r agonists and DPP-IV inhibitors are consistent with what is known about the incretin system. GLP-1r agonists can be given in pharmacologic amounts and result in the equivalence of very high levels of GLP-1r signaling. It may be that this causes the nausea and weight loss seen with these agents but not DPP-IV inhibitors. Interestingly, even though DPP-IV inhibitors only increase plasma GLP-1 into the high normal or supraphysiologic range, they seem to be as effective as exenatide for lowering HbA1c. Both classes of drugs have unique properties—in particular weight loss with exenatide and related drugs, and safety/tolerability with DPP-IV inhibitors—that add to the current choices for diabetes therapy. In addition, since both classes of drug act through novel mechanisms there are potential synergies with other agents used to treat diabetes.

One potential benefit of drugs that work through the incretin signaling systems that could determine the overall impact of DPP-IV inhibitors and GLP-1 mimetics is any effect to protect or enhance β-cell mass. Both GIP and GLP-1 have been shown to activate signaling pathways related to cell growth and death, and to stimulate replication and inhibit apoptosis *in vitro*. Importantly some of the effects of both GLP-1 agonists and DPP-IV inhibitors to increase islet mass have also been demonstrated in rodent models. There are currently no known diabetes drugs that affect β-cell mass, and this would add a very attractive mechanism to the spectrum through which these drugs work. Currently available treatments, including diet, metformin, sulfonylureas, thiazolidenediones, and insulin tend to lose effectiveness and over the course of 2 to 3 years most patients must have treatment amplified (72). It is important to realize that (*i*) there is no scientific evidence yet that GLP-1r agonists or DPP-IV inhibitors affect β-cell mass in humans, (*ii*) determination of β-cell mass in living humans can only be inferred from functional studies that are inexact, and (*iii*) trials to determine whether incretin based drugs provide a durable effect on HbA1c relative to other trials are probably the most direct way to determine effects on β-cell growth and apoptosis.

UNRESOLVED QUESTIONS AND FUTURE DIRECTIONS

Because of the recent application of the incretins to pharmacotherapy there has been a surge in research in this area and much new information has been obtained only recently. Nonetheless there are several fundamental questions that are still unanswered. It is still not clear how GLP-1 secretion is mediated; the conundrum of rapid stimulation by nutrients of a peptide that is predominantly made in the lower gut is still unresolved. Likewise the regulation of GLP-1 secretion in the brain has not been fully explained. There is increasing evidence that many of the actions attributed to GLP-1 are mediated not by traditional endocrine action but through neuro-endocrine pathways, and the architecture of this system still needs to be determined. The biology of GLP-1 in the heart has important clinical implications but research in this area is still in a nascent stage. Finally, the role of the incretins in diabetes is an area that bears continued attention. It is not clear whether the defect in the incretin effect reported in persons with type 2 diabetes is an essential component of the disease, or if it might be reversible. In addition, the difference between GLP-1 and GIP action in the type 2 diabetic islet has the potential to provide key insights into the pathogenesis of insulin secretion in this condition.

There are many unanswered questions that will go a long way toward determining the ultimate role of GLP-1 mimetics and DPP-IV inhibitors in therapeutics. While both classes of drugs appear to be safe and tolerable from the clinical trials reported, this impression is based on exposure of a relatively small numbers of subjects. The ultimate safety, efficacy and therapeutic role of incretin based therapies are issues that will play out in the clinic in the coming years.

REFERENCES

1. Tillil H, Shapiro ET, Miller MA, et al. Dose-dependent effects of oral and intravenous glucose on insulin secretion and clearance in normal humans. Am J Physiol 1988; 254(3 Pt 1):E349–E357.
2. D'Alessio DA. Incretins: Glucose-dependent insulinotropic polypeptide and glucagon-like peptide 1. In: Porte D, Baron A, Sherwin RS, eds. Ellenberg and Rifkin's Diabetes Mellitus. 6th ed. New York: McGraw-Hill; 2003:85–96.
3. Drucker DJ. The biology of incretin hormones. Cell Metab 2006; 3(3):153–165.
4. Kieffer TJ, Habener JF. The glucagon-like peptides. Endocr Rev 1999; 20(6):876–913.
5. Ahren B, Holst JJ. The cephalic insulin response to meal ingestion in humans is dependent on both cholinergic and noncholinergic mechanisms and is important for postprandial glycemia. Diabetes 2001; 50(5):1030–1038.
6. Nauck MA, Homberger E, Siegel EG, et al. Incretin effects of increasing glucose loads in man calculated from venous insulin and C-peptide responses. J Clin Endocrinol Metab 1986; 63(2):492–498.
7. Nauck M, Stockmann F, Ebert R, Creutzfeldt W. Reduced incretin effect in type 2 (non-insulin-dependent) diabetes. Diabetologia 1986; 29(1):46–52.
8. Perley MJ, Kipnis DM. Plasma insulin responses to oral and intravenous glucose: Studies in normal and diabetic subjects. J Clin Invest 1967; 46(12):1954–1962.
9. Greenbaum CJ, Prigeon RL, D'Alessio DA. Impaired beta-cell function, incretin effect, and glucagon suppression in patients with type 1 diabetes who have normal fasting glucose. Diabetes 2002; 51(4):951–957.
10. Muscelli E, Mari A, Natali A, et al. Impact of incretin hormones on beta-cell function in subjects with normal or impaired glucose tolerance. Am J Physiol Endocrinol Metab 2006; 291(6):E1144-E1150.

11. Henchoz E, D'Alessio DA, Gillet M, et al. Impaired insulin response after oral but not intravenous glucose in heart- and liver-transplant recipients. Transplantation 2003; 76(6):923–929.

12. Wolfe MM, Boylan MO, Kieffer TJ, Tseng C-C. Glucose-dependent insulinotropic polypeptide (GIP): Incretin vs Enterogastrone. In: Greeley GH, ed. Gastrointestinal Endocrinology. Totowa, NJ: Humana Press; 1999:439.

13. Schirra J, Katschinski M, Weidmann C, et al. Gastric emptying and release of incretin hormones after glucose ingestion in humans. J Clin Invest 1996; 97(1):92–103.

14. Ebert R, Creutzfeldt W. Gastrointestinal peptides and insulin secretion. Diabetes Metab Rev 1987; 3(1):1–26.

15. Kieffer TJ, McIntosh CH, Pederson RA. Degradation of glucose-dependent insulinotropic polypeptide and truncated glucagon-like peptide 1 in vitro and in vivo by dipeptidyl peptidase IV. Endocrinology 1995; 136(8):3585–3596.

16. Creutzfeldt W, Nauck M. Gut hormones and diabetes mellitus. Diabetes Metab Rev 1992; 8(2):149–177.

17. Irwin N, Gault VA, Green BD, et al. Effects of short-term chemical ablation of the GIP receptor on insulin secretion, islet morphology and glucose homeostasis in mice. Biol Chem 2004; 385(9):845–852.

18. Tseng CC, Kieffer TJ, Jarboe LA, Usdin TB, Wolfe MM. Postprandial stimulation of insulin release by glucose-dependent insulinotropic polypeptide (GIP). Effect of a specific glucose-dependent insulinotropic polypeptide receptor antagonist in the rat. J Clin Invest 1996; 98(11):2440–2445.

19. Miyawaki K, Yamada Y, Yano H, et al. Glucose intolerance caused by a defect in the entero-insular axis: A study in gastric inhibitory polypeptide receptor knockout mice. Proc Natl Acad Sci USA 1999; 96(26):14843–14847.

20. Ehses JA, Casilla VR, Doty T, et al. Glucose-dependent insulinotropic polypeptide promotes beta-(INS-1) cell survival via cyclic adenosine monophosphate-mediated caspase-3 inhibition and regulation of p38 mitogen-activated protein kinase. Endocrinology 2003; 144(10):4433–4445.

21. Kim SJ, Winter K, Nian C, Tsuneoka M, Koda Y, McIntosh CH. Glucose-dependent insulinotropic polypeptide (GIP) stimulation of pancreatic beta-cell survival is dependent upon phosphatidylinositol 3-kinase (PI3 K)/protein kinase B (PKB) signaling, inactivation of the forkhead transcription factor Foxo1, and down-regulation of bax expression. J Biol Chem 2005; 280(23):22297–22307.

22. Miyawaki K, Yamada Y, Ban N, et al. Inhibition of gastric inhibitory polypeptide signaling prevents obesity. Nat Med 2002; 8(7):738–742.

23. Gault VA, Irwin N, Green BD, et al. Chemical ablation of gastric inhibitory polypeptide receptor action by daily (Pro3)GIP administration improves glucose tolerance and ameliorates insulin resistance and abnormalities of islet structure in obesity-related diabetes. Diabetes 2005; 54(8):2436–2446.

24. Nauck MA, Heimesaat MM, Orskov C, Holst JJ, Ebert R, Creutzfeldt W. Preserved incretin activity of glucagon-like peptide 1 [7-36 amide] but not of synthetic human gastric inhibitory polypeptide in patients with type-2 diabetes mellitus. J Clin Invest 1993; 91(1):301–307.

25. Lynn FC, Pamir N, Ng EH, McIntosh CH, Kieffer TJ, Pederson RA. Defective glucose-dependent insulinotropic polypeptide receptor expression in diabetic fatty Zucker rats. Diabetes 2001; 50(5):1004–1011.

26. Meier JJ, Gallwitz B, Kask B, et al. Stimulation of insulin secretion by intravenous bolus injection and continuous infusion of gastric inhibitory polypeptide in patients with type 2 diabetes and healthy control subjects. Diabetes 2004; 53 (Suppl 3):S220–S224.

27. Rocca AS, Brubaker PL. Role of the vagus nerve in mediating proximal nutrient-induced glucagon-like peptide-1 secretion. Endocrinology 1999; 140(4):1687–1694.

28. Mentlein R, Gallwitz B, Schmidt WE. Dipeptidyl-peptidase IV hydrolyses gastric inhibitory polypeptide, glucagon-like peptide-1(7-36)amide, peptide histidine methionine and is responsible for their degradation in human serum. Eur J Biochem 1993; 214(3):829–835.

29. Deacon CF, Johnsen AH, Holst JJ. Degradation of glucagon-like peptide-1 by human plasma in vitro yields an N-terminally truncated peptide that is a major endogenous metabolite in vivo. J Clin Endocrinol Metab 1995; 80(3):952–957.

30. Vahl TP, Paty BW, Fuller BD, Prigeon RL, D'Alessio DA. Effects of GLP-1-(7-36)NH2, GLP-1-(7-37), and GLP-1- (9-36)NH2 on intravenous glucose tolerance and glucose-induced insulin secretion in healthy humans. J Clin Endocrinol Metab 2003; 88(4):1772–1779.

31. Meier JJ, Gethmann A, Nauck MA, et al. The glucagon-like peptide-1 metabolite GLP-1-(9-36) amide reduces postprandial glycemia independently of gastric emptying and insulin secretion in humans. Am J Physiol Endocrinol Metab 2006; 290(6):E1118 – E1123.

32. Thorens B. Expression cloning of the pancreatic beta cell receptor for the gluco-incretin hormone glucagon-like peptide 1. Proc Natl Acad Sci USA 1992; 89(18):8641–8645.

33. Bullock BP, Heller RS, Habener JF. Tissue distribution of messenger ribonucleic acid encoding the rat glucagon-like peptide-1 receptor. Endocrinology 1996; 137(7):2968–2978.

34. Nakagawa A, Satake H, Nakabayashi H, et al. Receptor gene expression of glucagon-like peptide-1, but not glucose-dependent insulinotropic polypeptide, in rat nodose ganglion cells. Auton Neurosci 2004; 110(1):36–43.

35. Gromada J, Holst JJ, Rorsman P. Cellular regulation of islet hormone secretion by the incretin hormone glucagon-like peptide 1. Pflugers Arch 1998; 435(5):583–594.

36. MacDonald PE, Salapatek AM, Wheeler MB. Glucagon-like peptide-1 receptor activation antagonizes voltage-dependent repolarizing K(+) currents in beta-cells: A possible glucose-dependent insulinotropic mechanism. Diabetes 2002; 51 (Suppl 3):S443–S447.

37. Wang Y, Perfetti R, Greig NH, et al. Glucagon-like peptide-1 can reverse the age-related decline in glucose tolerance in rats. J Clin Invest 1997; 99(12):2883–2889.

38. Wang Q, Brubaker PL. Glucagon-like peptide-1 treatment delays the onset of diabetes in 8 week-old db/db mice. Diabetologia 2002; 45(9):1263–1273.

39. Xu G, Stoffers DA, Habener JF, Bonner-Weir S. Exendin-4 stimulates both beta-cell replication and neogenesis, resulting in increased beta-cell mass and improved glucose tolerance in diabetic rats. Diabetes 1999; 48(12):2270–2276.

40. Bulotta A, Hui H, Anastasi E, et al. Cultured pancreatic ductal cells undergo cell cycle re-distribution and beta-cell-like differentiation in response to glucagon-like peptide-1. J Mol Endocrinol 2002; 29(3):347–360.

41. Scrocchi LA, Brown TJ, MaClusky N, et al. Glucose intolerance but normal satiety in mice with a null mutation in the glucagon-like peptide 1 receptor gene. Nat Med 1996; 2(11):1254–1258.

42. Ling Z, Wu D, Zambre Y, et al. Glucagon-like peptide 1 receptor signaling influences topography of islet cells in mice. Virchows Arch 2001; 438(4):382–387.

43. Li Y, Hansotia T, Yusta B, Ris F, Halban PA, Drucker DJ. Glucagon-like peptide-1 receptor signaling modulates beta cell apoptosis. J Biol Chem 2003; 278(1):471–478.

44. De Leon DD, Deng S, Madani R, Ahima RS, Drucker DJ, Stoffers DA. Role of endogenous glucagon-like peptide-1 in islet regeneration after partial pancreatectomy. Diabetes 2003; 52(2):365–371.

45. Creutzfeldt WO, Kleine N, Willms B, Orskov C, Holst JJ, Nauck MA. Glucagonostatic actions and reduction of fasting hyperglycemia by exogenous glucagon-like peptide I(7-36) amide in type I diabetic patients. Diabetes Care 1996; 19(6):580–586.

46. Schirra J, Nicolaus M, Roggel R, et al. Endogenous glucagon-like peptide 1 controls endocrine pancreatic secretion and antro-pyloro-duodenal motility in humans. Gut 2006; 55(2):243–251.

47. Schirra J, Houck P, Wank U, Arnold R, Goke B, Katschinski M. Effects of glucagon-like peptide-1(7-36)amide on antro-pyloro-duodenal motility in the interdigestive state and with duodenal lipid perfusion in humans. Gut 2000; 46(5):622–631.

48. Delgado-Aros S, Kim DY, Burton DD, et al. Effect of GLP-1 on gastric volume, emptying, maximum volume ingested, and postprandial symptoms in humans. Am J Physiol Gastrointest Liver Physiol 2002; 282(3):G424–G431.

49. Schirra J, Wank U, Arnold R, Goke B, Katschinski M. Effects of glucagon-like peptide-1(7-36)amide on motility and sensation of the proximal stomach in humans. Gut 2002; 50(3):341–348.

50. Imeryuz N, Yegen BC, Bozkurt A, Coskun T, Villanueva-Penacarrillo ML, Ulusoy NB. Glucagon-like peptide-1 inhibits gastric emptying via vagal afferent-mediated central mechanisms. Am J Physiol 1997; 273(4 Pt 1):G920–G927.

51. Turton MD, O'Shea D, Gunn I, et al. A role for glucagon-like peptide-1 in the central regulation of feeding. Nature 1996; 379(6560):69–72.

52. Flint A, Raben A, Astrup A, Holst JJ. Glucagon-like peptide 1 promotes satiety and suppresses energy intake in humans. J Clin Invest 1998; 101(3):515–520.

53. Prigeon RL, Quddusi S, Paty B, D'Alessio DA. Suppression of glucose production by GLP-1 independent of islet hormones: A novel extrapancreatic effect. Am J Physiol Endocrinol Metab 2003; 285(4):E701–E707.

54. Balkan B, Li X. Portal GLP-1 administration in rats augments the insulin response to glucose via neuronal mechanisms. Am J Physiol Regul Integr Comp Physiol 2000; 279(4):R1449– R1454.

55. Burcelin R, Da Costa A, Drucker D, Thorens B. Glucose competence of the hepatoportal vein sensor requires the presence of an activated glucagon-like peptide-1 receptor. Diabetes 2001; 50(8):1720–1728.

56. Ionut V, Hucking K, Liberty IF, Bergman RN. Synergistic effect of portal glucose and glucagon-like peptide-1 to lower systemic glucose and stimulate counter-regulatory hormones. Diabetologia 2005; 48(5):967–975.

57. Vahl T, Tauchi M, Durler T, et al. Glucagon-like peptide-1 (GLP-1) receptors expressed on nerve terminals in the portal vein mediate the effects of endogenous GLP-1 on glucose tolerance in rates. Endocrinology 2007; 148 (10):4965–4973.

58. Gros R, You X, Baggio LL, et al. Cardiac function in mice lacking the glucagon-like peptide-1 receptor. Endocrinology 2003; 144(6):2242–2252.
59. Nikolaidis LA, Elahi D, Hentosz T, et al. Recombinant glucagon-like peptide-1 increases myocardial glucose uptake and improves left ventricular performance in conscious dogs with pacing-induced dilated cardiomyopathy. Circulation 2004; 110(8):955–961.
60. Nikolaidis LA, Mankad S, Sokos GG, et al. Effects of glucagon-like peptide-1 in patients with acute myocardial infarction and left ventricular dysfunction after successful reperfusion. Circulation 2004; 109(8):962–965.
61. Bose AK, Mocanu MM, Carr RD, Brand CL, Yellon DM. Glucagon-like peptide 1 can directly protect the heart against ischemia/reperfusion injury. Diabetes 2005; 54(1):146–151.
62. Nikolaidis LA, Doverspike A, Hentosz T, et al. Glucagon-like peptide-1 limits myocardial stunning following brief coronary occlusion and reperfusion in conscious canines. J Pharmacol Exp Ther 2005; 312(1):303–308.
63. Ahren B, Schmitz O. GLP-1 receptor agonists and DPP-4 inhibitors in the treatment of type 2 diabetes. Horm Metab Res 2004; 36(11-12):867–876.
64. Kolterman OG, Buse JB, Fineman MS, et al. Synthetic exendin-4 (exenatide) significantly reduces postprandial and fasting plasma glucose in subjects with type 2 diabetes. J Clin Endocrinol Metab 2003; 88(7):3082–3089.
65. Agerso H, Jensen LB, Elbrond B, Rolan P, Zdravkovic M. The pharmacokinetics, pharmacodynamics, safety and tolerability of NN2211, a new long-acting GLP-1 derivative, in healthy men. Diabetologia 2002; 45(2):195–202.
66. Herman GA, Bergman A, Stevens C, et al. Effect of single oral doses of sitagliptin, a dipeptidyl peptidase-4 inhibitor, on incretin and plasma glucose levels after an oral glucose tolerance test in patients with type 2 diabetes. J Clin Endocrinol Metab 2006; 91(11):4612–4619.
67. Aschner P, Kipnes MS, Lunceford JK, Sanchez M, Mickel C, Williams-Herman DE. Effect of the dipeptidyl peptidase-4 inhibitor sitagliptin as monotherapy on glycemic control in patients with type 2 diabetes. Diabetes Care 2006; 29(12):2632–2637.
68. Charbonnel B, Karasik A, Liu J, Wu M, Meininger G. Efficacy and safety of the dipeptidyl peptidase-4 inhibitor sitagliptin added to ongoing metformin therapy in patients with type 2 diabetes inadequately controlled with metformin alone. Diabetes Care 2006; 29(12):2638–2643.
69. Rosenstock J, Brazg R, Andryuk PJ, Lu K, Stein P. Efficacy and safety of the dipeptidyl peptidase-4 inhibitor sitagliptin added to ongoing pioglitazone therapy in patients with type 2 diabetes: A 24-week, multicenter, randomized, double-blind, placebo-controlled, parallel-group study. Clin Ther 2006; 28(10):1556–1568.
70. Ahren B, Gomis R, Standl E, Mills D, Schweizer A. Twelve- and 52-week efficacy of the dipeptidyl peptidase IV inhibitor LAF237 in metformin-treated patients with type 2 diabetes. Diabetes Care 2004; 27(12):2874–2880.
71. Ahren B, Landin-Olsson M, Jansson PA, Svensson M, Holmes D, Schweizer A. Inhibition of dipeptidyl peptidase-4 reduces glycemia, sustains insulin levels, and reduces glucagon levels in type 2 diabetes. J Clin Endocrinol Metab 2004; 89(5):2078–2084.
72. Kahn SE, Haffner SM, Heise MA, et al. Glycemic durability of rosiglitazone, metformin, or glyburide monotherapy. N Engl J Med 2006; 355(23):2427–2443.

8

Pharmacotherapy of Obesity

Parimal Misra and Ranjan Chakrabarti

Metabolic Disorder Group, Dr. Reddy's Laboratories Ltd., Discovery Research, Hyderabad, India

INTRODUCTION

Obesity is a disorder of energy imbalance, wherein energy input exceeds output. Excess energy is stored in the form of triglycerides in the adipose tissue. Increased adipose cell size causes hypertrophic obesity and increased cell number causes hyperplastic obesity characteristic of a more severe condition. The key causes of obesity are the increased consumption of energy-rich but nutrient-poor diets (like saturated fats and sugars) and reduced physical activity. 65% of the U.S.A. population is overweight, defined as body mass index (BMI) greater than 25, and approximately 25% of the population is obese, defined as BMI >30 (1). The prevalence of obesity has increased dramatically over the last decade (2), a trend seen in many industrialized countries (3). According to the World Health Organization, there are more than one billion overweight adults in the world, of which at least 300 million are clinically obese. The health care burden of obesity is significant due to associated secondary chronic diseases such as type 2 diabetes, hypertension, stroke, cardiovascular diseases, respiratory disorders, gallbladder disease, osteoarthritis, and certain cancers (4). The increasing evidence that severe obesity has a genetic basis, resulting in the maintenance and defence of elevated weight (5) may explain why long-term weight loss is very difficult to achieve. This has strengthened the argument that severe obesity should be treated with pharmacological agents along with conventional diet and exercise regimes. To date, approved therapeutics have met with only moderate success and have had side effects, leaving an unmet need for effective and safe pharmacotherapy that poses a challenge to the pharmaceutical industry.

Energy homeostasis is a complex process involving multiple interacting mechanisms primarily coordinated by the brain, which receives feedback signals from the periphery through hormones and neurons and sends efferent signals to higher brain centers and the autonomic nervous system. Classic examples of hypothalamic targets include the leptin receptor, melanocortin-4 receptor and neuropeptide Y (NPY) receptors, which have been reviewed extensively (6,7).

Multiple CNS and peripheral pathways interact with each other to achieve a delicate homeostatic balance in energy intake and expenditure, exemplified by pharmacological perturbation. Thus, nonselective opioid antagonists (e.g., naloxone) inhibit agouti–related protein-induced hyperphagia (8), chronic treatment with morphine down-regulates melanocortin-4 receptor mRNA (9) and agents that act on the 5-hydroxytryptamine (5-HT) pathway, modify NPY and melanocortin systems (10,11).

Nonhomeostatic mechanisms also play an important role in controlling feeding behavior, especially in humans. Such mechanisms may initiate food intake, but because they are nonresponsive to feedback control from the body's fuel store, food intake is uncontrolled. Food as a reward is a nonhomeostatic over-ride with substantial impact on human feeding behavior. Although eating for reward is a social behavior, it nevertheless has a neurochemical template in the dopamine and the endocannabinoid systems (12).

Total energy expenditure is the sum of basal metabolism, the constant obligatory energy expenditure required for survival, and a variable portion needed for physical activity and adaptive thermogenesis. Adaptive thermogenesis means the ability of body to adapt to prolonged cold exposure or overfeeling. Biogenesis of mitochondria and the induction of specific mitochondrial proteins that control the efficiency of oxidative phosphorylation are the key cellular processes of adaptive thermogenesis (13). Thus treatments of obesity should target both homeostatic and nonhomeostatic mechanisms.

APPROVED DRUGS

The major antiobesity drugs in the market today are orlistat and sibutramine. Orlistat works by inhibiting the action of lipase enzymes in the stomach and small intestine to prevent the breakdown of fat and thereby reducing the amount of fat absorbed. Adverse effects are therefore related to fat malabsorption and include oily fecal spoting, flatus with discharge, fecal urgency, and oily/fatty stool (14). Sibutramine is a selective serotonin and noradrenaline re-uptake inhibitor, which induces considerable weight loss by increasing satiety as well as energy expenditure in a dose-dependent manner (15). Chronic administration in ob/ob mice not only reduces weight gain but serum free fatty acid concentrations, hyperinsulinemia, and insulin resistance (16). One interesting feature of sibutramine is that patients who do not respond can be easily identified during the first weeks of treatment, avoiding unnecessary long-term treatment of nonresponders. In the STORM (Sibutramine Trial of Obesity Reduction and Maintenance) trial, the group randomized to sibutramine after weight loss maintained their reduced weight for up to 18 months, whereas the placebo group regained weight. Sibutramine use is associated with a predictable small increase in blood pressure and pulse and some patients may be very sensitive to this cardiostimulatory effect (17).

The cannabinoid (CB1) receptor and its endogenous ligands, the endocannabinoids (18–20), have been shown to be involved in the control of weight and energy balance via a dual mechanism of food intake modification and the regulation of energy expenditure (21). The first-in-class CB1 receptor inverse agonist is rimonabant, which has been approved in Europe as an adjunct to diet and exercise for the treatment of obese (BMI >30) or overweight (BMI >27) patients with associated risk factors such as type 2 diabetes and dyslipidemia. Rimonabant is a "multi-impact" drug, acting on both the central nervous system to reduce food intake, as well as on adipocytes to increase adiponectin secretion, glucose tolerance, and high-density lipoprotein (HDL) levels, and reduce insulin resistance and triglyceride levels. The RIO (Rimonabant In Obesity) trial concluded that 20 mg of rimonabant reduced waist circumference by 7.5 cm (3.4 cm for placebo) and body weight by 7.2 kg (2.5 kg for placebo). More importantly, 39% of the patients taking 20 mg of rimonabant were able to lose 10% of body weight in one year and 32% maintained that loss for 2 years. HDL-cholesterol increased by 24.5% (16.8% for placebo) and triglycerides decreased by 8.8% (6.3% for placebo). The number of patients who met metabolic syndrome criteria was reduced by 50% in the rimonabant 20 mg arm, compared to 20% in the placebo arm. In the RIO Diabetes trials the average body weight loss was around 5.6 kg for the 20 mg arm and the average glycosylated hemoglobin level decreased 0.6% from a baseline value of 7.3%. Thus rimonabant may have a beneficial effect on some of the cardiovascular, diabetic, and dyslipidemic comorbidities associated with obesity. However, given its pharmacology, there is growing concern regarding its neuropsychiatric effects of anxiety and depression. Some CB1 antagonists currently under development are claimed to be safer than rimonabant, based on their high degree of specificity relative to a panel of brain receptors and enzymes and high selectivity for CB1 versus CB2 class receptors. Additionally, in an effort to alleviate some of the safety concerns related to the central action of rimonabant, drugs currently in early stages of discovery and development are targeted more on rimonabant's action on peripheral tissues. There is also a shift towards identification of neutral CB1 antagonists rather than the classical CB1 inverse agonists, as the former are likely to have a less complex pharmacology. Thus, when administered by themselves, such compounds would only have effects in regions of the cannabinoid system in which there is ongoing release of endogenous cannabinoids but would leave the constitutive activity of the system unchanged.

EMERGING THERAPEUTIC TARGETS

The challenge in developing drugs for obesity is the sheer complexity of the mechanisms for regulating body weight. Better understanding of these will identify new targets as a basis of drug development (Fig. 1).

Potential antiobesity drugs being investigated by different companies can be classified into four broad categories.

1. Agents that primarily decrease appetite through central nervous system action, e. g., cannabinoid receptor antagonists, selective 5-HT2c agonists, MC4 receptor agonists, melanin concentrating hormone (MCH) antagonists and NPY antagonists,.
2. Agents that primarily increase metabolic rate or affect metabolism through peripheral action, e.g., selective β_3-adrenergic receptor agonists, lipase inhibitors, and inhibitors of lipid metabolizing enzymes (diacyl glycerol acyltransferase, fatty acid synthase, acetyl-CoA carboxylase, stearoyl-CoA desaturase).
3. Agents that act on gastrointestinal tract, e.g., glucagon-like peptide-1 receptor agonists, CCK-A agonists and ghrelin antagonists.
4. Agents that not only affect obesity but also overall metabolic syndrome, e.g., peroxisome proliferator-activated receptor (PPAR) modulators,

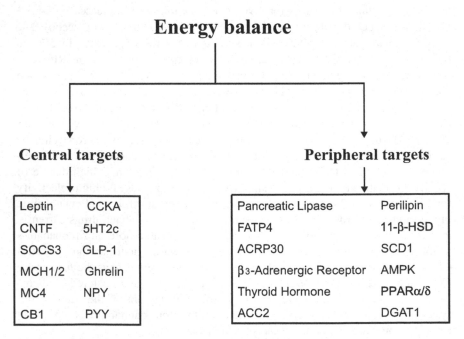

Figure 1   Targets for development of anti-obesity therapeutics.

carboxypeptidase inhibitors, protein tyrosine phosphatase inhibitors and AMP kinase modulators.

Agents That Primarily Decrease Appetite Through Central Nervous System Action

Selective 5-HT$_{2c}$ Agonists

There is a consensus that serotonergic neurotransmission modulates appetite. In particular, selective 5-HT receptor subtype 2c (5-HT$_{2c}$) agonists may induce satiety. Previously approved and clinically used nonselective 5-HT receptor agonists such as fenfluramine and related compounds were effective in reducing body weight. However, these drugs were withdrawn from the market following heart valve abnormalities possibly related to nonselectivity for 5-HT$_{2b}$ receptors in peripheral tissues (22,23). 5-HT$_{2c}$ receptors are low in density or absent in peripheral tissues but are expressed at high density in the hypothalamus. Thus, development of 5-HT$_{2c}$ agonists devoid of 5-HT$_{2b}$ actions could represent a novel class of anorectic agents without undesirable side effects. Recently, mice with targeted disruption of the selective 5-HT$_{2c}$ receptor, were found to develop hyperphagia, mild obesity, and reduced sensitivity to insulin and leptin (24,25). Based on these findings, 5-HT$_{2c}$ receptor agonists are expected to be useful antiobesity drugs. Lorcaserin (compound APD-356) from Arena Pharmaceuticals is presently in Phase III clinical trials. In a phase Ib trial, the drug was well tolerated and displayed predictable pharmacokinetics. This randomized, double blind, placebo-controlled, multiple ascending dose study enrolled 27 subjects (15 males and 12 females) with BMIs in the range 25 to 58. Participants were administered 3, 10, and 20 mg doses of APD-356 or placebo in successive cohorts of 9 subjects (6 APD-356, 6 placebo). Most common side effects reported were headache, nausea, and vomiting, all of which were generally mild.

Melanocortin-4 (MC4) Receptor Agonists

The MC4 receptor is another CNS target that has received much attention for the treatment of obesity because of human genetic validation (26). Hypothalamic corticotropin-releasing hormone stimulates production of pro-opimelanocortin in the anterior pituitary, where it undergoes proteolytic cleavage to produce adrenocorticotropin hormone (ACTH) and α-melanocyte-stimulating hormone (α-MSH), which binds to MC receptors. To date, MC receptors have been classified into five classes, MC1 to MC5. In contrast to other MC receptors, the MC4 receptor is found only in brain (27). Food intake is inhibited when α-MSH binds to the MC4 receptor. It was reported that a targeted mutation of MC4 receptor caused hyperphagia and adult-onset obesity with, hyperinsulinemia and hyperglycemia, similar to the agouti–obesity syndrome (28). Many companies are making efforts to develop low-molecular weight MC4 receptor agonists.

Melanin-Concentrating Hormone (MCH) Antagonist

MCH is a cyclic 19-amino acid peptide that regulates feeding behavior and energy homeostasis via interaction with the central melanocortin system (29). Two MCH receptors, both members of the G-protein–coupled receptor (GPCR) family, have so far been identified. The MCH-1 receptor is expressed in several brain regions in rodents and higher mammals (30–34). Transgenic mice overexpressing MCH are susceptible to insulin resistance and obesity (35), while mice lacking the gene are hypophagic and lean with elevated metabolic rates (36). MCH-1 receptor antagonists with oral activity have been described. For example, T-226296 from Takeda exhibited >90% suppression of MCH-stimulated–food intake in lean rats (37). Preclinical evidence describing hypophagia and weight loss with small molecular weight and peptidal antagonists in rodents is limited but suggests that MCH-1 receptor antagonism may be a valid approach for the treatment of human obesity and metabolic syndrome.

NPY Receptor Antagonists

NPY is the most abundant neuropeptide yet identified in the brain, and its diffuse localization suggests that it has a diverse range of actions. The orexigenic effects of NPY are probably the most spectacular, since it is the most powerful stimulator of food intake so far identified (38). Chronic intracerebral administration of NPY results in a glucocorticoid-dependent obesity in animals with many characteristics of metabolic syndrome (39). Six NPY receptor subtypes (Y1–Y6) have so far been identified, of which five (Y1, Y2, Y4, Y5, Y6) have been cloned and belong to the superfamily of GPCRs with seven transmembrane spanning domains (40). Several NPY1 and NPY5 antagonists have been synthesized but their effects in humans are unknown, and it is not clear whether antagonists can be synthesized with sufficient selectivity. NPY receptors are expressed in other areas of the body, and so the side-effect profile of antagonists is likely to be an issue.

Agents That Primarily Increase Metabolic Rate or Affect Metabolism Through Peripheral Action

Selective β_3-Adrenergic Receptor Agonists

β_3-adrenergic receptors have been shown to mediate thermogenesis and have therapeutic potential for obesity. β_3-adrenoreceptors are present and functional in the human heart (41), and expression has been reported in skeletal muscle and adipose tissue (42). They mediate both catecholamine-stimulated lipolysis in white and brown adipose tissue (BAT) and theromogenesis in BAT. It appears that BAT thermogenesis is primarily responsible for the removal of stored fat in animal models (43). There are significant differences between human and animal β_3-receptor isoforms. Because of the lack of selectivity, most agonists shown to be effective in rodents have modest effects in humans and are not always free from side effects (44).

Lipid Metabolizing Enzyme Inhibitors

Lipase inhibitors

Lipases (acylglycerol acylhydrolases) initiate the catabolism of fats and oils by hydrolyzing the fatty ester bonds of acylglycerols. Lipases differ from one another in their biochemical features and are selective in respect of the length and the level of saturation of the fatty acid chains (45). At present the only lipase inhibitor in the market is Orlistat. Alizyme, in collaboration with Takeda in Japan, is developing cetilistat (ATL-962)—an oral, nonabsorbed synthetic lipase inhibitor, derived from Alizyme's pancreatic lipase inhibitor research program, which has been in phase II clinical trials (46). All dose levels of cetilistat (60, 120, and 240 mg) demonstrated a significant reduction in weight, compared to placebo. The frequency of severe adverse events was comparable with placebo, although gastrointestinal adverse events were increased.

Diacylglycerol acyltransferase (DGAT)

DGAT catalyses the final step in mammalian triacylglycerol synthesis that merges the monoGAT and glycerol-3-phosphate pathways (47). In contrast to MGAT enzymes, which are predominantly expressed in tissues involved in dietary fat absorption, both DGAT1 and DGAT2 are widely expressed in range of tissues (48,49). Several natural products from various microorganisms have been reported to inhibit DGAT activity (50), although the specificity of these compounds has not yet been confirmed against cloned DGAT enzymes.

Fatty acid synthase (FAS)

Mammalian FAS catalyses the de novo synthesis of saturated fatty acids, such as myristate, plamitate, and stearate, using acetyl- and malonyl-CoA. It functions as a homodimer of a multifunctional protein that contains seven catalytic domains and a site for the prosthetic group 4′-phosphopantetheine (51). The enzyme is abundantly expressed in lipogenic tissues such as liver, adipose, and lactating breast (52). In coordination with carnitine palmitoyl transferase (CPT) and acetyl CoA carboxylase (ACC), FAS is believed to play an important role in maintaining energy homeostasis by converting excess food into lipids for storage and providing energy by upregulating the rate of β-oxidation (53).

An understanding of the role of FAS comes from investigations using two FAS inhibitors: cerulenin and C75. Administration of C75 caused a dose-dependent decrease in food intake in BALB/c mice and blocked the fasting-induced upregulation of orexigenic neuropeptides and the downregulation of anorexigenic neuropeptides in the hypothalamus (54,55). Similar results were observed with cerulenin, although with much less efficacy (54). Intraventricular injection of C75 resulted in dose-dependent inhibition of feeding, which could be circumvented by intraventricular injection of NPY (54). The effect of inhibiting FAS on food intake is so profound that there must be one or several natural counter-regulatory mechanisms if the pathway is truly operational in vivo (56).

Acetyl-CoA carboxylase (ACC)

This enzyme catalyses the carboxylation of acetyl-CoA to malonyl-CoA, which is a crucial regulator of mitochondrial fatty acid oxidation, through its inhibition of CPT1. In mammals, ACC exists in two isoforms, ACC1 and ACC2, encoded by different genes. ACC1 is the principal isoform in lipogenic tissues like adipose, whereas ACC2 is predominantly expressed in oxidative tissues like heart and skeletal muscle. Both isoforms are expressed in liver, where fatty acid synthesis and oxidation co-exist (57). ACC1 is believed to regulate fat synthesis in lipogenic tissues and ACC2 controls the rate of lipid oxidation (58) in oxidative tissues. Further analysis has also confirmed an important role of ACC2 in the malonyl-CoA/CPT1 axis, evidenced by an increase in CPT1 activity of hepatocytes isolated from ACC2-null mice. Surprisingly, CPT1 activity in skeletal muscle was not changed significantly by ACC2 deficiency (59). The knockout mice have a normal life span with no apparent pathophysiological condition caused by ACC2 deficiency.

One of the mammalian ACC inhibitors, CP-640186, has IC_{50} values of 50 nM for both the isoforms (60). Another compound, CP-610431, has also shown dual inhibition of both ACC1 and ACC2 with IC_{50} values of 0.107 and 0.112 nM, respectively. When tested in vivo, several inhibitors reduced triacylglycerol synthesis and increased fatty acid oxidation in rats, with a concurrent reduction in malonyl-CoA levels in the liver, muscle, and heart (61,62). In chronic (up to 8 weeks) studies in rats, CP-640186 led to reductions in liver, skeletal muscle, and adipose tissue triglycerides and subsequently reduced body weight due to selective reduction of body fat (62,63). A three dimensional structure of the carboxyltransferase domain of yeast ACC has been reported which shows features that are likely to be common among eukaryotic ACCs, including dimerization and conserved residues for substrate binding (64). Hopefully, this three dimensional structure will aid development of next generation ACC inhibitors for the potential treatment of obesity.

Steroyl-CoA desaturase (SCD)

SCD catalyses the rate-limiting step in the biosynthesis of mono-unsaturated fatty acids, particularly oleate and palmitoleate, which are the main mono-unsaturates of membrane phospholipids, cholesterol esters, waxes, and triglycerol (65), the preferred substrates being steraroyl-CoA. Mice with the targeted disruption of SCD1 isoform have reduced adiposity, increased energy expenditure and up-regulated expression of several genes, which encode enzymes of fatty acid β-oxidation in the liver (66). The SCD1 mutation also has increased adenosine monophosphate activated protein kinase (AMPK) phosphorylation and activity, and increased ACC phosphorylation in leptin-deficient ob/ob mice. Lower malonyl-CoA concentrations are known to de-repress CPT1. In SCD1 null mice, CPT1, and CPT2, activities were significantly increased thereby stimulating the oxidation of mitochondrial palmitoyl-CoA. Mice that lack SCD1 are lean, hypermetabolic and resistant to diet-induced obesity. Inactivation of SCD1 also improves the lipid metabolic profile (65,67) and insulin sensitivity, and attenuates the obese phenotype caused by leptin deficiency in ob/ob mice (68).

One of the main concerns in the development of SCD1 inhibitors as antiobesity and triacylglycerol lowering agents is the potential for side effects on the skin and eye, which are observed in SCD1-deficient mice (67). The pathological effect of the loss of SCD1 on cutaneous function is not compensated for by the other SCD isoforms, which are abundantly expressed in the skin (69).

Agents That Act on the Gastrointestinal Tract

Targeting appetite mechanisms to reduce food intake is the most popular pharmacological approach to obesity, but blocking the absorption of nutrients is a logical alternative. This is one of the mechanisms by which gastric bypass surgery produces weight loss, but pharmacological approaches would obviously be less invasive. Many peptides are synthesized and released from the gut, and several are known to modulate eating behavior. They respond to nutrients within the gastrointestinal tract by interacting with specific receptors to regulate appetite. Many of these circulating peptides have direct access to the hypothalamic region of brain, which regulates food intake. They may also function peripherally to modulate the activity of neurons such as, the vagus.

Glucogon-like Peptide-1 (GLP-1) Receptor Agonists

GLP-1, a gut incretin peptide hormone induced by glucose and other nutrients, has multiple actions which include delaying gastric emptying and stimulating β-cell–glucose transporter-2, glucokinase expression, insulin biosynthesis-secretion, and decreasing α-cell glucagon secretion (70). GLP-1 may mediate its anorectic action via the GLP-1 receptor in the CNS and is rapidly degraded by dipeptidyl peptidase-IV (DPP-IV). Exendin, a naturally occurring DPP-IV-resistant GLP-1 analog, has recently been approved for the treatment of type 2 diabetes. Chronic SC administration of GLP-1 to obese type 2 diabetes patients for 6 weeks led to an average 1.9 kg decrease in body weight; twice daily SC injection led to 4.7-kg weight loss over 2 years (70). Another GLP-1 analog, liraglutide, reduced plasma glucose for 24 h, lowered HbA1c and controlled body weight by a once daily injection (70,71). Therefore, although the interest in GLP-1 agonists to date is focused on the treatment of diabetes, GLP-1 agonists could act as weight reducing agents in obese diabetic patients. More research is needed however to fully clarify the role of GLP-1 in feeding.

Cholecystokinin-A (CCK-A) Agonists

CCK is a hormone released from the intestine in response to meals that plays an important role in termination of feeding (72). Two CCK receptor subtypes are known, CCK-A and CCK-B, for which selective ligands have been developed (73). Endogenous CCK acts as a satiety factor to curtail food intake and the development of CKK agonists has been disclosed. Using subtype-selective agonists and antagonists, it was shown that the effect of CCK on feeding is mostly mediated through the peripheral CCK-A receptor, confirming it as a target for the treatment of obesity (74).

Initially, most CCK agonists were peptide derivatives (75). A-71378 was found to be a potent and selective CCK-A agonist (76). Several additional hexapeptide CCK-A agonists have been reported (77), of which, ARL-15849 was found to be 6600-fold selective over CCK-B with improved stability and longer duration (78). This compound inhibited food intake at nanomolar potency following intraperitoneal administration in fasted rats, but so far, no orally active peptides have been reported.

Ghrelin Antagonists

Ghrelin, the only known circulating appetite stimulant, has generated widespread scientific interest and antagonists of its receptor are being developed by the pharmaceutical industry to treat obesity (79). Ghrelin is an acylated 28-amino acid peptide, considered to be a ligand for the growth hormone secretagogue receptor. It was isolated from the stomach and is localized to specific subpopulations of neurons (80). It enhances appetite in humans (81). In the Zucker fa/fa rat model, it stimulates feeding and increases body weight (82). Ghrelin in energy balance (83) and in the regulation of appetite and body weight (79) has been reviewed. Recently, Cytos Biotechnology ended development of an anti-ghrelin vaccine to treat obesity, as it failed to demonstrate an effect on weight loss in a phase III trial, raising doubts about this therapeutic strategy.

Agents That Not Only Affect Obesity but Overall Metabolic Syndrome

Obesity is associated with other disorders, such as insulin resistance, diabetes, dyslipidemia, and hypertension (84). This clustering in an individual has been termed the "metabolic syndrome" (also called syndrome X, insulin resistance syndrome, Reaven syndrome, and metabolic cardiovascular syndrome). It is prudent to emphasize that the ultimate therapeutic goal in the treatment of obesity is not only weight loss, but also a reduction in morbidity and mortality from associated disorders. This consideration favors new antiobesity agents that not only affect weight control, but also improve metabolic and cardiovascular disorders.

Peroxisome Proliferator Activated Receptor (PPAR) Modulators

PPARs, members of super family of nuclear hormone receptors, are major targets of drug discovery for treating obesity and associated disorders. PPAR-γ agonists, thiazolidinedione (TZD) drugs, are effective for diabetes and PPAR-α agonists, fibrates, for type IV/V dyslipidemia. Surprisingly, while controversial, recent reports suggest increased cardiovascular risk among subjects taking at least one of the commonly prescribed TZDs (Rosiglitazone). (REF: Nissen SE, Wolski KN, Engl J Med. 2007 Jun 14;356(24)2457–71.) Three PPAR isoforms, α, γ, and δ, are known. PPAR-γ antagonism has been considered as a strategy for obesity treatment, although the concept is relatively new (85). SR-202, a PPAR-γ

antagonist, inhibits adipocyte differentiation (86). Wild-type mice, fed at weaning for 10 weeks with SR-202 in a standard diet or high-fat diet had lesser weight gain, and lesser accumulation of both white adipose tissue accumulation and BAT than untreated mice. SR-202-treated mice on the standard diet had smaller adipocytes, whereas those on the high-fat diet had less adipocyte hypertrophy than in untreated mice (86). Several other PPAR-γ antagonists have recently been reported. GW-0072 and LG-100641 are among several that antagonize TZD-induced adipocyte differentiation (87,88), suggesting potential for the treatment of obesity.

PPAR-α agonists induce lipid catabolism through β-oxidation—a well-known pathway for energy expenditure (85). PPAR-α agonists decrease body weight in both leptin receptor-deficient fa/fa rats and high-fat fed rodents (89,90). The concept that a PPAR-α, γ dual activator with a significant PPAR-α component can induce body weight loss is supported by recent evidence with the compound DRF-2655 (91). This showed euglycemic and hypolipidemic activities in the insulin-resistant, hyperlipidemic genetic rodent models, db/db mice, and zucker fa/fa rats, and in fat-fed hyperlipidemic rats and hamsters. It reduced body weight in db/db mice, fat-fed hamsters, and also monosodium glutamate-induced obesity in Swiss albino mice (85). Body weight lowering might be mediated by the induction of target enzymes involved in lipid catabolism, through PPAR-α modulation. The concept of PPAR-α modulation for obesity has been strengthened by a study of oleylethanolamide (OEA), a naturally occurring lipid that regulates satiety and body weight (92). Mice lacking PPAR-α do not respond to OEA. The authors further hypothesized that the ability of OEA to reduce endothelial nitric oxide synthase expression through PPAR-α may contribute to the persistent satiety-inducing actions of this lipid modulator. Potent and specific PPAR-α activation is therefore a potential therapy for obesity and associated disorders.

PPAR-δ, less explored so far, has a potential role in several disease conditions including obesity. Animal studies have shown that activation of PPAR-δ induces fatty acid oxidation and energy dissipation, which in turn leads to an improved lipid profile and less obesity (93). Studies with a PPAR-δ agonist also showed insulin sensitization in monkeys (94). These data suggest that PPAR-δ activation may improve several features of the metabolic syndrome.

Carboxypeptidase Inhibitors

Carboxypeptidase has an important role in regulating metabolism. Knockout of this enzyme in mice protects against diet-induced obesity and enhances insulin sensitivity. MLN-4760, synthesized by Millennium, potently and selectively inhibits the enzyme and entered clinical development with completion of a phase I trial in 2003. The compound was found to be safe and well tolerated but further development in collaboration with Abbott was terminated.

Protein Tyrosine Phosphatase Inhibitors

Protein tyrosine phosphatase 1B (PTP1B) is an enzyme that removes phosphates from active insulin receptors thereby reducing the effects of insulin and possibly contributing to insulin resistance. Reduction in PTP1B activity could increase insulin sensitivity, reduce the "obesity metabolic cycle" of hyperinsulinemia followed by insulin resistance and perhaps increase energy expenditure. Merck Frost Canada and McGill University made a PTP1B knockout mouse model that is resistant to weight gain, when fed a high-fat diet and high-carbohydrate diet (95). Several companies have claimed novel PTP1B inhibitors as antidiabetic agents, and an antisense inhibitor of the RNA encoding for PTP1B is being developed as an antiobesity drug (96).

AMP-Activated Protein Kinase (AMPK) Modulators

AMP activated protein kinase (AMPK) is a phylogenetically conserved intracellular energy sensor that has been implicated as a major regulator of glucose and lipid metabolism in mammals. It is widely expressed and comprises catalytic α-subunits. It can be activated by phosphorylation at Thr 172 of the catalytic subunit by AMPK kinase, a protein that has so far eluded molecular characterization. In addition, the allosteric binding of AMP to AMPK enhances both its activity as well the stability of its phosphorylated state (97). AMPK was initially described as a kinase that phosphorylates and inactivates HMG-CoA reductase and acetyl-CoA carboxylase, thereby decreasing the rates of cholesterol and fatty acid biosynthesis, respectively (97). Subsequent studies have led to the idea that AMPK acts as an intracellular energy sensor stimulated by the increased intracellular AMP/ATP ratio, when cells are stressed by conditions such as hypoxia/ischemia in the heart and excessive contraction in skeletal muscle. Activated AMPK accelerates ATP-producing pathways, such as fatty acid and glucose oxidation, while reducing ATP consumption, ultimately leading to the preservation or restoration of adequate high-energy phosphates (98). Much attention is centered on the role of AMPK in both short- and long-term response to exercise (—99–101). Two adipocyte-derived hormones, leptin and adiponectin, which regulate energy homeostasis and glucose and lipid metabolism, induce the activation of AMPK. Leptin stimulates phosphorylation and activation of the α2-subunit of AMPK in skeletal muscle, invoked as a principal means of stimulating fatty acid oxidation (102). Adiponectin promotes phosphorylation and activation of AMPK in both liver and skeletal muscle, and this has also been suggested to account for the stimulatory effect of adiponectin on glucose utilization and fatty acid oxidation (103,104).

While the importance of AMPK to control lipid metabolism in liver and muscle is well established, its role in regulating lipolysis in adipose tissue has remained controversial. The β-adrenergic signaling pathway represents a prime regulator of triglyceride breakdown, acting via the accumulation of cAMP and subsequent protein kinase A-dependent phosphorylation of hormone sensitive lipase (HSL). The activity of HSL, the rate-limiting enzyme that catalyzes the hydrolysis of triglyceride to diglyceride and monoglyceride, is regulated by both phosphorylation and translocation to the lipid droplet (105,106). In 1989, Garton and coworkers (107) reported that AMPK phosphorylates HSL at Ser 565 in vitro without any direct effect on HSL activity, but this abolished the further phosphorylation of HSL by PKA at Ser 563. 5-amino-1,32-β-D-ribofuranosylimidazole-4-carboxamide

(AICAR), a cell permeable adenosine analog that can be phosphorylated to form 5-aminoimidazole-4-carboxamide-1-β-D-ribofuranosyl-5′-monophsphate, stimulates AMPK activity and glucose uptake in both muscle and adipose tissues (—108–111). Preincubation of isolated rat adipocyltes with AICAR reduced the response of these cells to the lipolytic β receptor agonist, isoproterenol (112,113). These observations led to the hypothesis that AMPK antagonizes lipolysis in adipocytes, presumably to prevent futile cycling and depletion of ATP. Moule and Denton (114) reported that isoproterenol stimulated AMPK phosphorylation and kinase activity in isolated rat epididymal fat cells, an observation seemingly at odds with an antilipolytic role for AMPK. To clarify the role of AMPK in regulating lipolysis in adipose tissue, Yin and coworkers (115) used 3T3-L1 adipocytes as a model system, measuring AMPK phosphorylation and activity after the treatment with different activators and/or inhibitors of the components along the β-adrenergic signaling pathway. Their findings support the idea that β-adrenergic agents activate AMPK via an intermediary rise in cAMP, which in turn enhances the lipolytic rate.

Tissue-selective inhibition of AMPK is a potential antiobesity strategy. Lab Servier reported novel imidazopyridine inhibitor compounds (116). In ob/ob mice one of these compounds, at 125 mg/kg, reduced serum triglyceride concentration to the same level as the traditional antidiabetes agent, metformin, administered at 250 mg/kg. α-Lipoic acid is a naturally occurring short chain fatty acid and powerful antioxidant that has been shown to have potent antiobesity properties in animals by suppressing hypothalamic AMPK (117). Added to the standard chow of Sprague Dawley rats for 2 weeks, α-lipoic acid (0.25%, 0.5%, and 1% weight/weight) reduced body weight and food intake in a dose-dependent manner. The reduced food intake was greater during the first few days of treatment. On cessation of treatment, body weight increased. This finding raises the interesting option of suppressing AMPK activation in the brain as opposed to peripheral tissues, for the treatment of obesity.

CLINICAL CONSIDERATIONS

Draft United States Food and Drug Administration (FDA) guidelines for the approval of weight loss therapies (http://www.fda.gov/cder/guidance/obesity.pdf) propose that a suitable efficacious drug intended for long-term use will demonstrate:

1. that the proportion of subjects who reach and maintain a loss of at least 5% of their initial body weight is significantly greater than placebo; or
2. that the drug effect is significantly better than the placebo effect and the mean drug-associated weight loss exceeds the mean placebo weight loss by at least 5%.

Such effects on weight should be maintained for at least 12 months after the initiation of treatment.

An important consideration in developing antiobesity drugs that act centrally is the potential for abuse and/or effect on other behavioral characteristics. The FDA requires substantial safety data before approving such drugs, which can only be obtained by long and expensive trials.

Recent apparent failures of several new drugs based on novel targets have raised questions about the translation to humans of animal studies. Leptin is now a classic example. The initial discovery that a mutation in the leptin gene resulted in morbid obesity in ob/ob mice led to the development of leptin protein as a treatment for obesity. The ability of leptin to induce greater weight loss in leptin-deficient ob/ob mice than in obese humans is often cited as evidence that rodent models are unreliable for predicting human response. Nevertheless, careful analysis of the data reveals that leptin has similar efficacy in leptin-deficient humans. On the other hand, both obese humans and older diet-induced obese rodents have a limited response to leptin therapy (118). A further example is the β3 adrenergic receptor agonists. Current data suggest that the chronic effects of these agonists on body composition are weaker in humans than in rodents (119). However, the understanding of this target is still limited, and further studies of selective agonists in subsets of obese humans are required. The problem with knockout or transgenic mice is that each reflects a subset of the human obese population. It is advisable that a new drug be checked in different animal models to help predict the potential dosing and treatment schedule in different subset of the human population.

CONCLUSION

It is indeed a challenge to understand pathophysiological mechanisms of increasing, epidemic incidence of obesity and develop appropriate new strategies including drugs. The development of new drugs lags considerably behind the increased incidence of obesity, and very few drugs are at a late stage of development. Current drugs are not optimal and have undesirable side effects. Despite some pessimism, recent advances in our understanding of the central and peripheral mechanisms involved in regulating energy homeostasis, and of signal transduction pathways by which peptides or hormones work, provide key knowledge for a platform of rational drug design. New targets are being investigated but safe and efficacious pharmacotherapy remains a promise. Moreover, pharmacotherapy alone is undesirable without changing human behavior through education and environmental modification, to encourage healthy and regular exercise. Compensatory mechanisms are undoubtedly engaged to counteract weight gain and any drug-induced weight loss is likely to engage countermeasures in homeostatic loops, maintaining energy balance. Further research is needed to understand these compensatory mechanisms and their impact on pharmacotherapy. Finally, it should be emphasized that the ultimate therapeutic goal in the treatment of obesity is not only weight loss but also a reduction in morbidity and mortality from associated disorders. This consideration favors antiobesity strategies that not only reduce weight but also improve metabolic and cardiovascular parameters.

REFERENCES

1. Flegal KM, Carroll MD, Ogden CL, et al. Prevalence and trends in obesity among US adults, 1999–2000. JAMA. 2002; 288(14):1723–1727.
2. Mokdad AH, Ford ES, Bowman BA, et al. Prevalence of obesity, diabetes, and obesity-related health risk factors, 2001. JAMA 2003; 289(1):76–79.
3. Kopelman PG. Obesity as a medical problem. Nature 2000; 404(6778):635–543.
4. Cooke D, Bloom S. The obesity pipeline: current strategies in the development of anti-obesity drugs. Nat Rev Drug Discov 2006; 5(11):919–131
5. Leibel RL, Rosenbaum M, Hirsch J. Changes in energy expenditure resulting from altered body weight. N Engl J Med 1995; 332(10):621–628.
6. Friedman JM. Modern science versus the stigma of obesity. Nat Med 2004; 10(6):563–569.
7. Barsh GS, Schwartz MW. Genetic approaches to studying energy balance: perception and integration. Nat Rev Genet 2002; 3(8):589–600.
8. Berridge KC. Motivation concepts in behavioral neuroscience. Physiol Behav 2004; 81(2):179–209.
9. Alvaro JD, Tatro JB, Quillan JM, et al. Laboratory of Molecular Psychiatry, Yale University School of Medicine, New Haven, Connecticut 06508, SA. Mol Pharmacol 1996; 50(3):583–591.
10. Dryden S, Frankish H, Wang Q, et al. Neuropeptide Y and energy balance: one way ahead for the treatment of obesity? Eur J Clin Invest 1994; 24(5):293–308.
11. Heisler LK, Cowley MA, Tecott LH, et al. Activation of central melanocortin pathways by fenfluramine. Science 2002; 297(5581):609–611.
12. Schultz G. Neuron 2002; 36:241.
13. Lowell BB. Adaptive thermogenesis: turning on the heat. Curr Biol 1998; 8(15):R517–R520.
14. Ballinger A. Orlistat in the treatment of obesity. Expert Opin Pharmacother 2000; 1(4):841–847.
15. Astrup A, Hansen DL, Lundsgaard C, et al. Sibutramine and energy balance. Int J Obes Relat Metab Disord. 1998; 22 Suppl 1:S30–S35; discussion S36–7, S42.
16. Day C, Bailey CJ. Effect of the antiobesity agent sibutramine in obese-diabetic ob/ob mice. Int J Obes Relat Metab Disord 1998; 22(7):619–23.
17. Ryan DH. Medeiros–Neto G, Halpern A, Bouchard C, Progress in Obesity Research: 9. Montrouge, France: John Libby Eurotext, 2003:1051–1057.
18. Di Carlo G, Izzo AA.Cannabinoids for gastrointestinal diseases: potential therapeutic applications. Expert Opin Investig Drugs 2003; 12(1):39–49.
19. Pertwee RG.Cannabinoid receptor ligands: clinical and neuropharmacological considerations, relevant to future drug discovery and development. Expert Opin Investig Drugs 2000; 9(7):1553–1571.
20. Xiang J-N, Lee JC. Ann Rep Med Chem 1999; 34:199.
21. Trillou RC, Arnone C, Gonalons N, et al. J Physiol Regul Integr Comp Physiol 2003; 284:345.
22. Rothman RB, Baumann MH, Savage JE, et al. Evidence for possible involvement of 5-HT(2B) receptors in the cardiac valvulopathy associated with fenfluramine and other serotonergic medications. Circulation 2000; 102(23):2836–2841.

23. Fitzgerald LW, Burn TC, Brown BS, et al. Possible role of valvular serotonin 5-HT(2B) receptors in the cardiopathy associated with fenfluramine. Mol Pharmacol 2000; 57(1):75–81.

24. Tecott LH, Sun LM, Akana SF, et al. Eating disorder and epilepsy in mice lacking 5-HT2c serotonin receptors. Nature 1995; 374(6522):542–546.

25. Nonogaki K, Strack AM, Dallman MF, et al. Leptin-independent hyperphagia and type 2 diabetes in mice with a mutated serotonin 5-HT2C receptor gene. Nat Med. 1998 Oct;4(10):1152–1156.

26. Gantz I, Fong TM. The melanocortin system. Am J Physiol Endocrinol Metab 2003; 284(3):E468–E474.

27. Proietto J, Fam BC, Ainslie DA et al. Novel anti-obesity drugs. Expert Opin Investig Drugs 2000; 9(6):1317–1326.

28. Huszar D, Lynch CA, Fairchild-Huntress V, et al. Targeted disruption of the melanocortin-4 receptor results in obesity in mice. Cell 1997; 88(1):131–141.

29. Qu D, Ludwig DS, Gammeltoft S, et al. A role for melanin-concentrating hormone in the central regulation of feeding behaviour. Nature 1996; 380(6571):243–247.

30. Chambers J, Ames RS, Bergsma D, et al. USA 1992; 89:1174.

31. Hervieu G, Dytko GM, Foley JJ, et al. Nature 1999; 400:261.

32. Lembo PM, Grazzini E, Cao J, et al. The receptor for the orexigenic peptide melanin-concentrating hormone is a G-protein-coupled receptor. Nat Cell Biol. 1999 Sep;1(5):267–271.

33. Lembo PM, Grazzini E, Cao J, et al. The receptor for the orexigenic peptide melanin-concentrating hormone is a G-protein-coupled receptor. Nat Cell Biol 1999; 1:267–271.

34. Saito Y, Nothacker HP, Wang Z, et al. Molecular characterization of the melanin-concentrating-hormone receptor. Nature 1999; 400(6741):265–269.

35. Ludwig DS, Tritos NA, Mastaitis JW, et al. Melanin-concentrating hormone over-expression in transgenic mice leads to obesity and insulin resistance. J Clin Invest 2001; 107(3):379–386.

36. Shimada M, Tritos NA, Lowell BB, et al. Mice lacking melanin-concentrating hormone are hypophagic and lean. Nature 1998; 396(6712):670–674.

37. Takekawa S, Asami A, Ishihara Y, et al. T-226296: a novel, orally active and selective melanin-concentrating hormone receptor antagonist. Eur J Pharmacol 2002; 438(3):129–135.

38. Wieland HA, Bradford SH, Krist B, et al. Exp Opin Invest Drugs 2000; 9:1327.

39. Zarjevski N, Cusin I, Vettor R, et al. Chronic intracerebroventricular neuropeptide-Y administration to normal rats mimics hormonal and metabolic changes of obesity. Endocrinology 1993; 133(4):1753–1738.

40. Wieland HA, Bradford SH, Krist B, et al. Opin Invest Drugs 2000; 9:1327.

41. Gauthier C, Tavernier G, Charpentier F, et al. Functional beta3-adrenoceptor in the human heart. J Clin Invest 1996; 98(2):556–562.

42. Chamberlain PD, Jennings KH, Paul F, et al. The tissue distribution of the human beta3-adrenoceptor studied using a monoclonal antibody: direct evidence of the beta3-adrenoceptor in human adipose tissue, atrium and skeletal muscle. Int J Obes Relat Metab Disord 1999; 23(10):1057–1065.

43. Himms-Hagen J. Brown adipose tissue thermogenesis and obesity. Prog Lipid Res 1989;28(2):67–115.

44. Weyer C, Gautier JF, Danforth E Jr. Diabetes Metab. 1999; 25:11.
45. Haas MJ, Cichowicz DJ, Bailey DG. Lipids 1992; 27:571.
46. Fong TM. Advances in anti-obesity therapeutics. Expert Opin Investig Drugs 2005; 14(3):243–250.
47. Coleman RA, Lee DP. Enzymes of triacylglycerol synthesis and their regulation. Prog Lipid Res 2004; 43(2):13476.
48. Cases S, Smith SJ, Zheng YW, et al. Identification of a gene encoding an acyl CoA:diacylglycerol acyltransferase, a key enzyme in triacylglycerol synthesis. Proc Natl Acad Sci U S A 1998; 95(22):13018–13023.
49. Cases S, Stone SJ, Zhou P, et al. Cloning of DGAT2, a second mammalian diacylglycerol acyltransferase, and related family members. J Biol Chem 2001; 276(42):38870–38876.
50. Tomoda H, Namatame I, Omura S. Proc Jpn Acad Ser BPhys Biol Sci 2002; 78: 217.
51. Smith S, Witkowski A, Joshi AK. Structural and functional organization of the animal fatty acid synthase. Prog Lipid Res 2003; 42(4):289–317.
52. Jayakumar A, Tai M-H, Huang W-Y, et al. Human fatty acid synthase: properties and molecular cloning. Proc Natl Acad Sci U S A 1995; 92(19):8695–8699.
53. Shi Y, Burn P. Lipid metabolic enzymes: emerging drug targets for the treatment of obesity. Nat Rev Drug Discov 2004; 3(8):695–710.
54. Loftus TM, Jaworsky DE, Frehywot GL et al. Reduced food intake and body weight in mice treated with fatty acid synthase inhibitors. Science 2000; 288(5475):2379–2381.
55. Shimokawa T, Kumar MV, Lane MD. Effect of a fatty acid synthase inhibitor on food intake and expression of hypothalamic neuropeptides. Proc Natl Acad Sci U S A 2002; 99(1):66–71.
56. Bouchard C. N Engl J Med 2000; 343:1888.
57. Abu-Elheiga L, Almarza-Ortega DB, Baldini A, et al. Human acetyl-CoA carboxylase 2. Molecular cloning, characterization, chromosomal mapping, and evidence for two isoforms. J Biol Chem 1997; 272(16):10669–10677.
58. Abu-Elheiga L, Brinkley WR, Zhong L, et al. The subcellular localization of acetyl-CoA carboxylase 2. Proc Natl Acad Sci U S A 2000; 97(4):1444–1449.
59. Abu-Elheiga L, Oh W, Kordari P, et al. Acetyl-CoA carboxylase 2 mutant mice are protected against obesity and diabetes induced by high-fat/high-carbohydrate diets. Proc Natl Acad Sci U S A 2003; 100(18):10207–10212.
60. Perry DA, Harwood HJ Jr. PCT Patent WO2003072197, 2003; Chem Abstr 2003;139:230625.
61. Arbeeny CM, Meyers DS, Bergquist KE, et al. Inhibition of fatty acid synthesis decreases very low density lipoprotein secretion in the hamster. J Lipid Res 1992; 33(6):843–351.
62. Harwood HJ Jr, Petras SF, Shelly LD et al. Isozyme-nonselective N-substituted bipiperidylcarboxamide acetyl-CoA carboxylase inhibitors reduce tissue malonyl-CoA concentrations, inhibit fatty acid synthesis, and increase fatty acid oxidation in cultured cells and in experimental animals. J Biol Chem 2003; 278(39):37099–37111.
63. Harwood HJ Jr. Treating the metabolic syndrome: acetyl-CoA carboxylase inhibition. Expert Opin Ther Targets 2005; 9(2):267–281.

64. Zhang H, Yang Z, Shen Y, et al. Crystal structure of the carboxyltransferase domain of acetyl-coenzyme A carboxylase. Science 2003; 299(5615):2064–2067.

65. Ntambi JM, Miyazaki M. Recent insights into stearoyl-CoA desaturase-1. Curr Opin Lipidol 2003; (3):255–261.

66. Dobrzyn P, Dobrzyn A, Miyazaki M et al. Stearoyl-CoA desaturase 1 deficiency increases fatty acid oxidation by activating AMP-activated protein kinase in liver. Proc Natl Acad Sci U S A 2004; 101(17):6409–6414.

67. Miyazaki M, Man WC, Ntambi JM. Targeted disruption of stearoyl-CoA desaturase1 gene in mice causes atrophy of sebaceous and meibomian glands and depletion of wax esters in the eyelid. J Nutr 2001; (9):2260–2268.

68. Cohen P, Miyazaki M, Socci ND et al. Role for stearoyl-CoA desaturase-1 in leptin-mediated weight loss. Science 2002; 297(5579):240–243.

69. Shi Y, Burn P. Lipid metabolic enzymes: emerging drug targets for the treatment of obesity. Nat Rev Drug Discov 2004; 3(8):695–710

70. Rondinone CM Diabetes: the latest developments in inhibitors, insulin sensitisers, new drug targets and novel approaches. October 18–19, 2004, The Hatton, London, UK. Expert Opin Ther Targets 2005; 9(2):415–418.

71. Das SK, Chakrabarti R. Non-insulin dependent diabetes mellitus: present therapies and new drug targets. Mini Rev Med Chem 2005; 5(11):1019–1034.

72. Moran TH, Schwartz GJ. Neurobiology of cholecystokinin. Crit Rev Neurobiol 1994; 9(1):1–28.

73. Dunlop J. CCK receptor antagonists. Gen Pharmacol 1998; (4):519–524.

74. Szewczyk JR, Laudeman C. CCK1R agonists: a promising target for the pharmacological treatment of obesity. Curr Top Med Chem 2003; 3(8):837–854.

75. Holladay MW, Bennett MJ, Tufano MD et al. Synthesis and biological activity of CCK heptapeptide analogues. Effects of conformational constraints and standard modifications on receptor subtype selectivity, functional activity in vitro, and appetite suppression in vivo. J Med Chem 1992, 35(16):2919–2928.

76. Lin CW, Holladay MW, Witte DG, et al. A71378: a CCK agonist with high potency and selectivity for CCK-A receptors. Am J Physiol 1990; 258(4 Pt 1):G648–G651.

77. Pierson ME, Comstock JM, Simmons RD, et al. Synthesis and biological evaluation of potent, selective, hexapeptide CCK-A agonist anorectic agents. J Med Chem 1997; 19;40(26):4302–4307.

78. Simmons RD, Blosser JC, Rosamond JD. Pharmacol Biochem Behav 1994; 47: 701.

79. Cummings DE, Overduin J, Foster-Schubert KE. Curr Opin Endocrinol Diabetes 2005; 12:72.

80. Kojima M, Hosoda H, Date Y, et al. Ghrelin is a growth-hormone-releasing acylated peptide from stomach. Nature 1999; 402(6762):656–660.

81. Ludwig DS, Tritos NA, Mastaitis JW, et al. Melanin-concentrating hormone over-expression in transgenic mice leads to obesity and insulin resistance. J Clin Invest 2001; 107(3):379–386.

82. Shimada M, Tritos NA, Lowell BB, et al. Mice lacking melanin-concentrating hormone are hypophagic and lean. Nature 1998; 396(6712):670–674.

83. Cummings DE, Foster-Schubert KE, Overduin J. Ghrelin and energy balance: focus on current controversies. Curr Drug Targets 2005; (2):153–169.

84. Barton M, Carmona R, Ortmann J et al. Obesity-associated activation of angiotensin and endothelin in the cardiovascular system. Int J Biochem Cell Biol 2003; 35(6):826–837.

85. Chakrabarti R, Rajagopalan R. Curr Med Chem Immun Endoc Metab Agents 2004; 4:67.

86. Doggrell S. Exp Opin Invest Drugs 2003; 12:713.

87. Oberfield JL, Collins JL, Holmes CP et al. A peroxisome proliferator-activated receptor gamma ligand inhibits adipocyte differentiation. Proc Natl Acad Sci U S A 1999; 96(11):6102–6106.

88. Mukherjee R, Hoener PA, Jow L et al. A selective peroxisome proliferator-activated receptor-gamma (PPARgamma) modulator blocks adipocyte differentiation but stimulates glucose uptake in 3T3-L1 adipocytes. Mol Endocrinol 2000; 14(9):1425–1433.

89. Chaput E, Saladin R, Silvestre M, et al. Fenofibrate and rosiglitazone lower serum triglycerides with opposing effects on body weight. Biochem Biophys Res Commun 2000; 271(2):445–450.

90. Mancini FP, Lanni A, Sabatino L, et al. Fenofibrate prevents and reduces body weight gain and adiposity in diet-induced obese rats. FEBS Lett 2001; 491(1–2):154–158.

91. Vikramadithyan RK, Hiriyan J, Suresh J, et al. DRF 2655: a unique molecule that reduces body weight and ameliorates metabolic abnormalities. Obes Res 2003; 11(2):292–303.

92. Fu J, Gaetani S, Oveisi F, et al. Oleylethanolamide regulates feeding and body weight through activation of the nuclear receptor PPAR-alpha. Nature 2003; 425(6953):90–93.

93. A Peters JM, Lee SST, Li W, et al. Mol Cell Biol 2000; 20:5119.

94. A Wang Y-X, Lee C-H, Tiep S, et al. Cell 2003; 113:159.

95. Kennedy B, Payette P, Gresser M, et al. PCT Patent WO200006712:2000; Chem Abstr 2000; 132:150278.

96. Bays H, Dujovne C. Anti-obesity drug development. Expert Opin Investig Drugs 2002; 11(9):1189–1204.

97. Hardie DG, Carling D, Carlson M. The AMP-activated/SNF1 protein kinase subfamily: metabolic sensors of the eukaryotic cell? Annu Rev Biochem 1998; 67:821–855.

98. Kemp BE, Mitchelhill KI, Stapleton D, et al. Dealing with energy demand: the AMP-activated protein kinase. Trends Biochem Sci 1999; 24(1):22–25.

99. Zong H, Ren JM, Young LH, et al. AMP kinase is required for mitochondrial biogenesis in skeletal muscle in response to chronic energy deprivation. Proc Natl Acad Sci U S A 2002; 99(25):15983–15987.

100. Winder WW, Hardie DG. AMP-activated protein kinase, a metabolic master switch: possible roles in type 2 diabetes. Am J Physiol 1999; 277(1 Pt 1):E1–E10.

101. Mu J, Brozinick JT Jr, Valladares O, et al. Mol Cell 2002; 7:1085.

102. Minokoshi Y, Kim YB, Peroni OD, et al. Leptin stimulates fatty-acid oxidation by activating AMP-activated protein kinase. Nature 2002; 415(6869):339–343.

103. Tomas E, Tsao TS, Saha AK, et al. Enhanced muscle fat oxidation and glucose transport by ACRP30 globular domain: acetyl-CoA carboxylase inhibition and AMP-activated protein kinase activation. Proc Natl Acad Sci U S A, 2002; 99(25):16309–16313.

104. Yamauchi T, Kamon J, Minokoshi Y, et al. Nat Med 2002; 8:1288.

105. Londos C, Brasaemle DL, Schultz CJ, et al. On the control of lipolysis in adipocytes. Ann N Y Acad Sci 1999; 892:155–168

106. Holm C, Osterlund T, Laurell H et al. Molecular mechanisms regulating hormone-sensitive lipase and lipolysis. Annu Rev Nutr 2000;20:365–393.

107. Garton AJ, Campbell DG, Carling D et al. Phosphorylation of bovine hormone-sensitive lipase by the AMP-activated protein kinase. A possible antilipolytic mechanism. Eur J Biochem 1989;179(1):249–254.

108. Bergeron R, Russell RR III, Young LH, et al. Am J Physiol 1999; 276:E938.

109. Hayashi T, Wojtaszewski JF, Goodyear LJ. Exercise regulation of glucose transport in skeletal muscle. Am J Physiol 1997; 273(6 Pt 1):E1039–E1051.

110. Merrill GF, Kurth EJ, Hardie DG, et al. AICA riboside increases AMP-activated protein kinase, fatty acid oxidation, and glucose uptake in rat muscle. Am J Physiol 1997;273(6 Pt 1):E1107–E1112

111. Salt IP, Connell JM, Gould GW. 5-aminoimidazole-4-carboxamide ribonucleoside (AICAR) inhibits insulin-stimulated glucose transport in 3T3-L1 adipocytes. Diabetes 2000 49(10):1649–1656.

112. Sullivan JE, Brocklehurst KJ, Marley AE, et al. Inhibition of lipolysis and lipogenesis in isolated rat adipocytes with AICAR, a cell-permeable activator of AMP-activated protein kinase. FEBS Lett 1994; 353(1):33–36.

113. Corton JM, Gillespie JG, Hawley SA, et al. 5-aminoimidazole-4-carboxamide ribonucleoside. A specific method for activating AMP-activated protein kinase in intact cells? Eur J Biochem 1995 229(2):558–565.

114. Moule SK, Denton RM. The activation of p38 MAPK by the beta-adrenergic agonist isoproterenol in rat epididymal fat cells. FEBS Lett 1998; 439(3):287–290.

115. Yin W, Mu J, Birnbaum MJ. Role of AMP-activated protein kinase in cyclic AMP-dependent lipolysis In 3T3-L1 adipocytes. J Biol Chem 2003; 278(44):43074–43080.

116. Rault S, Lancelot J-C, Kopp M, et al. PCT Patent WO20040439572004. Chem Abstr 2004; 140:375173.

117. Kim MS, Park JY, Namkoong C, et al. Anti-obesity effects of alpha-lipoic acid mediated by suppression of hypothalamic AMP-activated protein kinase. Nat Med 2004; 10(7):727–733.

118. Heymsfield SB, Greenberg AS, Fujioka K, et al. Recombinant leptin for weight loss in obese and lean adults: a randomized, controlled, dose-escalation trial. JAMA 1999 282(16):1568–1575.

119. Larsen TM, Toubro S, van Baak MA, et al. Effect of a 28-d treatment with L-796568, a novel beta(3)-adrenergic receptor agonist, on energy expenditure and body composition in obese men. Am J Clin Nutr 2002 76(4):780–788.

9

Reducing the Burden of Diabetic Vascular Complications

Mark E. Cooper and Michael Brownlee

*JDRF Einstein Centre for Diabetic Complications,
Diabetes and Metabolism Division, Baker Heart Research Institute,
Melbourne, Victoria, Australia*

OVERVIEW

The major burdens of diabetic vascular complications are debilitating morbidity and increased mortality. For people with both type 1 and type 2 diabetes, reduced quality of life and shortened lifespan are consequences of both the classical microvascular complications of retinopathy and nephropathy, and accelerated macrovascular disease. Fortunately, the outlook for these complications has improved over the last 20 years, with more precisely, timed laser photocoagulation for vision-threatening retinopathy, more rigorous management of blood pressure in those with or at risk of renal disease, including widespread use of agents which interrupt the renin–angiotensin system (RAS), and more intensive risk factor reduction, particularly liberal use of lipid lowering agents in this high-risk population for cardiovascular disease. With increasing elucidation of the underlying causes of diabetic complications (1) it is predicted that over the next two decades even better therapeutic strategies will be implemented to not only treat but also to retard and prevent the development of diabetic vascular complications.

DIABETIC RETINOPATHY

Diabetic retinopathy remains the leading cause of blindness in the working population. After 15 years of type 1 diabetes, more than 80% of individuals will have evidence of retinal disease and up to 25% are at risk of proliferative retinopathy (2). Diabetic retinopathy is characterized by progressive alterations in the retinal microvasculature, including pericyte loss, basement membrane thickening, and changes in retinal blood flow (3). This is followed by the appearance of microaneurysms (4). These microvascular changes lead to areas of retinal nonperfusion, increased microvascular permeability, and pathologic intraocular proliferation of retinal vessels. Neovascularization, the hallmark of proliferative diabetic retinopathy , and macular edema secondary to increased permeability, can both result in severe and permanent visual loss. Macular edema appears to be more prevalent in type 2 diabetes. Now, with appropriate medical and ophthalmologic care, more than 90% of visual loss resulting from proliferative diabetic retinopathy can be prevented. Treatment of macular edema, however, is not yet as efficacious.

DIABETIC NEPHROPATHY

Diabetic nephropathy is characterized by hypertension, proteinuria, and declining renal function (5). It remains the major cause of end-stage renal failure in the Western World, accounting in some countries for more than 50% of patients requiring dialysis and/or renal transplantation. Fortunately, this life-threatening condition only occurs in a minority of patients and its incidence appears to be on the decrease. The reason for this apparent reduction in the proportion of diabetic subjects developing overt renal disease, remains unexplained (6). Injury to the kidney in diabetes affects not only the glomerulus but also tubules and the interstitium (7). In the glomerulus, all three major cell types, the podocyte (glomerular epithelial cell), the mesangial cell, and the endothelial cell, appear to be damaged. The classical morphological changes include mesangial matrix expansion, glomerular basement membrane thickening, and tubulointerstitial fibrosis (8). The natural history of nephropathy has been particularly well characterized in type 1 diabetes (9). This includes the initial hyperfiltration/hypertrophy phase where there is an increase in the glomerular filtration rate in association with renal and in particular glomerular hypertrophy. This is followed by a second phase, in which renal morphological changes occur without an increase in urinary albumin excretion. This is followed by the incipient nephropathy stage with modest elevations in urinary albumin excretion, known as "microalbuminuria," generally with normal renal function (9). In the majority of patients with microalbuminuria, the nephropathic process progresses to the overt stage with further increases in systemic blood pressure, increasing proteinuria and a progressively declining glomerular filtration rate. Finally, often after 20 years of diabetes, the disease progresses to end-stage renal failure. Fortunately, early and aggressive intensive glycemic control and early introduction of antihypertensive agents that interrupt the RAS appear to delay the onset of microalbuminuria and overt renal disease in type 1 diabetes (10). Similar benefits from optimized glycemic control and blood pressure control have also been demonstrated in type 2 diabetes. Although aggressive therapy can double the time until dialysis or kidney transplantation is needed, once on dialysis, the survival rate for people with diabetes remains half that of people without diabetes.

CARDIOVASCULAR DISEASE

Cardiovascular disease represents the major burden of complications in both forms of diabetes. Indeed, even in type 1 diabetes, the major cause of reduced lifespan is cardiovascular disease. All type 1 diabetic patients in a recent study had significant coronary artery atheroma by their early 40s, and the severity was correlated with HbA1c levels (11). In type 1 patients with persistent proteinuria due to diabetic nephropathy, the risk of coronary disease is nearly 15 times higher than in those without proteinuria (12). Pathologically, atherosclerosis in diabetes resembles macrovascular disease in people without diabetes, but is more extensive and progresses more rapidly. People with diabetes have more rapidly progressive and extensive coronary artery disease, with a greater incidence of multivessel disease and a greater number of diseased vessel segments than do people without diabetes. Although dyslipidemia and hypertension occur with greater frequency in type 2 diabetic populations, there is still excess risk of atherosclerosis after adjusting for these other risk factors. In fact, diabetes itself is now considered a heart attack equivalent, since the risk of myocardial infarction in this population has been reported to be the same as that for nondiabetic individuals who have already suffered a myocardial infarction (13).

The underlying explanations for the earlier onset and more diffuse nature of atherosclerosis in diabetes remain to be fully delineated. Indeed, it is not known if atherosclerosis in diabetes represents an accelerated form of the disease or is a specific form of this disorder. It is already evident that many of the pathways induced by hyperglycemia, such as increased reactive oxygen species generation, advanced glycation end-product accumulation, and local activation of the RAS are implicated in the vascular changes seen in diabetes (14,15).

Mortality from diabetic heart disease is not limited to premature atherosclerosis presenting clinically as ischemic heart disease, but is also due to an increased risk of heart failure. Although initially the two- to threefold increase in heart failure seen in diabetes was attributed to the high-atherosclerotic burden, it is now considered that there may be a diabetes-specific "cardiomyopathy" (16) characterized by abnormalities in mitochondrial function, diastolic dysfunction, and cardiac fibrosis (17). This area of research has been relatively neglected, but with increasing understanding of mitochondrial dysfunction and prosclerotic pathways associated with the hyperglycemic milieu, it is likely that new advances in this field will be made over the next decade.

PATHOGENESIS OF DIABETIC VASCULAR COMPLICATIONS

It is clearly evident from studies in both type 1 and type 2 diabetes that the two clinical features most closely linked to the development of diabetic microvascular complications are poor glycemic control and elevated blood pressure (18,19), while lipoprotein abnormalities, as well as elevated blood pressure and poor glycemic control, are linked to the development of diabetic macrovascular complications. These clinical clues have greatly assisted in delineating at the biochemical, molecular, and cellular levels, how glucose and increased blood pressure, both systemic and local, promote the development and progression of end-organ injury. Cells damaged by diabetes are those that cannot prevent intracellular hyperglycemia by down-regulating their rate of glucose transport in the face of systemic hyperglycemia (20). Intracellular hyperglycemia is a critical stimulus, activating key signaling pathways to induce expression of cytokines and other mediators, ultimately leading to organ damage (1). Historically, the first pathway to be characterized linking glucose to end-organ injury was the polyol pathway (21). In spite of its role in diabetic complications being first investigated, almost 40 years ago, inhibition of polyol accumulation, despite the development of aldose reductase inhibitors, has not ultimately been clinically efficacious.

Another glucose-dependent pathway is the biochemical process of advanced glycation (22). Via the generation of early glycated products and intermediates such as methylglyoxal and 3-deoxyglucosone, a range of long-lived, glucose-induced modifications of proteins, lipids, and nucleic acids results in a family of diverse chemical moieties known as advanced glycated end-products (AGEs) (Fig. 1). Some of AGEs interact with a range of binding proteins, the best characterized being the receptor for AGE (RAGE) (23), while others directly affect the function of intracellular proteins. The AGE/RAGE interaction activates a range of intracellular signaling pathways, as well as promoting expression of growth factors and proinflammatory molecules, leading to end-organ injury. Different therapeutic approaches have been considered to inhibit the deleterious effects of these AGEs (24). They include inhibitors of AGE formation such as aminoguanidine (25), thiazolium compounds that are postulated to cleave pre-formed AGEs (26), inhibitors of the AGE/RAGE interaction such as soluble RAGE (14), and more recently small molecules that act as antagonists to the receptor. Despite a large body of research as well as clinical trials with several of these putative AGE inhibitors, none has yet been recommended for routine clinical practice. This is due to a number of factors including side effects and inadequate clinical efficacy in clinical trials such as the ACTION-1 trial (27).

High intracellular glucose also increases the formation of diacylglycerol, which then activates various isoforms of the enzyme, protein kinase C (PKC)(1). Furthermore, it is likely that other glucose-derived products such as polyols and AGEs also activate PKC (28,29). Although mammalian cells express at least 12 different isoforms, in the setting of diabetes most interest has focused on the α and β1/β2 isoforms (30). It remains to be determined which isoforms predominate in the diabetic context but studies from the Joslin Diabetes Center have emphasized the role of the β isoform (30). Indeed, this research led to the development of a relatively specific PKC-β–isoform inhibitor, LY 333531, now known as ruboxistaurin (31). Initial experimental studies first on retinopathy and then nephropathy

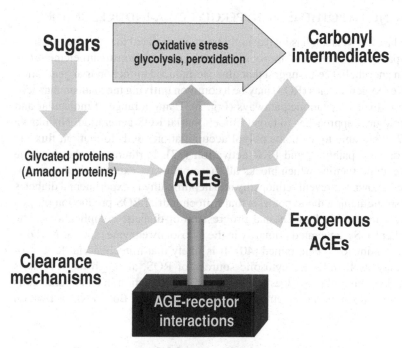

Figure 1 Potential sources and fate of advanced glycated endproducts (AGEs).

provided evidence of an end-organ protective role for this compound (31). Subsequently, relatively large clinical trials have suggested moderate benefit in diabetic macular edema but not proliferative retinopathy. (32). A role for ruboxistaurin in other complications such as nephropathy and neuropathy is even less well delineated (33).

Other researchers have suggested that other PKC isoforms such as PKC-α may play a more important role in nonretinal complications. Indeed, in studies performed in PKC-α knockout mice, induction of diabetes was associated with less renal injury including less albuminuria, in association with reduced renal expression of vascular endothelial growth factor (34). Furthermore, there was a lack of depletion of the slit pore protein, nephrin, which is implicated in the trans-glomerular permeability of albumin in these PKC-α knockout mice (35).

Finally, the other major intracellular glucose-dependent pathway considered to have a role in diabetic complications is the hexosamine pathway (1). Increased glucose flux through this pathway via the enzyme, glutamine fructose-6-phosphate aminotransferase, has been shown to enhance renal extracellular matrix accumulation (36). Unfortunately, a lack of specific inhibitors of enzymes involved in this pathway has made it difficult to determine its relative importance in diabetic complications.

A UNIFYING HYPOTHESIS OF HYPERGLYCEMIA-INDUCED INJURY

Over the last few years, it has increasingly been appreciated that the four glucose-induced pathways referred to above, may have a common upstream element (1). Studies in endothelial cells suggest that glucose-induced mitochondrial generation of reactive oxygen species (ROS) may be a common unifying mechanism that activates these diverse metabolic pathways (Fig. 2). Using a range of molecular and pharmacological approaches to target mitochondrial ROS generation, Nishikawa et al. (37) were able to attenuate polyol accumulation, AGE formation, flux via the hexosamine pathway, and PKC activation (37). Furthermore, the thiamine derivative, benfotiamine which blocks all these pathways except polyol accumulation, was shown to prevent retinopathy and nephropathy in experimental diabetes (38,39), strengthening the hypothesis that mitochondrial ROS production plays a central role in the development and progression of diabetic complications. The role of other ROSs, generated primarily in the cytosol by enzymes such as NADPH oxidase, remains to be determined (40). It is likely that mitochondrial ROS production may itself influence cytosolic sources of ROS, although the reverse is unlikely, since high glucose does not induce ROS production in endothelial cells lacking the mitochondrial electron transport chain (20). Both PKC activation

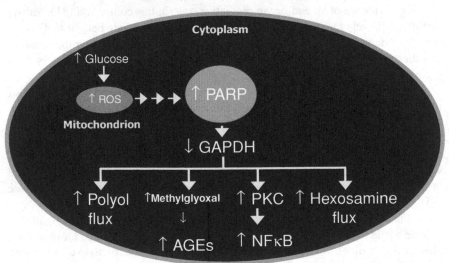

Figure 2 A unifying hypothesis proposed and validated by Brownlee and colleagues that emphasizes the central role of mitochondrial reactive oxygen species generation in the development of hyperglycemia-induced organ injury. *Source*: Adapted from Refs. 1, 37.

and the AGE/RAGE interaction appear to activate NADPH oxidase (41), further enhancing ROS generation and thus promoting end-organ injury. Over the next decade diabetes-induced ROS generation will be further characterized and investigators will be in a better position to rationally design new strategies to specifically inhibit local ROS generation as an approach to prevention of complications.

VASOACTIVE HORMONE PATHWAYS

Although most researchers have focused on glucose-induced pathways in diabetic complications, it is clear that other pathways, particularly those related to regulation of blood pressure, also play an important role (42). Most interest has been on the vasoactive hormone pathway known as the renin-angiotensin system (RAS), which is essentially a cascade of enzymatic reactions leading to the generation of the powerful vasoconstrictor and trophic hormone, angiotensin II (AII). Indeed, more than 20 years ago, Brenner's group demonstrated in normotensive diabetic rats that a reduction in intraglomerular pressure by inhibition of angiotensin converting enzyme (ACE) reduced albuminuria and led to less renal structural injury (43). These beneficial effects, subsequently reproduced by AII receptor antagonists (44), were initially attributed to their hemodynamic effects on both glomerular and systemic hypertension. However, it is now appreciated that these drugs have many other effects, including suppression of a range of AII-mediated nonhemodynamic actions. These include a reduction in expression of various growth factors, reduced signaling by key mediators of injury including PKC, MAP kinase, and NF-κB, and effects on other pathways such as the advanced glycation pathway. Indeed, ACE inhibitors have been shown to not only inhibit AGE formation but to modulate expression of soluble RAGE, an endogenous antagonist to the AGE/RAGE interaction (45). These effects may reflect the ability of agents which interrupt the RAS to reduce ROS formation (46). It is likely that other vasoactive hormones also play a role, including vasoconstrictors such as endothelin and urotensin II. This area of research continues to be actively pursued; with the added benefit various nonpeptide antagonists of these vasoactive pathways are already available to be employed.

INTERACTIONS BETWEEN HEMODYNAMIC AND METABOLIC PATHWAYS

As outlined above, there appear to be important interactions among the various pathways implicated in diabetic complications. A number of metabolic and hemodynamic pathways have been described (Fig. 3) which appear to confer end-organ effects via common signaling pathways such as PKC and NF-κB (42). However, recent studies suggest that metabolic mediators such as AGEs and hemodynamic mediators including AII directly influence each other (47). For example, infusion of AII promotes the formation of AGEs, and this effect can be attenuated by AII receptor antagonists. Furthermore, AGEs can directly modulate various components of the RAS including increasing AT1 receptor and ACE expression. This

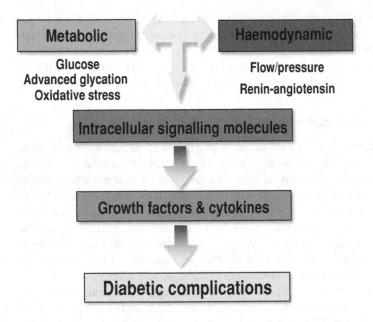

Figure 3 Potential interactions between hemodynamic and metabolic pathways in promoting the development of diabetic complications. *Source*: From Ref. 42.

bidirectional effect of AII and AGEs can be considered an important mechanism whereby hemodynamic and metabolic stimuli directly interact with each other to perpetuate and amplify end-organ injury. Some of these effects may reflect the ability of ACE inhibitors to reduce ROS formation. It has also been suggested that high blood pressure increases the expression of glucose transporters (48), thereby increasing intracellular glucose concentrations. The clinical observations that unilateral stenosis of the ophthalmic artery prevents diabetic retinopathy in the affected eye and that unilateral renal artery stenosis prevents diabetic glomerular disease in the affected kidney are consistent with this idea. In the future, optimal organ protection in diabetes may depend on targeting the key upstream mechanism of injury, such as mitochondrial ROS production (1). Currently, however, a regimen of multiple drugs that inhibits each of the separate pathways is regarded as the optimal strategy. This has been employed to reduce injury in both normotensive and hypertensive models of diabetic nephropathy. Indeed, both blockade of the RAS and reduction in tissue AGE accumulation appear to confer superior renoprotection than monotherapy (49,50).

HYPERGLYCEMIC MEMORY

One of the major unresolved clinical issues in the field of diabetic complications is "hyperglycemic memory." Based on a follow-up of the Diabetes Control and

Complications Trial (DCCT) known as the Epidemiology of Diabetes Interventions and Complications (EDIC) study, it has become apparent that subjects in the DCCT with long-term exposure to hyperglycemia remained more susceptible to complications despite subsequent lowering of hyperglycemia (51). In contrast, lower levels of glycemia made subjects more resistant to damage from subsequent higher levels. How could a finite period of different degrees of hyperglycemia result in different susceptibilities to complications? The discovery of the molecular and cellular basis of both types of metabolic memory is urgently needed so that solutions can be designed to prevent or reverse the damaging "memory" of prior hyperglycemia, and to mimic or induce the protective "memory" of lower levels of glucose.

In studies examining the long-term cardiovascular events in the DCCT/EDIC cohort, it has been postulated that AGEs may represent a biochemical mechanism whereby cumulative effects of more severe hyperglycemia lead to end-organ injury years after better control is established (52). This does not explain the protective type of hyperglycemic memory and likely does not fully explain the damage of "hyperglycemic memory." Recent discoveries in molecular biology, particularly in the fields of genetics and epigenetics, will lead to new advances and a better understanding of the mechanisms that confer both types of metabolic memory. Indeed, it has been postulated that glucose-induced superoxide production may induce mutations in mitochondrial DNA leading to defective encoding of electron transport complex subunits, which would then result in ongoing enhanced superoxide production (53). This would promote the pathways described earlier even in the absence of hyperglycemia. On the other hand, exposure to lower levels of hyperglycemia and ROS may cause compensatory changes such as increased antioxidant gene expression, which in response to lower glucose levels may explain the protective type of hyperglycemic memory.

CLINICAL TRIALS

Diabetic microvascular complications occur only in a minority of subjects and take many years to appear; and therefore, it has been difficult to design adequately powered clinical trials to determine if certain treatments confer adequate end-organ protection. Because of this, most studies have been secondary rather than primary prevention studies. For example, the RENAAL study, which demonstrated renoprotection in type 2 diabetes subjects with advanced renal disease, had to recruit more than 1500 subjects with existing nephropathy and follow them up for more than 3 years (54). With current treatments for retinopathy and nephropathy, such as laser photocoagulation and RAS blockade, respectively, now considered routine and unethical to withhold in clinical trials, the rates of progression of complications are now even slower, further reducing the power of trials. Over the last few years, several large studies have been performed to explore the potential role of the PKC inhibitor, ruboxistaurin (32,33). These trials, both retinal and renal, have had to be performed with subjects concomitantly receiving state-of-the-art medical care. Despite positive findings from some of the studies, the FDA has not approved this agent for diabetic retinopathy and has requested a further very large clinical study for more than at least 3 years before further considering registration of this drug. With respect to nephropathy, the FDA currently only recognizes a reduction in the development of end-stage renal failure as a reason to register a drug for renoprotection. This endpoint is particularly difficult to achieve with the widespread use of RAS blockers, which reduce the rate of decline in renal function. It is hoped that over the next few years surrogate markers of renal injury such as albuminuria will be accepted, thus enhancing the power of the clinical trials and allowing investigators to recruit fewer patients and to follow them for shorter periods.

The expense of clinical trials in this area limits their conduct to major pharmaceutical companies. This has resulted in a lack of adequate clinical investigation of agents, which, although potentially very useful, would not be financially viable to develop. One example is benfotiamine, which has been shown experimentally to reduce retinal and renal injury in diabetes (38,39). Indeed, in various small studies of diabetic neuropathy, this drug appears to show promise (55). Alternative approaches to traditional clinical trials are needed to evaluate such agents clinically, to increase the armamentarium of clinicians in treating and preventing diabetic complications.

FUTURE PERSPECTIVES

It still remains to be determined, if all vascular complications should be treated in a similar manner. It is possible that renal disease may be best managed by focusing on interruption of blood pressure-dependent pathways, whereas other complications may require increased focus on glucose-dependent pathways. Currently, aggressive glycemic control appears to be effective in slowing down microvascular complications in both type 1 and type 2 diabetes (18), whereas macrovascular disease has been more difficult to retard with intensified insulin therapy. The explanation for this phenomenon remains to be determined. It is possible that comorbid factors such as dyslipidemia and hypertension may be more important than glucose, although at this stage this cannot be directly tested because current strategies to normalize hyperglycemia in type 1 or type 2 diabetes are not particularly effective. Indeed, it is likely that glucose-induced pathways play a key role in diabetic macrovascular complications, with the most recent follow-up studies of the DCCT/EDIC demonstrating a clear-cut reduction in carotid intima-media thickness, coronary artery calcification, and cardiovascular events with intensive glycemic control (52,56). Therefore, it is likely that over the next decade, with improved understanding of how glucose confers its deleterious effects on the macro as well as the microvasculature, clinicians will be given the tools to reduce the burden associated with diabetic complications. At present, though, it should be emphasized that while intensive treatment of hyperglycemia, hypertension, dyslipidemia, and urinary albumin excretion can reduce the risk of cardiovascular disease by up to 50% in type 2 diabetes (57,58), perhaps only 7% of all patients currently meet goals set by the American Diabetes Association for HbA1c, blood pressure, and LDL-cholesterol levels (59). Since the majority of people with diabetes die from coronary heart disease, widespread implementation of these goals by clinicians would reduce the burden of diabetic vascular complications substantially.

REFERENCES

1. Brownlee M. Biochemistry and molecular cell biology of diabetic complications. Nature 2001; 414:813–820.
2. Roy MS, Klein R, O'Colmain BJ, et al. The prevalence of diabetic retinopathy among adult type 1 diabetic persons in the United States. Arch Ophthalmol 2004; 122:546–551.
3. Bursell SE, Clermont AC, Kinsley BT, et al. Retinal blood flow changes in patients with insulin-dependent diabetes mellitus and no diabetic retinopathy. Invest Ophthalmol Vis Sci 1996; 37:886–897.
4. Stitt AW, Gardiner TA, Archer DB. Histological and ultrastructural investigation of retinal microaneurysm development in diabetic patients. Br J Ophthalmol 1995; 79:362–367.
5. Cooper ME. Pathogenesis, prevention, and treatment of diabetic nephropathy. Lancet 1998; 352:213–219.
6. Cooper ME. Is diabetic nephropathy disappearing from clinical practice? Pediatr Diabetes 2006; 7:237–238.
7. Gilbert RE, Cooper ME. The tubulointerstitium in progressive diabetic kidney disease: More than an aftermath of glomerular injury? [Review]. Kidney Internat 1999; 56:1627–1637.
8. Mauer S, Steffes M, Ellis E, et al. Structural-functional relationships in diabetic nephropathy. J Clin Invest 1984; 74:1143–1155.
9. Mogensen CE, Christensen C K, Vittinghus E. The stages in diabetic renal disease. With emphasis in the stage of incipient diabetic nephropathy. Diabetes 1983; 32:64–78.
10. Cooper ME, Jandeleit-Dahm K, Thomas MC. Targets to retard the progression of diabetic nephropathy. Kidney Int 2005; 68:1439–1445.
11. Larsen J, Brekke M, Sandvik L, et al. Silent coronary atheromatosis in type 1 diabetic patients and its relation to long-term glycemic control. Diabetes 2002; 51:2637–2641.
12. Borch-Johnsen K, Andersen PK, Deckert T. The effect of proteinuria on relative mortality in type 1 (insulin-dependent) diabetes mellitus. Diabetologia 1985;28:590–596.
13. Haffner SM, Lehto S, Ronnemaa T, et al. Mortality from coronary heart disease in subjects with type 2 diabetes and in nondiabetic subjects with and without prior myocardial infarction. N Engl J Med 1998; 339:229–234.
14. Bucciarelli LG, Wendt T, Qu W, et al RAGE blockade stabilizes established atherosclerosis in diabetic apolipoprotein E-null mice. Circulation 2002; 106:2827–2835.

15. Candido R, Jandeleit-Dahm KA, Cao Z, et al. Prevention of accelerated atherosclerosis by angiotensin-converting enzyme inhibition in diabetic apolipoprotein E-deficient mice. Circulation 2002; 106:246–253.

16. Poornima IG, Parikh P, Shannon RP. Diabetic cardiomyopathy: The search for a unifying hypothesis. Circ Res 2006; 98:596–605.

17. Candido R, Forbes JM, Thomas MC, et al. A breaker of advanced glycation end products attenuates diabetes-induced myocardial structural changes. Circ Res 2003; 92:785–792.

18. Diabetes Control and Complications Trial Research Group. The effect of intensive treatment on the development and progression of long-term complications in insulin-dependent diabetes mellitus. N Engl J Med 1993; 329:977–986.

19. Adler AI, Stratton IM, Neil HAW, et al. Association of systolic blood pressure with macrovascular and microvascular complications of type 2 diabetes (UKPDS 36): Prospective observational study. Br Med J 2000; 321:412–419.

20. Brownlee M. The pathobiology of diabetic complications: A unifying mechanism. Diabetes 2005; 54:1615–1625.

21. King GL, Brownlee M. The cellular and molecular mechanisms of diabetic complications. Endocrinol Metab Clin North Am 1996; 25:255–270.

22. Brownlee M. Lilly Lecture 1993. Glycation and diabetic complications. Diabetes 1994; 43:836–841.

23. Neeper M, Schmidt AM, Brett J, et al. Cloning and expression of a cell surface receptor for advanced glycosylation end products of proteins. J Biol Chem 1992; 267:14998–15004.

24. Goldin A, Beckman JA, Schmidt AM, et al. Advanced glycation end products: Sparking the development of diabetic vascular injury. Circulation 2006; 114:597–605.

25. Brownlee M, Vlassara H, Kooney A, et al. Aminoguanidine prevents diabetes-induced arterial wall protein cross-linking. Science 1986; 232:1629–1632.

26. Vasan S, Zhang X, Zhang X, et al. An agent cleaving glucose-derived protein crosslinks in vitro and in vivo. Nature 1996; 382:275–278.

27. Bolton WK, Cattran DC, Williams ME, et al. Randomized trial of an inhibitor of formation of advanced glycation end products in diabetic nephropathy. Am J Nephrol 2004; 24:32–40.

28. Kapor-Drezgic J, Zhou X, Babazono T, et al. Effect of high glucose on mesangial cell protein kinase C-delta and -epsilon is polyol pathway-dependent. J Am Soc Nephrol 1999; 10:1193–1203.

29. Scivittaro V, Ganz MB, Weiss MF. AGEs induce oxidative stress and activate protein kinase C-beta(II) in neonatal mesangial cells. Am J Physiol Renal Physiol 2000; 278:F676–683.

30. Sheetz MJ, King GL. Molecular understanding of hyperglycemia's adverse effects for diabetic complications. JAMA 2002; 288:2579–2588.

31. Ishii H, Jirousek MR, Koya D, et al. Amelioration of vascular dysfunctions in diabetic rats by an oral PKC beta inhibitor. Science 1996; 272:728–731.

32. Aiello LP, Davis MD, Girach A, et al. Effect of ruboxistaurin on visual loss in patients with diabetic retinopathy. Ophthalmology 2006; 113:2221–2230.

33. Tuttle KR, Bakris GL, Toto RD, et al. The effect of ruboxistaurin on nephropathy in type 2 diabetes. Diabetes Care 2005; 28:2686–2690.

34. Menne J, Park JK, Boehne M, et al. Diminished loss of proteoglycans and lack of albuminuria in protein kinase C-alpha-deficient diabetic mice. Diabetes 2004; 53:2101–2109.

35. Menne J, Meier M, Park JK, et al. Nephrin loss in experimental diabetic nephropathy is prevented by deletion of protein kinase C-alpha signaling in-vivo. Kidney Int 2006; 70:1456–1462.

36. Kolm-Litty V, Sauer U, Nerlich A, et al. High glucose-induced transforming growth factor beta1 production is mediated by the hexosamine pathway in porcine glomerular mesangial cells. J Clin Invest 1998; 101:160–169.

37. Nishikawa T, Edelstein D, Du XL, et al. Normalizing mitochondrial superoxide production blocks three pathways of hyperglycemic damage. Nature 2000; 404:787–790.

38. Hammes HP, Du X, Edelstein D, et al. Benfotiamine blocks three major pathways of hyperglycemic damage and prevents experimental diabetic retinopathy. Nat Med 2003; 9:294–299.

39. Babaei-Jadidi R, Karachalias N, Ahmed N, et al. Prevention of incipient diabetic nephropathy by high-dose thiamine and benfotiamine. Diabetes 2003; 52:2110–2120.

40. Gorin Y, Block K, Hernandez J, et al. Nox4 NAD(P)H oxidase mediates hypertrophy and fibronectin expression in the diabetic kidney. J Biol Chem 2005; 280:39616–39626.

41. Wautier MP, Chappey O, Corda S, et al. Activation of NADPH oxidase by AGE links oxidant stress to altered gene expression via RAGE. Am J Physiol Endocrinol Metab 2001; 280:E685–E694.

42. Cooper ME. Interaction of metabolic and haemodynamic factors in mediating experimental diabetic nephropathy. Diabetologia 2001; 44:1957–1972.

43. Zatz R, Dunn BR, Meyer TW, et al. Prevention of diabetic glomerulopathy by pharmacological amelioration of glomerular capillary hypertension. J Clin Invest 1986; 77:1925–1930.

44. Allen TJ, Cao Z, Youssef S, et al. The role of angiotensin II and bradykinin in experimental diabetic nephropathy: functional and structural studies. Diabetes 1997; 46:1612–1618.

45. Forbes JM, Thorpe SR, Thallas-Bonke V, et al. Modulation of soluble receptor for advanced glycation end products by angiotensin-converting enzyme-1 inhibition in diabetic nephropathy. J Am Soc Nephrol 2005; 16:2363–2372.

46. Dandona P, Kumar V, Aljada A, et al. Angiotensin II receptor blocker valsartan suppresses reactive oxygen species generation in leukocytes, nuclear factor-kappa B, in mononuclear cells of normal subjects: Evidence of an anti-inflammatory action. J Clin Endocrinol Metab 2003; 88:4496–4501.

47. Thomas MC, Tikellis C, Burns WM, et al. Interactions between renin angiotensin system and advanced glycation in the kidney. J Am Soc Nephrol 2005; 16:2976–2984.

48. Gnudi L, Viberti G, Raij L, et al. GLUT-1 overexpression: Link between hemodynamic and metabolic factors in glomerular injury? Hypertension 2003; 42:19–24.

49. Davis BJ, Forbes JM, Thomas MC, et al. Superior renoprotective effects of combination therapy with ACE and AGE inhibition in the diabetic spontaneously hypertensive rat. Diabetologia 2004; 47:89–97.

50. Coughlan MT, Thallas-Bonke V, Pete J, et al. Combination therapy with the AGE cross-link breaker, alagebrium, and angiotensin converting enzyme inhibitors in diabetes: Synergy or redundancy? Endocrinology 2007; 148:886–895.

51. Writing Team for the Diabetes Control and Complications Trial/Epidemiology of Diabetes Interventions and Complications Research Group. Effect of intensive therapy on the microvascular complications of type 1 diabetes mellitus. JAMA 2002; 287:2563–2569.

52. Nathan DM, Lachin J, Cleary P, et al. Intensive diabetes therapy and carotid intima-media thickness in type 1 diabetes mellitus. N Engl J Med 2003;348:2294–2303.

53. Ballinger SW, Patterson C, Yan CN, et al. Hydrogen peroxide- and peroxynitrite-induced mitochondrial DNA damage and dysfunction in vascular endothelial and smooth muscle cells. Circ Res 2000; 86:960–966.

54. Brenner BM, Cooper ME, de Zeeuw D, et al. Effects of losartan on renal and cardiovascular outcomes in patients with type 2 diabetes and nephropathy. N Engl J Med 2001; 345:861–869.

55. Haupt E, Ledermann H, Kopcke W. Benfotiamine in the treatment of diabetic polyneuropathy–A three-week randomized, controlled pilot study (BEDIP study). Int J Clin Pharmacol Ther 2005; 43:71–77.

56. Cleary PA, Orchard TJ, Genuth S, et al. The effect of intensive glycemic treatment on coronary artery calcification in type 1 diabetic participants of the Diabetes Control and Complications Trial/Epidemiology of Diabetes Interventions and Complications (DCCT/EDIC) Study. Diabetes 2006; 55:3556–3565.

57. Gaede P, Vedel P, Larsen N, et al. Multifactorial intervention and cardiovascular disease in patients with type 2 diabetes. N Engl J Med 2003; 348:383–393.

58. Saydah SH, Fradkin J, Cowie CC. Poor control of risk factors for vascular disease among adults with previously diagnosed diabetes. JAMA 2004; 291:335–342.

59. Buse JB, Ginsberg HN, Bakris GL, et al. Primary prevention of cardiovascular diseases in people with diabetes mellitus: A scientific statement from the American Heart Association and the American Diabetes Association. Diabetes Care 2007; 30:162–172.

10

Diabetic Retinopathy: Translating Discoveries to Treatments

Thomas W. Gardner, Gregory R. Jackson, David A. Quillen, and
Ingrid U. Scott

*Departments of Ophthalmology and Cellular and Molecular Physiology,
Pennsylvania State College of Medicine, Hershey, Pennsylvania, U.S.A.*

DIABETIC RETINOPATHY: WHERE ARE WE NOW?

Retinopathy is one of the most dreaded complications of diabetes because blindness is a greater fear than loss of a limb or death (www.lionsclubs.org/EN/content/news_news_release58.shtml). Fortunately, advances in the control of blood pressure, hyperglycemia, and hyperlipidemia have reduced the risk of vision-threatening retinopathy in persons with diabetes in each of the succeeding decades from the 1960s to the 1990s (1,2). Nevertheless, the number of persons with diabetes is expected to double by the year 2030 particularly in the developing world (3,4), so fundamentally new approaches are urgently needed to prevent more visually impaired persons, particularly in countries with limited access to medical care. Diabetic retinopathy has been viewed from a surgical perspective and ophthalmologists have employed destructive photocoagulation using halogen light or laser sources for 50 years (5). Photocoagulation remains the primary treatment for diabetic retinopathy in the 21st century. It effectively reduces the risk of blindness but is destructive, expensive, and can be uncomfortable. Its mechanism of action is similar to that of gamma radiation for tumors; i.e., to destroy diseased tissue. Photocoagulation does not address the metabolic processes that lead to the development retinopathy and vision loss. Many patients are reluctant to undergo the treatment, and those who have already loss vision often do not fully regain their sight.

Vision impairment from diabetes ranges from a difficulty seeing in dim illumination impaired blue or green color sensitivity, or glare, even in patients with normal visual acuity on a standard Snellen eye chart. These symptoms may be due to cataracts or dysfunction of the retina in the absence of overt microangiopathy. When visual acuity drops to the 20/30 to 20/40 range driving, reading, and filling insulin syringes can be difficult. If the visual acuity drops to 20/60-20/80 driving, working, and gainful employment are very difficult. Visual acuity 20/200 (the big "E") or less is deemed "legal blindness" and is a usually a late manifestation of diabetic eye disease. Diabetic eye disease can be very asymmetric so patients can have good vision in one eye and very little or no vision in the other eye. Combined with the added morbidity of peripheral neuropathy, patients with diabetic retinopathy have trouble with a wide variety of sensory inputs and can be frustrated with simple tasks. For example, persons with retinopathy often have dysfunction of the spinal cord posterior columns, and greater risk of falls and fractures (6,7). Taken together, diabetic eye disease is a crucial part of the overall long-term toll inflicted by diabetes and it is important to consider the eye in context of other manifestations.

The original description of diabetic retinopathy by von Graefe in 1856 was based on ophthalmoscopically visible vascular changes in the retina (8), and for the ensuing 150 years diabetic retinopathy has generally considered to be a "microvascular" disorder. The other major chronic complications of diabetes, nephropathy, and peripheral neuropathy, have likewise been considered in this light to form a triad of manifestations that cause clinical disability. The vascular lesions in the retina include the well-known features of microaneurysms, intraretinal hemorrhages, lipid exudates, venous beading, and neovascularization. These vascular features are readily detectable on clinical examination because blood vessels contain pigmented erythrocytes, and with fluorescein angiography. These clinical features have corresponding cellular and histological lesions, including focal areas of endothelial cell perforation in microaneurysms, acellular capillaries, pericyte "ghosts", hemorrhages, and lipid deposits within the retina, basement membrane thickening, and new vessels growing through inner retinal surface into the vitreous gel.

By contrast, the retina (a network) is normally transparent like a window and invisible to standard clinical evaluation methods. For this reason the involvement of the retina by diabetes has received relatively little attention. The retinal parenchyma is comprised of five general classes of cells (9). Neurons (photoreceptors, bipolar cells, horizontal cells, amacrine cells, and ganglion cells) perform the sensory functions that enable vision. Glial cells, including astrocytes and Müller cells, provide essential metabolic support to maintain nutrient supply and waste removal from neuronal metabolism and maintain the extracellular ionic environments needed for action potentials and vision. Microglial cells are resident macrophages within the central nervous system that sense the local environment and respond to metabolic stresses, ranging from infections, to trauma, to retinal detachment. Vascular endothelial cells and pericytes are a fourth class of retinal cells that comprise less than 5% of the total mass or volume of the retina. In fact, the retina has a relative paucity of blood vessels because the hemoglobin would otherwise interfere with light transmission and visual function. A fifth class of cells, the retinal pigment epithelium, interdigitates with and supports the function of photoreceptors. Taken together, even on strictly anatomical basis it is evident that the vascular cells comprise a minority of the retina. Therefore, it is essential to recognize how diabetes impacts the entire retina.

The first recognition of retinal involvement in diabetes was published in the early 1960s (10,11) but these observations received little attention because the trypsin digest method of histologic analysis and fluorescein angiography that were developed contemporaneously corresponded more closely with the clinical picture. Early evidence for functional changes in the retina was provided by Simonsen in 1969 (12), who showed impaired electrical responses to light stimulation (electroretinogram). Bresnick (13,14) provided evidence for the importance of the neural retina 20 years later when he showed electroretinographic (ERG) responses predicted the progression of retinopathy better than did ophthalmoscopic findings. These findings had limited impact on the field because of optimism that laser photocoagulation could prevent vision loss from diabetes, and the cellular changes related to impaired ERG alterations were not understood. Ophthalmologists focused on the needs to save vision in those persons who were at greatest short-term risk and less on long-term prevention of complications, a matter beyond their immediate control. Over the last decade it has become increasingly evident that while laser photocoagulation reduces the risk of blindness, it does not prevent visual impairment and is unappealing to patients.

THE STATE OF THE ART IN DIABETIC RETINOPATHY RESEARCH

Diabetic Retinopathy Is a Neurovascular Disease

The cellular features of early, preclinical diabetic retinopathy have largely been investigated by studies in rodents, including streptozotocin- or alloxan-treated rodents and dogs, genetically altered rodents, and spontaneously diabetic, obese monkeys. Most studies have emphasized leakage, occlusion, or death of endothelial cells and pericytes (15–19). These findings correlate closely with features seen on clinical ophthalmoscopy and fluorescein angiography, including microaneurysms and nonperfused capillaries. These findings do not however, determine the temporal sequence of cellular changes, their cause(s), or the means by which vision is impaired.

By contrast, recent work has revealed involvement of the entire retina and ushered in a new perspective of how diabetes impacts the retina. Numerous clinical and laboratory studies now show clearly that diabetic retinopathy is a neurovascular degeneration or retinal neuropathy, and that all retinal cell types are affected by diabetes. Retinal neurons die by apoptosis (20,21); astrocyte and Müller cell functions are impaired as evidenced by impaired interconversion of glutamate to glutamine (22), cytokine expression (23–25), and reactive gliosis (26,27). Microglial cells in the inner retina become activated (28–30) and are a source of inflammatory cytokines and phagocytose dying neurons, so their involvement in diabetes is similar to other neurodegenerations, such as multiple sclerosis and Parkinson's disease. It is not known currently which of these changes begin first, how alterations in any cell type affects other cells, or how these changes lead to the clinical phenotype or impair visual function.

These findings clearly show that the clinically visible retinal microvascular lesions are only the tip of the diabetic retinopathy iceberg. They also imply the long-held concept of a primary "microvascular" complication incompletely describes the full spectrum of diabetic retinopathy. Diabetes affects the parenchyma of kidneys, nerves, the heart, brain, and even bone. Hence, nephropathy, neuropathy, cerebral dysfunction, cardiomyopathy, and osteopenia involve the whole organ, not merely their respective blood vessels. There are, to the best of our knowledge, no empirical data from animal or human studies that prove the primary impact of diabetes is on the microcirculation. Therefore, the term "microvascular disease" is inadequate, misleading, and should be replaced by a more comprehensive definition of "retinopathy," "nephopathy," and "neuropathy" that includes the full spectrum of functional and structural changes, not just those that are visible to by standard clinical examination. This change in the conceptual framework is needed because after three decades of research, the "microvascular" approach has yielded no Food and Drug Administration-approved treatments for diabetes complications. A protein kinase C beta inhibitor, ruboxistaurin (Arxxant™, Eli Lilly, Indianapolis, IN) reduces the risk of vision loss in persons with diabetes (31–33) but has failed to win Food and Drug Administration approval as of this writing (May, 2007). In fact, protein kinase C ß is expressed throughout the neural retina in normal rat retina (Todd Fox, T. Gardner, unpublished data) so in addition to affecting retinal vascular permeability (34), a PKC ß inhibitor may also directly affect the neural retina. Protein kinase C beta expression increases in retinas of diabetic rats and PKC beta inhibition reduces VEGF-induced retinal vascular permeability and normalizes retinal blood flow changes in diabetic rats and humans (33,35). Indeed, ruboxistaurin reduces the risk of vision loss in patients without thickening of the central macula, as well as those with central macular thickening (32). This observation suggests that ruboxistaurin may work in part by nonvascular mechanisms and/or the patients tested had sub-clinical macular edema.

Taken together, we argue that a more comprehensive view of the impact of diabetes on multiple tissues is more likely to yield improved means to prevent and treat complications. For example, a comprehensive definition of "diabetic retinopathy" would be "functional and structural impairment of the retina due to diabetes." This definition does not limit the concept to the changes that are visible clinically and would allow inclusion of various parameters that might be determined in the future. Similar approaches could be used for renal and nerve involvement.

When Does Diabetic Retinopathy Begin?

In light of the neurovascular concept of diabetic retinopathy we can consider the onset of the disease when retinal function is impaired, rather than when its structure is altered. Numerous animal and human studies have shown that indices of retinal function, including color vision, contrast sensitivity, dark adaptation, and electrical responses change before clinically evident vascular lesions (36,37) Diabetic peripheral neuropathy is diagnosed based on reduced nerve conduction velocities or decreased ability to sense vibrations of a flexible nylon filament. Thus, it is reasonable to consider at least a tentative diagnosis of retinopathy when retinal function, as reflected by ERG responses or the ability to see in dim illumination are impaired, even if the retina appears normal. The clinical implications of this perspective are discussed below.

What Initiates Diabetic Retinopathy?

Most concepts of diabetic retinopathy employ a linear view of events leading from initiation to phenotype. However, in spite of extensive work, it remains unclear which factor(s) in the diabetic milieu actually damage retinal function and structure. Given the complexity of metabolic derangements in diabetes it is exceedingly difficult to parse out the role of a specific metabolic pathway. Most studies have emphasized the roles of excess glucose as the primary metabolic injury and peptide growth factors, such as vascular endothelial growth factor and insulin-like growth factor I as mediators of vascular damage (reviewed in Ref. 38). Recent studies have begun to examine the roles of other key metabolic alterations of diabetes, such as hyperlipidemia, insulin resistance, or insulin deficiency in an integrated fashion to yield information on interactions of various parameters. Indeed, alterations in plasma lipids are closely associated with diabetic macular edema and the risk of vision loss (39,40). Systemic insulin resistance is also a major risk factor for the development of retinopathy and other complications in patients with type 1 and type 2 diabetes (41–44). These findings strongly suggest that the pathogenesis of retinopathy and other complications involves factors beyond simple hyperglycemia-induced vascular changes.

The role of tissue-specific contributions to insulin resistance and that brain-specific insulin resistance leads to neurodegeneration have been revealed with tissue-specific gene deletion studies (45–48), but similar approaches have not yet been employed widely in investigations of diabetic retinopathy. Integrative physiology approaches, such as hyperinsulinemic-euglycemic clamp studies that are standard for investigations of the role of the liver, muscle, and adipose also have yet to be applied to study the retina. Hence, there remains an opportunity to dissect the underlying cause(s) of complications with these techniques.

Recently we suggested a concept of a normal homeostatic equilibrium in which factors that promote retinal cell survival and function outweigh noxious influences that would threaten retinal viability (49) (Fig. 1). This concept assumes

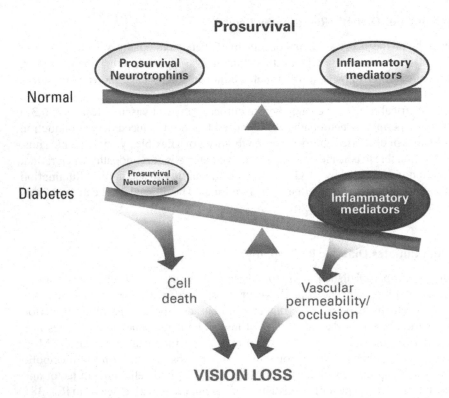

Figure 1   Diabetes disturbs the homeostatic equilibrium of the retina. Under normal conditions there is an equilibrium in which pro-survival and anti-inflammatory stimuli maintain retinal cell survival and function. In diabetes, pro-survival (neurotrophic) inputs may be reduced and pro-inflammatory cytokines, chemokines, and cellular responses increase. Together, these processes accelerate retinal cell death and increase vascular permeability and occlusion, thus impairing vision. Treatments may be directed at augmenting neurotrophic inputs and decreasing pro-inflammatory responses so that repair processes can predominate.

that various hormones, including insulin/IGF-1, brain-derived neurotrophic factor (BDNF), and perhaps VEGF, provide trophic stimuli to maintain retinal neural and vascular cell survival in the postmitotic state. In diabetes, trophic inputs from insulin/IGF-1 receptor (50) or BDNF (51) signaling are impaired, and may induce a physiologic adaptive response to maintain neural cell function and survival when normal rophic inputs are lost. VEGF-stimulated cell survival (and proliferation) is mediated via Akt kinase, as is insulin receptor stimulated cell survival (52). The various "growth factors" up-regulated in the retina in diabetes (38) exert pro-survival effects (53) but when present in high concentrations or for prolonged periods, may also have adverse inflammatory effects, including vascular leakage and proliferation. In this way the normal homeostatic equilibrium shifts to one that leads to cell death and dysfunction. This disequilibrium begins shortly after the onset of diabetes when the retina still appears normal. This concept may be useful to design therapeutic strategies by increasing neuroprotective and decreasing pro-inflammatory factors.

The Role of Visual Function Studies in Understanding of Diabetic Retinopathy

Viewing diabetic retinopathy as a neurovascular disease creates a renewed interest in visual function studies that can play an important role in elucidating the disease mechanisms and validating animal models. A careful characterization of the visual function impairments associated with different diabetic retinopathy stages may provide inferences to the underlying mechanisms and permit evaluation of the validity of current mechanistic hypotheses. For example, diabetic retinopathy is generally thought to predominantly affect the inner retina because the microvascular insults occur to the inner retinal blood supply. However, documented insults to visual function such as impaired adaptation in dark conditions (dark adaptation) are largely attributable to impaired outer retina function including the retinal pigment epithelium and choroidal blood supply. This observation implies that diabetes and diabetic retinopathy may insult the retina in a more generalized fashion than currently believed. Regardless of the cause of this impairment, these results must be reconciled with current mechanistic theories of disease pathogenesis. Information regarding human disease–related visual dysfunction can be used to validate animal models. Comprehensive animal models of diabetic retinopathy and affected patients should exhibit similar visual dysfunction. Models that more closely resemble the phenotypes of human patients are preferred for mechanistic studies and may provide a better platform to predict drug discovery outcomes. Models that lack these characteristic visual function impairments may not generalize as well to humans. Comparisons of phenotypic changes in animal and human models should facilitate more rapid understanding of key pathogenic changes and accelerate discovery and validation of therapeutic targets. A concept of how clinical and animal studies may be integrated is shown in Figure 2.

CURRENT LIMITATIONS IN THE FIELD

Corroboration of Laboratory and Clinical Research

Comprehensive understanding of disease mechanisms and development of curative or preventive strategies is greatly facilitated by the availability of human tissue for biochemical and pathological analysis. Whereas biopsies can be readily obtained from kidneys, nerves, myocardium, and even brain, the retina is unique in that biopsy samples of living tissues are never available. Postmortem eyes are useful for pathological studies and some cellular studies have been reported (23,54,55), but are not useful for biochemical studies because of the interval between death and

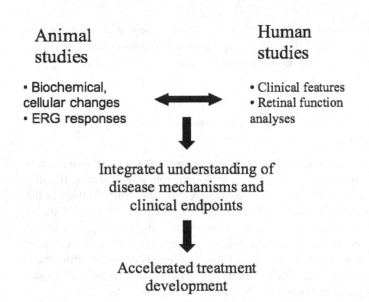

Figure 2 A strategy to integrate clinical and animal studies of diabetic retinopathy. Animal models provide vital information regarding biochemical and cellular processes, and of retinal electroretinographic (ERG) responses but not direct analysis of retinal function. Human studies provide direct measures of cell-layer–specific changes in retinal function that will provide unbiased information about retinal changes in animal models. Together, these complementary approaches can provide an integrated understanding of disease mechanisms and clinical endpoints and accelerate development and implementation of new treatments.

availability for studies. Therefore retinopathy researchers have relied on rodent and canine models that appear to reflect most of the recognized abnormalities of early stage disease. However, they lack maculas and rodents are usually inbred strains devoid of the genetic heterogeneity of humans. Non-human primates have been studied to a limited degree (18,56) but the eyes are not usually available for biopsies. Therefore, while rodent models continue to be used widely it is uncertain how predictive the results may be in humans.

Over 20 different pharmacologic interventions have been shown to reduce some aspect of retinal lesions in rodent models, ranging from inhibitors of aldose reductase, protein kinase C, advanced glycation end-products, VEGF, platelet aggregation, oxidative or nitrative stress, inflammation (steroids, nonsteroidal anti-inflammatory agents, ICAM-1 and TNF blockers, minocycline), and angiotensin 2 receptors. In humans, intensive metabolic control, blood pressure, and lipid lowering are the only interventions with demonstrable efficacy, but at present no complications-specific therapies are available. Thus, it is imperative that transla-tional research be conducted in a coordinated fashion to maximize the chance to achieve benefits for patients.

What Are the Key Research Questions?

The underlying mechanisms that initiate and perpetuate retinopathy remain unclear, partly because so many parameters change in response to this complex metabolic disease. A change in a protein, metabolite, or pathway does not prove that it is causative for the disease since it may also represent a physiologic adaptation or be part of broad-spectrum response. The most secure information currently available regarding diabetic retinopathy is provided by the Diabetes Control and Complications Trial (DCCT) (57), which showed that intensive treatment reduced the risk of retinopathy development and progression. This study has beeen interpreted as demonstrating the role of excess glucose but since the intensive therapy was achieved by more continuous insulin therapy, it might also reasonably be interpreted as an insulin response trial (49). Indeed, the DCCT was not designed or capable of demonstrating the reason for the response (58). Therefore, the first key question is to determine the mechanism and the effect of intensive therapy. Is it due to lowering blood metabolite levels or a direct effect of insulin on target tissues?

The risk of hypoglycemia is rate-limiting for the use of intensive therapy (59), so another important question is how can the benefits of intensive therapy be achieved without increasing hypoglycemia? Local delivery of drugs to the eye is successful for cytomegalovirus retinitis so similar but less-invasive approaches might be used to deliver drugs to the retina. Local drug delivery to the retina is under intense investigation and may provide means to provide adjunctive therapies via minimally invasive procedures with little systemic risk (60,61).

A third question is how to detect and follow retinal changes in diabetes in order to shorten clinical trials so that new drugs can reach patients in a timely fashion as discussed below.

Identification and Validation of New Clinical Trial Endpoints

Treatment of the earliest stages of diabetic retinopathy is hampered by the lack of suitable clinical trial endpoints. Currently, the FDA-accepted primary endpoints are based on progression on a fundus imaging grading scale or a clinically significant change in vision, and most studies require 2 to 3 years and several hundred patients to detect a change. The visible lesions associated with diabetic retinopathy progress slowly in the earliest stages of the disease and may not even be visible when retinal dysfunction begins early in the disease process. Vision is defined solely as acuity, the resolving power of the center of the macula, a region only 100 μm in diameter. Visual acuity has severe limitations as an endpoint in the evaluation of potential therapies targeted at diabetic retinopathy, especially in the earliest stages of the disease because disease can progress without change in acuity or vice versa. Evaluation of early stage interventions with a visual acuity endpoint requires long study durations and large numbers of patients enrolled because a sufficient number of patients must demonstrate the visual acuity change during the trial to allow statistical evaluation of the intervention. For example, in the ruboxistaurin diabetic retinopathy studies, the rate of "significant" (3-lines of acuity) change was only 9.9% in the placebo-treated group vs 6.7% in the drug-treated group (32) so it is difficult to show a strong therapeutic effect. The burden imposed by visual acuity as the main clinical endpoint renders impractical clinical trials aimed at early disease. Therefore, more sensitive clinical trial endpoints are needed that will shorten the duration and enhance the feasibility of clinical trials and permit evaluation of treatments aimed at interventions earlier in the disease process, thereby allowing the identification of treatments that may prevent the vision loss associated with later stages of the disease.

How do we move forward in the development of new endpoints? It is a reasonable first step to evaluate visual function tests other than acuity as potential clinical trial endpoints. This will require that clinicians, industry, and regulatory agencies recognize that vision encompasses more than central visual acuity. Indeed, use of patient self-administered quality of life measures, such as the visual function index (VF-14), (62) indicate the need for broad measures of vision. The community's acceptance of alternative quantitative and validated visual function measurements is a requisite step to develop outcome measurements that enable the study of treatments aimed at early treatment and preserving vision. The benefit of early treatment is that acuity will be preserved as well as other important aspects of vision, which will provide vastly better patient outcomes than are possible today.

Potential endpoints are plentiful because a wide variety of visual functions are impaired in diabetes even before the manifestation of clinically apparent disease. Solid comparative studies examining the diagnostic test characteristics of these tests are needed to identify the best potential endpoints. The goal is to identify clinically important endpoints that are sensitive to changes in early stage disease. Endpoints should be evaluated in well-defined cohorts to allow direct comparisons between the potential outcome measurements. Unfortunately, comparing the performance of these tests from previously published literature is uninformative because of variable definitions of disease severity, lack of standardization in patient testing, and because the purpose of most studies was not to evaluate the diagnostic capabilities of the tests. However, the prior literature is useful in identifying potential tests to evaluate. Dark adaptation (ability to see in dim light after exposure to a bright light), scotopic (dim-light) sensitivity, and white stimulus light-on-white background perimetry (visual fields) to name a few have been shown to be impaired in diabetic patients without retinopathy (63–65), and in patients with varying levels of diabetic retinopathy severity (63,65–69). White-on-white perimetry (the standard clinical tool for visual field quantification) correlates better to diabetic retinopathy severity than visual acuity (69). In addition to psychophysical tests (dark adaptation, scotopic sensitivity, perimetry), electrophysiological tests such as electroretinography may be considered as candidate endpoints because humans with diabetes have impaired ERG responses, most prominently in the oscillatory potential and latency of the b-wave (36,37). The use of electroretinography as an endpoint would facilitate the decision to

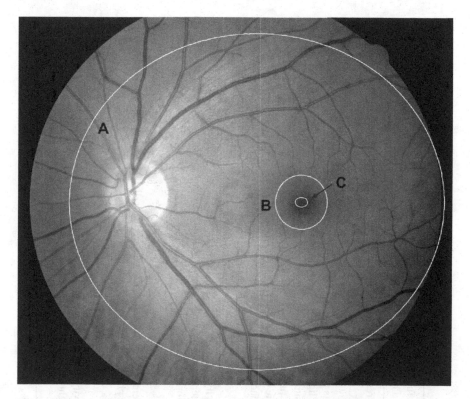

Figure 3 Retinal regions assessed by retinal functional tests. The circles outline the regions that the various functional tests evaluate. Circle A: 24° radius from the fovea; tested by white-on-white perimetry, frequency doubling perimetry and scotopic sensitivity. Circle B: Perifoveal region (5° around center of fovea) tested by dark adaptometry. Circle C (*arrow*) central 1 of the fovea tested by visual acuity and contrast sensitivity. Thus, the proposed new measures of retinal function (items 3–5 in Table 2) provide much greater information about the retina than do standard tests such as visual acuity.

move candidate treatments into human studies because electroretinography is also easily assessed in animals, unlike psychophysical measurements. However, electroretinography is unlikely to be useful as a clinical trial endpoint because it is difficult to standardize between clinics and diabetes-induced changes are of small magnitude (<30%). However, other tests shown in Table 1 and Figure 3 may have effect sizes >100% which would greatly increase sensitivity and reduce the number of subjects required for sufficiently powered studies. These potential tests are now under evaluation.

Once promising endpoints have been identified translational research is needed to adapt these tests for clinical trial usage. Most psychophysical tests conducted for research purposes are unsuited for clinical trial usage. Often the equipment is not commercially available and not standardized. In addition the

Table 1 Comparison of Retinal Function Tests

Retinal functional test	Region of retina tested	Retinal function reflected by test	Clinical correlates	Importance to patients
1. Visual acuity	Foveal cone photoreceptors	Spatial resolution	Center-involving macular edema	Debilitating loss of quality of life
2. Dark adaptometry	Perifoveal macular function	Speed by which retina adapts to darkness after light exposure; measures rod and cone function	Metabolic insults to the retina and vasculature such as ischemia, hypoxia, and nutritional deprivation	Difficulty with night driving and adapting to different lighting environments
3. Scotopic sensitivity	Central 24° of the visual field	Absolute threshold of rod photoreceptors	Very sensitive test to retinal hypoxia and ischemia. Photoreceptor dysfunction and death	Difficulty with night driving, and mobility in dim illumination or in the dark.
4. Frequency doubling perimetry	Magnocellular ganglion cells of inner retina responsible for the central 24° of visual field	Sensitivity to the frequency doubling illusion	Damage to the magnocellular pathway	Screening test for glaucoma
5. Photopic visual sensitivity (white-on-white perimetry)	Central 24° of the visual field	Increment threshold of cone photoreceptors	Sensitive to retinal cell death and metabolic insults to the retina	Difficulty with a wide variety of activities of daily living
6. Contrast sensitivity	Foveal cone photoreceptors	Sensitivity to differences in light intensity	Depressed in a wide variety of retinal diseases that comprise retinal integrity	Difficulty with a wide variety of activities of daily living

protocols are usually of long duration and have high operator and patient burden. The temptation is to only evaluate tests that are clinically suitable at the outset, which is a mistake. More elaborate methodology often provides a fuller understanding of the disease. Using the information gained from elaborate protocols, the task is to distill out the essential aspect of the promising test into a device and protocol that is clinically acceptable, chiefly by developing short duration, simple protocols, and standardized economical equipment.

Once a clinically useful endpoint is developed, validation as a primary endpoint can only be achieved by including the endpoints into clinical trials as secondary or adjunctive endpoints. This is a necessary step to evaluate the endpoint's utility as a clinical trial endpoint. Cross-sectional studies can establish the underlying biological plausibility of the endpoint, reliability, sensitivity, and other diagnostic test characteristics, but cannot establish the endpoints' predictive value or responsiveness to intervention. The validation of an endpoint is not a clear process, but widespread clinical acceptance and extensive experience with the endpoint in relevant clinical trials are necessary. Researchers and industry will have to commit the resources required to evaluate promising endpoints in clinical trials.

When new treatments for the earliest stages of diabetic retinopathy are approved based on these novel endpoints, the next challenge is to change clinical practice. Screening versions of the clinical trial endpoints will be required to identify patients that would benefit from treatment and monitor the effectiveness of therapy. Risk factor assessments will have to be conducted to determine which patients should be screened, and reimbursement issues will have to be resolved.

THE ROLE OF OPHTHALMOLOGY DEPARTMENTS IN THE EFFORT TO CONQUER DIABETIC RETINOPATHY

As our understanding of the underlying mechanisms of diabetic retinopathy has expanded, a fundamental theme has emerged: we must improve our diagnostic and therapeutic capabilities to detect and treat diabetic retinopathy at a much earlier stage in the disease process. The current paradigm of waiting for visible retinopathy to become severe enough to warrant surgery is no longer acceptable. Academic departments of ophthalmology must lead this transformation by prioritizing clinical and translational research along with the more traditional missions of patient care, basic science research, and education. This broad approach is fairly straightforward for eye-specific diseases such as glaucoma or macular degeneration, whereas diabetic retinopathy is but one component of a multifactorial systemic metabolic disease with genetic components.

Diabetic retinopathy research is evolving rapidly and becoming increasingly complex; as a result, it is impossible to conduct meaningful basic science and clinical research in isolation. Departments of ophthalmology must cultivate communities of eye and vision researchers within their organizations by removing the arbitrary barriers that exist between ophthalmology and other clinical and basic science departments. Two of the most important initiatives in medical science research, the NIH Roadmap for Medical Research and the Clinical and Translational Science Awards, emphasize the importance of interdisciplinary, team-oriented research (70,71). This same principle applies to facilitating collaborative relationships between clinicians and basic scientists. The success of future clinical research initiatives depends on our ability to effectively link clinicians and basic scientists to facilitate the translation of basic science discovery into better eye care; i.e., significantly reduced risk of vision impairment in persons with diabetes.

General aspects of this transformational approach are discussed in Chapter 1 by Drs. Greenbaum and Harrison. Here we consider challenges specific to ophthalmology where the many of its practitioners are interested in surgery rather than in disease prevention or treatment by nonsurgical means.

First, we must recall that the patient is the most important component of any clinical research endeavor. Ultimately, the goal of an effective clinical research program is to enable patients to reduce their risk of impairment by receiving the most advanced care possible in a controlled setting that minimizes potential risks. Patient schedulers, ophthalmic technicians, and faculty must be knowledgeable about the clinical research initiatives in order to promote awareness about the available clinical trials and direct appropriate patients to those trials. We must fully integrate the clinical research program into the patient care arena; clinical research is patient care, not an adjunct. Facilitating patient scheduling, ancillary testing, and therapeutic interventions are necessary to ensure clinical research functions as an integral part of the mission of an ophthalmology department. Recruitment and retention of faculty with clinical research expertise, study coordinators, and support personnel are essential components to a successful program. Clinical trial coordinators play a particularly important role in the process, serving as the critical link between the patient and the physician, the clinic, the regulatory bodies, the governmental and industry sponsors, and others.

Clinical research enables academic departments of ophthalmology to distinguish themselves within the communities they serve. Aggressively communicating clinical research opportunities to referring physicians and developing a simple process to enable referring physicians and their patients to access the clinical research system are essential. Regional clinical research networks provide an opportunity to expand the scope of the clinical research program beyond the walls of the academic health center and increase the number of patients available to participate in clinical trials.

Educational programs can be used to facilitate the exchange of ideas and skills sets among faculty members (72). In addition to the standard Grand Rounds and Visiting Professor Rounds offered at most academic centers, innovative forums designed to promote interaction between clinicians and basic scientists from multiple departments are essential. For example, regular interdisciplinary research conferences and research meetings are important to disseminate new information and stimulate discussions and collaborations among faculty members with different—and potentially complementary–perspectives.

These ambitious but vital initiatives require long-term financial investments that are difficult to support from clinical revenues so collaboration with foundations committed to public health are required.

Who Will Make the Discoveries?

The current and future implications of diabetic eye disease for patients and societies are enormous as diabetes becomes a pandemic even in developing countries (4). Currently, the number of researchers who devote their energies primarily to finding new treatments is small compared to the magnitude of the problem. In the United States fewer than 20 physicians have NIH grants focused on diabetic retinopathy and only one K08 training grant and two R43 grants for young physician –and scientists are listed on the NIH CRISP database under the search term, "diabetic retinopathy." Diabetic retinopathy is not currently a business line for most major pharmaceutical firms because of the high cost of investment and risk of failure. Young clinician and discovery investigators should be encouraged to enter the field by medical school department chairs and research administrators by encouraging interdisciplinary research and providing protected time required for long-term commitment to solving a complex problem.

Opportunities for the Future

Peptic ulcer disease was once the domain of abdominal surgeons who treated late-stage bleeding ulcers, but fundamental research has now led to specific treatments based on understanding of the disease etiology of *Helicobacter pylori* infection and acid overproduction. Dental cavities once assured that tooth loss and dentures was an inevitable part of aging but use of simple hygienic measures and fluoride supplementation now provide a high likelihood of healthy teeth for a lifetime. Diabetic retinopathy is the only major eye disease for which a disease-specific systemic intervention (intensive insulin therapy) has been shown to be effective to slow its onset and progression. These findings and the explosion of new information and potential therapies provides the real possibility that the management of diabetic retinopathy will shift from surgical intervention for late-stage disease to focus on prevention and early intervention prior to loss of vision. The potential for this outcome is demonstrated by the reduced risk of retinopathy in patients who were diagnosed in subsequent decades (2) and is due to improved control of diabetes, hypertension, and hyperlipidemia.

CONCLUSIONS

Future progress toward prevention of vision impairment from diabetes requires conceptual, organizational, and technological advances (Table 2). The conceptual advances include an understanding that "retinopathy" includes the entire retina, and that involvement of organs as "complications" may be but a continuum of the impact diabetes exerts on all tissues, rather than from distinct complications-specific mechanisms (49). Organizational advances will include improved means to fund and conduct bidirectional translational research designed to solve the needs

Table 2 Categories of Advances for a Curative Approach to Diabetic Retinopathy

Category	Examples
Conceptual	1. Diabetic retinopathy involves the entire retina. 2. Complications are part of a continuum of diabetes-induced metabolic injury
Organizational	Fund and conduct bidirectional translational research based on patient needs
Technological	1. Define the pathophysiology of retinopathy and mechanism of intensive control 2. Characterize retinal function across disease spectrum and develop new clinical endpoints 3. Develop minimally invasive ocular drug delivery

of patients and their families. Technological progress would include (*i*) defining the cellular and molecular pathophysiology underlying retinopathy initiation and progression, which will be related to understanding the mechanisms by which intensive control has its effects; (*ii*) unbiased characterization of retinal function over the spectrum of disease severity to reveal the topological sequence of cellular dysfunction and permit development of robust, quantitative, clinically useful tests that can also serve as clinical trial endpoints; and (*iii*) development of safe, effective, minimally invasive, long-term ocular drug delivery methods.

In many ways, diabetic retinopathy is an optimal disease target for an ambitious curative strategy because the population at risk is easily defined and generally motivated and knowledgeable about the potential for adverse outcomes; substantial private and public investment is available (NIH, Juvenile Diabetes Research Foundation, American Diabetes Association); and public health infrastructure is already involved in the problem (Centers for Disease Control and Prevention, World Health Organization, Prevent Blindness America). The key technological advances likely will be incremental because systemic and ocular therapies must develop in concert, and require the conceptual and organizational progress for the breakthroughs patients seek to relieve their fear of losing vision.

ACKNOWLEDGMENTS

Supported by the Juvenile Diabetes Research Foundation, the American Diabetes Association, and the Pennsylvania Lions Sight Conservation and Eye Research Foundation.

REFERENCES

1. Rossing K, Jacobsen P, Rossing P, Lauritzen E, Lund-Andersen H, Parving HH. Improved visual function in IDDM patients with unchanged cumulative incidence of sight-threatening diabetic retinopathy. Diabetes Care 1998; 21(11):2007–2015.

2. Hovind P, Tarnow L, Rossing K, et al. Decreasing incidence of severe diabetic microangiopathy in type 1 diabetes. Diabetes Care 2003; 26(4):1258–1264.
3. Wild S, Roglic G, Green A, Sicree R, King H. Global prevalence of diabetes: Estimates for the year 2000 and projections for 2030. Diabetes Care 2004; 27(5):1047–1053.
4. Hossain P, Kawar B, El Nahas M. Obesity and diabetes in the developing world—a growing challenge. N Engl J Med 2007; 356(3):213–215.
5. Meyer-Schwickerath G. Licktkoagulation. Buech Augenarzt 1959; 33:1–96.
6. Bonds DE, Larson JC, Schwartz AV, et al. Risk of fracture in women with type 2 diabetes: The Women's Health Initiative Observational Study. J Clin Endocrinol Metab 2006; 91(9):3404–3410.
7. Schwartz AV, Hillier TA, Sellmeyer DE, et al. Older women with diabetes have a higher risk of falls: A prospective study. Diabetes Care 2002; 25(10):1749–1754.
8. Fischer F. The First Case of Diabetic Retinopathy. Berlin: Springer-Verlag; 1989.
9. Gardner TW, Antonetti DA, Barber AJ, LaNoue KF, Levison SW. Diabetic retinopathy: More than meets the eye. Surv Ophthalmol 2002; 247 (Suppl 2):S253–S262.
10. Bloodworth JMB. Diabetic retinopathy. Diabetes 1962; 2:1–22.
11. Wolter J, R. Diabetic retinopathy. Am J Ophthalmol 1961; 51:1123–1139.
12. Simonsen SE. ERG in Juvenile Diabetics: A prognostic study. In: Goldberg MF, Fine SL, eds. Symposium on the Treatment of Diabetic Retinopathy. Arlington: US Department of Health, Education and Welfare; 1969:681–689.
13. Bresnick GH, Palta M. Predicting progression to severe proliferative diabetic retinopathy. Arch Ophthalmol 1987; 105(6):810–814.
14. Bresnick GH. Diabetic retinopathy viewed as a neurosensory disorder. Arch Ophthalmol 1986; 104(7):989–990.
15. Mizutani M, Kern TS, Lorenzi M. Accelerated death of retinal microvascular cells in human and experimental diabetic retinopathy. J Clin Invest 1996; 97(12):2883–2890.
16. Kern TS, Engerman RL. Vascular lesions in diabetes are distributed non-uniformly within the retina. Exp Eye Research 1995; 60(5):545–549.
17. Antonetti DA, Lieth E, Barber AJ, Gardner TW. Molecular mechanisms of vascular permeability in diabetic retinopathy. Semin Ophthalmol 1999; 14(4):240–248.
18. Kim SY, Johnson MA, McLeod DS, et al. Retinopathy in monkeys with spontaneous type 2 diabetes. Invest Ophthalmol Vis Sci 2004; 45(12):4543–4553.
19. Chakravarthy U, Hayes RG, Stitt AW, McAuley E, Archer DB. Constitutive nitric oxide synthase expression in retinal vascular endothelial cells is suppressed by high glucose and advanced glycation end products. Diabetes 1998; 47(6):945–952.
20. Barber AJ, Lieth E, Khin SA, Antonetti DA, Buchanan AG, Gardner TW. Neural apoptosis in the retina during experimental and human diabetes. Early onset and effect of insulin. J Clin Invest 1998; 102(4):783–791.
21. Martin PM, Roon P, Van Ells TK, Ganapathy V, Smith SB. Death of retinal neurons in streptozotocin-induced diabetic mice. Invest Ophthalmol Vis Sci 2004; 45(9):3330–3336.
22. Lieth E, LaNoue KF, Antonetti DA, Ratz M, Penn State Retina Research Group. Diabetes reduces glutamate oxidation and glutamine synthesis in the retina. Exp Eye Res 2000; 70(6):723–730.
23. Lutty GA, McLeod DS, Merges C, Diggs A, Plouét J. Localization of vascular endothelial growth factor in human retina and choroid. Arch Ophthalmol 1996; 114(8):971–977.

24. Gerhardinger C, Brown LF, Roy S, Mizutani M, Zucker CL, Lorenzi M. Expression of vascular endothelial growth factor in the human retina and in nonproliferative diabetic retinopathy. Am J Pathol 1998; 152(6):1453–1462.
25. Joussen AM, Poulaki V, Mitsiades N, et al. Suppression of Fas-FasL-induced endothelial cell apoptosis prevents diabetic blood-retinal barrier breakdown in a model of streptozotocin-induced diabetes. FASEB J 2003; 17(1):76–78.
26. Lieth E, Barber AJ, Xu B, et al. Glial reactivity and impaired glutamate metabolism in short-term experimental diabetic retinopathy. Näller Diabetes 1998; 47:815–820.
27. Mizutani M, Gerhardinger C, Lorenzi M. Müller cell changes in human diabetic retinopathy. Diabetes 1998; 47:445–449.
28. Rungger-Brandle E, Dosso AA, Leuenberger PM. Glial Reactivity, an early feature of diabetic retinopathy. Invest Ophthalmol Vis Sci 2000; 41(7):1971–1980.
29. Zeng XX, Ng YK, Ling EA. Neuronal and microglial response in the retina of streptozotocin-induced diabetic rats. Visual Neuroscience 2000; 17(3):463–471.
30. Krady JK, Basu A, Allen CM, et al. Minocycline reduces proinflammatory cytokine expression, microglial activation, and caspase-3 activation in a rodent model of diabetic retinopathy. Diabetes 2005; 54(5):1559–1565.
31. Anonymous. The effect of ruboxistaurin on visual loss in patients with moderately severe to very severe nonproliferative diabetic retinopathy. Initial results of the protein kinase Cbeta inhibitor diabetic retinopathy study (PKC-DRS) multicenter randomized clinical trial. Diabetes 2005; 54:2188–2197.
32. Aiello LP, Davis MD, Girach A, et al. Effect of ruboxistaurin on visual loss in patients with diabetic retinopathy. Ophthalmology 2006; 113(12):2221–2230.
33. Anonymous. Effect of ruboxistaurin in patients with diabetic macular edema: Thirty-month results of the randomized PKC-DMES clinical trial. Arch Ophthalmol 2007; 125(3):318–324.
34. Harhaj NS, Felinski EA, Wolpert EB, Sundstrom JM, Gardner TW, Antonetti DA. VEGF activation of protein kinase C stimulates occludin phosphorylation and contributes to endothelial permeability. Invest Ophthalmol Vis Sci 2006; 47:5106–5115.
35. Aiello LP. The potential role of PKC beta in diabetic retinopathy and macular edema. Survey Ophthalmol 2002; 47(Suppl 2):S263–S269.
36. Ghirlanda G, Di Leo MA, Caputo S, Cercone S, Greco AV. From functional to microvascular abnormalities in early diabetic retinopathy. Diabetes-Metabolism Rev 1997; 13(1):15–35.
37. Bearse MA, Jr., Han Y, Schneck ME, Adams AJ. Retinal function in normal and diabetic eyes mapped with the slow flash multifocal electroretinogram. Invest Ophthalmol Vis Sci 2004; 45(1):296–304.
38. Gariano RF, Gardner TW. Retinal angiogenesis in development and disease. Nature 2005; 438(7070):960–966.
39. Chew EY, Klein ML, Ferris FL, III, et al. Association of elevated serum lipid levels with retinal hard exudate in diabetic retinopathy. Early Treatment Diabetic Retinopathy Study (ETDRS) Report 22. Archi Ophthalmol 1996; 114(9):1079–1084.
40. Lyons TJ, Jenkins AJ, Zheng D, et al. Diabetic retinopathy and serum lipoprotein subclasses in the DCCT/EDIC cohort. Invest Ophthalmol Vis Sci 2004; 45(3):910–918.
41. Zhang L, Krzentowski G, Albert A, Lefebvre PJ. Risk of developing retinopathy in Diabetes Control and Complications Trial type 1 diabetic patients with good or poor metabolic control. Diabetes Care 2001; 24(7):1275–1279.

42. Orchard TJ, Chang YF, Ferrell RE, Petro N, Ellis DE. Nephropathy in type 1 diabetes: A manifestation of insulin resistance and multiple genetic susceptibilities? Further evidence from the Pittsburgh Epidemiology of Diabetes Complication Study. Kidney Int 2002; 62(3):963–970.

43. Chaturvedi N. Differing aspects of insulin resistance in diabetic complications: The shape of things to come. RD Lawrence lecture 2000. Diabetic Med 2002; 19:973–937.

44. Chaturvedi N, Sjoelie AK, Porta M, et al. Markers of insulin resistance are strong risk factors for retinopathy incidence in type 1 diabetes. Diabetes Care 2001; 24(2):284–289.

45. Michael MD, Kulkarni RN, Postic C, et al. Loss of insulin signaling in hepatocytes leads to severe insulin resistance and progressive hepatic dysfunction. Mol Cell 2000; 6(1):87–97.

46. Kido Y, Burks DJ, Withers D, et al. Tissue-specific insulin resistance in mice with mutations in the insulin receptor, IRS-1, and IRS-2. J Clin Invest 2000; 105(2):199–205.

47. Kulkarni RN, Bruning JC, Winnay JN, Postic C, Magnuson MA, Kahn CR. Tissue-specific knockout of the insulin receptor in pancreatic beta cells creates an insulin secretory defect similar to that in type 2 diabetes. Cell 1999; 96(3):329–339.

48. Schubert M, Gautam D, Surjo D, et al. Role for neuronal insulin resistance in neurodegenerative diseases. Proc Natl Acad Sci USA 2004; 101:3100–3105.

49. Antonetti DA, Barber AJ, Bronson SK, et al. Diabetic retinopathy: Seeing beyond glucose-induced microvascular disease. Diabetes 2006; 55(9):2401–2411.

50. Reiter CEN, Wu X, Sandirasegarane L, et al. Diabetes reduces basal retinal insulin receptor signaling: Reversal with systemic and local insulin. Diabetes 2006; 55:1148–1156.

51. Seki M, Tanaka T, Nawa H, et al. Involvement of brain-derived neurotrophic factor in early retinal neuropathy of streptozotocin-induced diabetes in rats: Therapeutic potential of brain-derived neurotrophic factor for dopaminergic amacrine cells. Diabetes 2004; 53(9):2412–2419.

52. Barber AJ, Nakamura M, Wolpert EB, et al. Insulin rescues retinal neurons from apoptosis by a phosphatidylinositol 3-kinase/Akt-mediated mechanism that reduces the activation of caspase-3. J Biol Chem 2001; 276(35):32814–32821.

53. Chaum E. Retinal neuroprotection by growth factors: A mechanistic perspective. J Cell Biochem 2003; 88(1):57–75.

54. Podesta F, Romeo G, Liu WH, et al. Bax is increased in the retina of diabetic subjects and is associated with pericyte apoptosis in vivo and in vitro. Am J Path 2000; 156(3):1025–1032.

55. Abu-El-Asrar AM, Dralands L, Missotten L, Al-Jadaan IA, Geboes K. Expression of apoptosis markers in the retinas of human subjects with diabetes. Invest Ophthalmol Vis Sci 2004; 45(8):2760–2766.

56. Johnson MA, Lutty GA, McLeod DS, et al. Ocular structure and function in an aged monkey with spontaneous diabetes mellitus. Exp Eye Res 2005; 80(1):37–42.

57. Anonymous. The effect of intensive treatment of diabetes on the development and progression of long-term complications in insulin-dependent diabetes mellitus. N Engl J Med 1993; 329:977–986.

58. Nathan DM. Relationship between metabolic control and long-term complications of diabetes. In: Kahn CR, Weir GC, King GL, Jacobson AM, Moses AC, Smith RJ,

eds. Joslin's Diabetes Mellitus. 14th ed. Philadelphia: Lippincott Williams & Wilkins; 2005:809–821.

59. Cryer PE. Hypoglycemia is the limiting factor in the management of diabetes. Diabetes/Metabol Res Rev 1999; 15(1):42–46.

60. Ghate D, Edelhauser HF. Ocular drug delivery. Expert Opin Drug Deliv 2006; 3(2):275–287.

61. Mac Gabhann F, Demetriades AM, Deering T, et al. Protein transport to choroid and retina following periocular injection: Theoretical and experimental study. Ann Biomed Eng 2007; 35(4):615–630.

62. Linder M, Chang TS, Scott IU, et al. Validity of the visual function index (VF-14) in patients with retinal disease. Arch Ophthalmol 1999; 117(12):1611–1616.

63. Henson DB, Williams DE. Normative and clinical data with a new type of dark adaptometer. Am J Optom Physiol Opt 1979; 56(4):267–271.

64. Abraham FA, Haimovitz J, Berezin M. The photopic and scotopic visual thresholds in diabetics without diabetic retinopathy. Metab Pediatr Syst Ophthalmol 1988; 11(1-2):76–77.

65. Mao WS, Hu Z, Pang GX. Study of diabetic eye complications other than diabetic retinopathy. Chin Med J (Engl) 1982; 95(8):579–582.

66. Holopigian K, Seiple W, Lorenzo M, Carr R. A comparison of photopic and scotopic electroretinographic changes in early diabetic retinopathy. Invest Ophthalmol Vis Sci 1992; 33(10):2773–2780.

67. Mantyjarvi M. Colour vision and dark adaptation in diabetic patients after photocoagulation. Acta Ophthalmol (Copenh) 1989; 67(2):113–118.

68. Agardh E, Stjernquist H, Heijl A, Bengtsson B. Visual acuity and perimetry as measures of visual function in diabetic macular oedema. Diabetologia 2006; 49(1):200–206.

69. Bengtsson B, Heijl A, Agardh E. Visual fields correlate better than visual acuity to severity of diabetic retinopathy. Diabetologia 2005; 48(12):2494–2500.

70. Zerhouni EA. Clinical research at a crossroads: The NIH roadmap. J Investig Med 2006; 54(4):171–173.

71. Zerhouni EA. US biomedical research: Basic, translational, and clinical sciences. JAMA 2005; 294(11):1352–1358.

72. Mallon WT. The benefits and challenges of research centers and institutes in academic medicine: Findings from six universities and their medical schools. Acad Med 2006; 81(6):502–512.

11

Transplant-Based Treatments for the Patient with Long-Standing Type 1 Diabetes

Mahfuzul Khan

*Endocrinology Training Program, Diabetes Branch, NIDDK,
National Institutes of Health (DHHS), Bethesda, Maryland, U.S.A.*

David M. Harlan

*Diabetes Branch, NIDDK, National Institutes of Health (DHHS),
and Professor of Medicine, Uniformed Services University of the
Health Sciences, Bethesda, Maryland, U.S.A.*

TYPE 1 DIABETES MELLITUS AND AUTOIMMUNITY

Type 1 diabetes (T1D) is an autoimmune disease thought to result from the activation of T lymphocytes specific for autoantigens in insulin-producing pancreatic beta cells. The T cell response leads to decreasing endogenous insulin production which becomes clinically manifest when the remaining beta cell mass can no longer produce sufficient insulin to maintain glucose homeostasis. This immunopathologic basis of T1D is supported by several complementary lines of evidence including the following:

- The presence of circulating antibodies to beta cell antigens that predict disease development (1).
- Genome-wide association studies have identified 10 genetic loci most strongly associated with T1D susceptibility, six of which either influence immune function (MHC, CTLA4, CD25, PTPN2, MDA5) or the insulin-specific T-cell repertoire (insulin VNTR) (2).

- The pathognomonic pancreatic islet lesion known as "insulitis," i.e., infiltrating macrophages and lymphocytes, predominantly T-cells, seen at postmortem examination of individuals with T1D.
- Recurrence within several weeks of both diabetes and islet autoimmunity (rising islet antibody titer and typical insulitis on biopsy) in the diabetic twin recipient of a segmental pancreas graft from the nondiabetic identical twin (3).

The relevance of islet autoimmunity to a discussion of transplantation as a treatment for T1D, as opposed to other end organ diseases treated with transplants, is that the immunological barrier may well be greater for T1D, for at least three reasons. First, there is an established and persistent islet autoimmune response against the very tissue being transplanted. In contrast, for the typical heart, kidney, or liver allograft recipient, there is no anti-cardiomyocyte, anti-nephron, or anti-hepatocyte autoimmune T-cell response. Second, the relevant cellular mass being transplanted is quite small. That is, while a transplanted heart, kidney, or liver weighs approximately 250 g, 150 g, and 1.5 kg, respectively, an islet allograft recipient receives only 5 to 10 g of tissue. It is not unreasonable to surmise that the immune system could more easily and quickly destroy 5 grams of tissue than an organ that weighs orders of magnitude more. Third, most current antirejection therapies rely on agents, e.g., cyclosporine or tacrolimus, that interfere with calcineurin phosphatase function, which is also known to interfere with beta-cell function (4).

T1D PROGNOSIS

Prior to the discovery of insulin in 1922, T1D was rapidly fatal with very few individuals surviving more than a few months. Over the years, however, and especially over the past 20 years, diabetes management has advanced considerably. The resulting dramatic improvement in T1D prognosis is an important consideration when discussing transplant-based treatments. The Diabetes Control and Complications Trial (DCCT) clearly demonstrated that tight glycemia control with intensive insulin therapy prevents or at least delays the onset of diabetic microvascular complications (5). Subsequently, the DCCT/EDIC found that intensive insulin therapy also prevented macrovascular complications (6). In addition to the improved prognosis stemming from better blood glucose control (achieved with improved insulin delivery capability, facilitated by blood glucose monitoring), greater emphasis on blood pressure control, lipid lowering with safe and effective agents, and smoking cessation, have together resulted in gratifyingly improved survival of people with T1D. For instance, the Pittsburgh Epidemiology of Diabetes Complications Study (7) recently reported findings based upon 906 individuals diagnosed with T1D between 1950 and 1980, stratified into five cohorts by year of diagnosis. As shown (Fig. 1), the all-cause 20-year mortality for individuals with T1D declined in each successive cohort since 1950 such that for the 179 individuals diagnosed between 1975 and 1980, the 20-year mortality was 3.5%. Similar findings have been reported by other groups

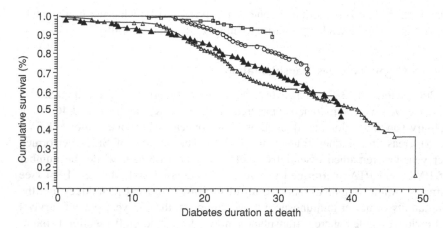

Figure 1 All-cause mortality by diagnosis cohort: the Pittsburgh EDC study. △, 1950–1959; ▲, 1960–1964; ○, 1965–1969; □,1970–1974; ■, 1975–1980. *Source*: Adapted from Ref. 7.

around the world (8–10). In an attempt to place this mortality in perspective, notwithstanding that good statistics are difficult to come by, the 20-year mortality for healthy children and young adults in the United States is about 1.5% (see http://www.cdc.gov/nchs/datawh/statab/unpubd/mortabs/lewk3_10.htm). Thus, T1D can be estimated to further increase a young person's mortality risk over the subsequent 20 years by approximately 2% or by about 0.1% per year. We know that individuals with T1D die predominately from premature cardiovascular disease and that renal failure is a major risk factor for atherosclerosis, so the reduced incidence of end-stage renal disease documented in the same studies tracking T1D mortality may underlie the improved survival. Even for patients with long-standing T1D sufficiently problematic to warrant transplant-based treatment, provided kidney function is preserved, the annual mortality is 1% or less (11).

TRANSPLANT-BASED APPROACHES

Since Joseph Murray performed the first successful therapeutic kidney transplant in 1954, transplant physicians and scientists have realized that the most formidable hurdle facing the field is a safe and effective way to prevent the recipient's immune system rejecting the allograft [reviewed in Ref. 12]. The inviolable *primum non nocere* principle underlying medical practice dictates that the risk must not outweigh the potential benefit gained. Life-preserving transplant procedures such as those for patients with end-stage heart, liver, or kidney failure have gained wide acceptance. However, because T1D is treatable in almost all patients, considerable controversy shrouds transplant-based treatments for this disease. Indeed, Dr. David Sutherland, a leading developer of pancreas transplantation, wrote in 1984 words that remain true today (3): "One of the principal drawbacks to pancreas transplantation is the necessity of permanent immunosuppression of the recipient. . . . This is of particular concern in a procedure which is not immediately life-saving, but is intended primarily to improve the quality of life."

Whole-Organ Pancreas Transplantation

In 2006, a total of 1387 pancreas transplants were performed in the United States; of these, 924 were simultaneous pancreas–kidney (SPK) allografts and 463 were solitary pancreas allografts defined as either pancreas transplants alone (PTAs) or pancreas after kidney transplants (PAKs). The number of SPKs performed per year has remained essentially stable for over a decade, while the number of PAKs and PTAs performed per year has increased sixfold since 1994 (see http://www.unos.org/data). As a result of improved surgical techniques and the availability of newer immunosuppressive regimens, the one-year patient survival following a whole pancreas transplant is now >95%, and graft function is maintained in >85% of patients.

Pancreas Transplantation: Metabolic Control

Most pancreas allograft recipients achieve insulin-independent normoglycemia. In fact, the mean glycated hemoglobin levels reported for patients 5 and 10 years after transplantation were lower (5.3% and 5.5%, respectively) than the DCCT target value (6.0%), and even within the DCCT less than half of the intensively treated group achieved that glycemia target (13,14). The obvious explanation for this observation is that the transplanted pancreas secretes insulin in a more physiologic manner in response to the prevailing blood glucose level. This could also explain why, compared to individuals treated with insulin, transplant recipients almost never suffer serious hypoglycemia and most report a better quality of life.

Pancreas Transplantation: Diabetes Complications and Survival

The goal of pancreas transplantation is to restore normoglycemia and thereby prevent the long-term complications of diabetes, so as to preserve life quality and duration. Thus, pancreas transplantation's success can be measured by its effect on life quality, diabetes complication rates, and on overall survival. While perhaps counterintuitive, early experience indicated that pancreas transplant did not improve proliferative retinopathy (15). One potential explanation is that the typical transplant recipient's proliferative retinal disease had progressed too far to be reversible. Indeed, advanced diabetic retinopathy is present in most patients at the time of pancreas transplantation. Nevertheless, more recent experience suggests that diabetic retinopathy stabilizes in the majority of pancreas-kidney allograft recipients (16,17).

Perhaps, the more important question is whether pancreas transplantation would prevent or improve the risk of end-stage renal disease in those considering solitary pancreas allografts (PTA or PKA). While no studies enrolling large patient numbers have been performed, the University of Minnesota investigators reported that histologically graded diabetic nephropathy was alleviated when kidney biopsies were studied from eight individuals with functioning pancreas allografts transplanted at least 10 years earlier (13,18). Even so, the renal function of each individual was worse than before their transplant 10 years earlier, presumably due to immunosuppressive-agent–associated nephrotoxicity. In a separate study, these investigators (18) also compared one group (n = 13) with successful pancreas allografts to a control group (n = 10), who had either lost graft function early or never received a transplant. Compared to the controls, the transplant group had worse kidney function at 5-year follow-up. In fact, the two patients in the study who subsequently required kidney transplants had both previously received a pancreas allograft. Although a small study, the outcome certainly questioned the benefit of solitary pancreas transplantation with regard to preserving kidney function. On the other hand, yet unanswered is the question whether pancreas transplantation preserves kidney function in patients with diabetes, who have undergone simultaneous pancreas-kidney (SPK) transplantation versus solitary kidney transplantation. In fact, long-term survival of SPK recipients (up to 8-year follow-up) was not significantly improved compared to recipients of a kidney only transplant from a living donor (20–22).

Does pancreas transplantation prolong the diabetic patient's life? The proper way to address this question would be a randomized controlled trial, but such a study is unlikely for practical reasons. Indeed, such a randomized trial has not been conducted even for the much more common kidney transplantation procedure. However, studies comparing the outcome of kidney allograft recipients to those on the waiting list for a kidney transplant have shown a significant survival benefit starting 8 months following the transplant (19). Using a similar retrospective, observational, cohort study design for pancreas transplantation, with data from 124 transplant centers across the United States, we found that solitary pancreas transplantation provided no survival benefit and may have actually have been associated with excess mortality. We examined the survival of patients after SPK, PAK, and PTA, compared with that for patients on the waiting list for these procedures (11). The study's key findings are as follows (Fig. 2):

- *Increased mortality in the immediate postoperative period.* In all groups (SPK, PAK or PTA), mortality was increased in the first three postoperative months.
- *Increased survival in SPK recipients.* Beyond the 3-month–postoperative period, SPK recipients enjoyed a survival advantage (RR of mortality 0.43). As discussed above, whether the pancreas transplant actually confers additional survival benefit over kidney transplant alone remains a matter of debate.
- *Increased mortality in isolated pancreas transplant groups.* Perhaps the most sobering finding was that for isolated pancreas allograft (PTA or PAK) recipients with preserved kidney function (either because they never lost kidney function or because they had previously received a kidney transplant), mortality for subjects who received a pancreas allograft was greater than for those

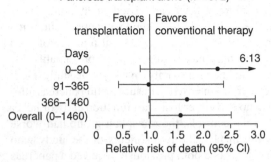

Pancreas transplant alone (*n* = 672)

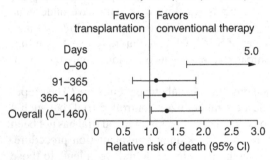

Pancreas-after-kidney transplant (*n* = 1398)

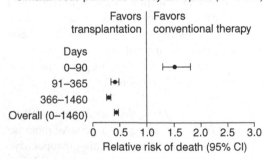

Simultaneous pancreas-kidney transplant (*n* = 9502)

Figure 2 Relative risk of mortality by transplant types. Days are posttransplant (recipients) or additional days waiting (patients not transplanted). Relative risk of 1.0 indicates that the risk of transplantation equals the risk of not being transplanted. *Source*: Adapted from Ref. 11.

who had not had a pancreas transplant (RR of 1.7 1-year posttransplant in the PTA group). The caveat is that because the analysis was retrospective, questions can be raised about comparability of treatment and control groups. It is also possible that a pancreas transplant–associated survival benefit takes more than 4 years to become evident.

- *Even patients with long-standing T1D have good prognosis.* As cited above, as long as kidney function is preserved, individuals with long-standing and difficult-to-control T1D (on the waiting list for pancreas transplant) have surprisingly good survival, with about a 1% mortality/year.

Pancreas Transplantation: Any Candidates?

Who should be considered as an appropriate whole-organ pancreas transplant candidate? The American Diabetes Association (ADA) recommends that "pancreas transplantation should be considered an acceptable therapeutic alternative to continued insulin therapy in diabetic patients with imminent or established end-stage renal disease who have had or plan to have a kidney transplant" (23). The available clinical data would appear to support this recommendation for patients with the opportunity to receive an SPK, but are less clear for PAK candidates. However, as indicated, an ever-diminishing proportion of people with T1D progress to end-stage kidney disease. Is there a role therefore for pancreas transplantation in patients with preserved kidney function? The ADA recommends that PTA should only be considered in patients who have:

1) Frequent, acute, and severe metabolic complications requiring medical attention,
2) Incapacitating clinical and emotional problems with exogenous insulin therapy, or
3) Experienced consistent failure of insulin-based management to avert acute complications.

Several caveats need to be considered with regard to these clinical practice recommendations. First, the most commonly cited reason for categorizing diabetes as uncontrolled is hypoglycemia unawareness, and we now know that this awareness can often be restored to most subjects by strictly avoiding hypoglycemia for a period of just 2 to 3 weeks (24). Second, the demands of a chronic disease and its management can affect the psyche, occasionally leading to clinically overt psychiatric illness. This impact of T1D cannot be ignored but surgery is not typically considered as a solution for psychosocial problems. Third, the increasing popularity and practicality of continuous glucose monitoring systems promises to markedly decrease hypoglycemia risk for the patient with T1D. Last, existing evidence indicates that PTA and PKA may not confer a survival benefit. As with all major surgical procedures then, caution should be exercised before referring the patient with T1D and preserved renal function for PTA and perhaps even for PAK procedures.

AN EMERGING ISSUE: RECURRENT AUTOIMMUNITY AND T1D IN PANCREAS TRANSPLANT RECIPIENTS

Recent evidence suggests that recurrent islet autoimmunity, despite continued immunosuppression, may be a common cause for graft failure in pancreas transplant recipients. Burke and associates (25) studied 254 simultaneous pancreas-kidney (SPK) allograft recipients for recurrence of autoimmunity. While the majority (52%) remained autoantibody negative or had pretransplant islet autoantibody titers that persisted (30%), 17% converted to autoantibody positivity during follow-up. Forty patients (16%) reverted to hyperglycemia and their beta-cell failure was associated with autoantibody conversion, strongly suggesting islet autoimmunity as the cause for the recurrent diabetes. The same investigators have recently reported that autoantibody prevalence among whole-organ donors is very low (3%) and even then donors typically have only one detectable antibody and are therefore at low risk for T1D (26). Hence, the recurrence of diabetes after SPK transplantation appears to be due to recurrent islet autoimmunity. Since SPK recipients with recurrent diabetes typically receive multiagent immunosuppression that maintains kidney allograft function (i.e., the recipient's pancreas allograft function is lost but the same donor's kidney continues to function), these observations suggest that the immunosuppression effectively prevents the allo-immune response but is less effective in controlling the autoimmune response. Further immunosuppressive regimen modification, including agents that target the humoral immune response, e.g., anti CD20 antibody and/or plasmapheresis, has been used to salvage graft function in a few patients.

ISOLATED ISLET TRANSPLANTATION

Isolated islet transplantation is very appealing as it enjoys some distinct advantages over whole-organ transplantation:

1) By transplanting only isolated islets (and not the greater than 95% of the pancreas unaffected by T1D), complications associated with whole-organ transplantation can be avoided.
2) Because isolated islets can be infused via a percutaneous catheter, most general anesthesia-associated and surgical complications can be avoided.
3) Islets can be procured from pancreata deemed unsuitable for organ transplantation.

Even so, the major hurdle limiting organ pancreas transplantation also applies to isolated islet transplantation, i.e., recipients still require life-long immunosuppressive therapy. Prior to 2000, isolated islet transplant outcomes did not compare favorably with whole-organ pancreas transplant outcomes. This appeared to change when Shapiro and colleagues from the University of Alberta reported their success with a modified protocol now widely referred to as the "Edmonton protocol"(27). The Edmonton investigators modified earlier approaches in four ways:

1) Infusion of more islets, recipients receiving islets from at least two donors.
2) Use of a novel and steroid-sparing immunosuppressive regimen shown to be effective in kidney allograft recipients (28).
3) Islet infusion as soon as possible following their isolation.
4) Avoidance of animal proteins, i.e., fetal bovine serum, during islet isolation.

Subsequent studies revealed that the key features of Edmonton's early success were the first two modifications, islet dose and steroid-sparing immunosuppression. Centers around the world soon adopted the Edmonton protocol, but the initial enthusiasm has dampened considerably (29,30). The format used above to evaluate pancreas transplantation will be used to evaluate the current status of islet transplantation.

Islet Transplantation: Metabolic Control

Even the most experienced centers have reported one-year insulin-independence rates that are much lower than for pancreas transplantation, and insulin independence rates fall off rapidly after the first year. For instance, a follow-up study of 64 Edmonton islet allograft recipients reported that about 65% remained insulin-independent at 1 year, but this declined to just under 10% at 5 years (31). The Immune Tolerance Network (ITN) trial, in which nine centers attempted to replicate Edmonton's early success, was also disappointing with only 44% of recipients being insulin independent at 1 year and only 14% (5 of the 36 patients) at 2 years (32). Thus, islet transplantation does not yet compare favorably to pancreas transplantation with regard to metabolic control achieved. On the other hand, the majority of patients from both the Edmonton (82% at 5 years) and ITN (66% at 2 years) trials continued to have detectable C-peptide secretion following islet transplantation. One of the DCCT's important lessons is that endogenous beta-cell function correlates directly with the safety and efficacy of insulin-based treatment regimens (5). It is therefore not surprising that recipients of islet allografts experience much less-frequent severe hypoglycemia and retain improved glycemia control even when they resume insulin therapy.

ISLET TRANSPLANTATION: DIABETES COMPLICATIONS

Recent findings indicate that like whole-pancreas transplantation islet transplantation stabilizes diabetic retinopathy in most patients (33). There is no clear evidence yet to suggest whether this procedure may reduce diabetes-associate macrovascular complications. The net effect of islet transplantation on recipient kidney function will be discussed below.

Islet Transplantation: Acute and Long-Term Complications

When compared to whole pancreas transplantation, islet transplantation is unquestionably safer in the short term, but the procedure is not free from serious complications. All centers performing islet transplantation have experienced potentially serious complications including major bleeding events requiring transfusions or lapatotomy, portal vein (branch) thrombosis, and gall bladder wall puncture (30–32). The most experienced centers report that they have overcome the bleeding and thrombotic complications. Even so, the immunosuppressive agents have resulted in mouth ulcers requiring debridement, bone marrow suppression leading to anemia and neutropenia, opportunistic infections, diarrhea, edema, nausea, acne, fatigue, and ovarian cysts in premenopausal women. Furthermore, isolated islets are infused into the recipient's portal vein and lodge in the liver, which can lead to structural changes in the surrounding liver parenchyma (34,35) of as yet unknown clinical significance.

As with all other transplant therapies, chronic immunosuppressive agent use (especially calcineurin phosphatase inhibitors) leads to declining renal function in islet transplant recipients (31,32,36). Among islet recipients in the Edmonton study followed for 3 years, glomerular filtration rate decreased in 92% of patients and both albuminuria and microalbuminuria tended to progress; e.g., for micro- or macroalbuminuria, 7 of 41 met criteria prior to transplant compared to 15 of 41 on follow-up (36). Recipients also more frequently required lipid-lowering agents and multiple blood pressure medications than prior to transplantation; and both hyperlipidemia and hypertension are known complications of tacrolimus plus rapamycin immunotherapy (31).

Recent studies have also raised concerns regarding the islet transplant recipient's risk of HLA sensitization. Since most islet allograft recipients require islets from multiple donors to achieve insulin independence, and since islets are allocated based solely on ABO compatibility (HLA matching would not be practical), recipients can become widely sensitized to multiple HLA antigens (37). Shapiro and colleagues (38) recently reported that among 98 individuals studied following islet transplantation, a third developed *de novo* HLA antibodies, the majority (52%) having donor-specific antibodies against both class 1 and class 2 HLA molecules. A greater risk of sensitization was documented with discontinuation of immunosuppression following graft failure. For example, although the anti-HLA antibodies appeared in most patients while they were on maintenance immunosuppression, the incidence of broad HLA-sensitization (defined as panel reactive activity >50%) rose abruptly following the complete cessation of immunosuppression. Of particular concern, younger patients were more likely to develop anti-donor HLA antibodies. Since this group is projected to have a long life expectancy, and thus may go on to develop renal failure arising from diabetic nephropathy or immunosuppression-related nephrotoxicity, such broad HLA-sensitization could severely restrict the kidney donor pool for their future renal replacement therapy.

Islet Transplantation: Cost

To achieve insulin independence, most islet recipients require islets from two or more donor organs. Further, the isolation procedure is imperfect such that islets suitable for clinical use are obtained from only about half the attempts. In the ITN trial, for example, islets suitable for transplant were isolated from 45% of donated organs, and recipients received islets from an average of 2.1 donors (32). Thus, a typical recipient would require four pancreata to obtain sufficient islets for a transplant designed to achieve insulin independence. To the cost of those four pancreata, one needs to add costs associated with the equipment, supplies, and personnel required to harvest organs and isolate islets, interventional radiology expenses for the portal vein cannulation, immunosuppressive agents and assays for monitoring their blood levels, prophylactic antibiotics, and clinic visits. In the United States then, the average estimated cost for each islet allograft recipient to be rendered insulin-independent for 1-year posttransplant is estimated to exceed $150,000.

Islet Transplantation: Any Candidates?

Identifying the suitable islet transplant candidate can be difficult. The clinician must weigh the potential short-term gain against procedure- and immunosuppression-related risks. The current ADA guidelines consider islet transplantation to be a "rapidly evolving technology that also requires immunosuppression and should be performed only within the setting of controlled research studies" (23).

New Directions for Islet Transplantation and Replacement Therapy

The insulin secretory capacity of insulin-independent islet allograft recipients is estimated to be only 20% to 40% normal (39). Starting from this low baseline, they then gradually lose islet function such that within a few years insulin therapy is required to maintain euglycemia. Thus, investigators are working to improve islet engraftment efficiency and to preserve islet function post-transplant. Since current estimates suggest that improved islet isolation procedures can only marginally increase isolated islet volume, efforts are focused on improving isolated islet quality. A recent review has estimated that only 10% to 20% of transplanted islets actually survive the infusion process (40), but others have suggested higher survival of 25% to 50% (41). For instance, Korsgren and associates (42) from Uppsala, Sweden labeled isolated porcine islets with 2-deoxy-2[F]fluoro-D-glucose (FDG), infused the islets into the recipient pig portal vein and then obtained serial PET/CT images. By measuring radioactivity loss, they surmised that almost 50% of the transplanted islets were destroyed within minutes after they were infused. The Uppsala group has also described a thrombotic reaction they call the instant blood-mediated inflammatory reaction (IBMIR), which occurs when purified human islets are incubated in ABO-compatible blood. They propose that IBMIR damages islets and leads to clot formation and leukocyte infiltration into the islets (43), and data from human islet recipients suggest that this process occurs *in vivo* (44). The group has initiated efforts to test, using their pig islet transplantation model, whether IBMIR can be overcome by conjugating preformed heparin complexes to the islet surface (45).

Several groups are also testing alternative islet implantation sites, including the omental pouch and skeletal muscle. For example, analogous to autotransplantation of parathyroid tissue into an intramuscular site following parathyroidectomy, isolated islets have been successfully transplanted into the forearm of a patient who underwent total pancreatectomy due to recurrent pancreatitis (42). Still many other groups are working to protect islets following their transplantation by encapsulating them. Islet encapsulation, if successful, would have two main benefits: (*i*) avoidance of toxic immunosuppression and (*ii*) the possibility that non-human islets could be used thus overcoming the limited supply of human cadaveric islets. A Phase I trial is currently underway in Italy using islets encapuslated with sodium alginate (AG) and poly-L-ornithine (PLO) (46).

Other efforts are focused on developing newer, safer, and more effective immunosuppressive agents, as well other means to stimulate beta-cell growth *in vivo*. While many agents have been shown to promote beta-cell replication and/or regeneration *in vitro* and in animal models, no data exist to suggest that this approach works in humans. For instance, Thompson and colleagues (47) from the University of British Columbia treated 11 islet allograft recipients with deteriorating glycemia control with the GLP-1 receptor agonist exenatide for 3 months. They reported that three patients either avoided insulin therapy or discontinued its usage; two were not on insulin at the start of the trial but would have been required to initiate it due to hyperglycemia and another was able to discontinue insulin while on exenatide. While on exenatide, most patients had decreased insulin requirements and most also lost weight, but their insulin requirements returned to baseline soon after exenatide was discontinued. Taken together, these findings suggest that exenatide did not have a trophic effect on the transplanted islets, but rather decreased insulin requirements by promoting weight loss.

CONCLUSIONS

Compared to a similar individual diagnosed just one generation ago, an individual diagnosed with T1D today has a dramatically better prognosis. Even so, people with T1D continue to develop disease complications and struggle with the rigorous treatment schedule that requires nearly constant attention to diet, exercise, weight, insulin administration, and frequent blood glucose monitoring. Simultaneous pancreas-kidney transplantation clearly benefits patients with T1D and kidney failure, although most of the survival benefit appears to derive from the transplanted kidney. Isolated pancreas transplantation on the other hand most likely increases mortality risk, although if successful it can also improve quality of life. Recurrent islet autoimmunity in the pancreas transplant recipient has now surfaced and represents a clinical challenge.

Enthusiasm surrounding isolated islet transplantation has dampened over time due to the procedure's rather limited clinical success, expense and immuno-suppressive agent-induced toxicity. Research focused on improving the islet isolation technique, islet engraftment, and on developing more effective, les-toxic immunosuppressive agents or perhaps protecting islets from immune destruction, e.g., via encapsulation or gene therapy, will be required to move islet transplantation beyond its present status as a promising experimental therapy.

Perhaps the greatest potential for a T1D treatment breakthrough lies in the detailed knowledge required to specifically abrogate the pathogenic anti-beta cell immune response. Quoting from an editorial written by Edwin Gale in 2002, ". . . a mature immune response is characterized by redundancy; raising concern that selective blockade of one potential pathway to disease may simply prompt others to take its place. The induction of tolerance seems to be the most promising way forward: we are more likely to win this particular war by gaining the insight needed to negotiate with the immune system than by seeking to bomb it into submission." (48).

REFERENCES

1. Achenbach P, Bonifacio E, Ziegler AG. Predicting type 1 diabetes. Curr Diab Rep 2005; 5(2):98–103.
2. Todd JA, Walker NM, Cooper JD, et al. Robust associations of four new chromosome regions from genome-wide analyses of type 1 diabetes. Nat Genet 2007; 39(7):857–864.
3. Sutherland DE, Sibley R, Xu XZ, et al. Twin-to-twin pancreas transplantation: Reversal and reenactment of the pathogenesis of type I diabetes. Trans Assoc Am Physicians 1984; 97:80–87.
4. Heit JJ, Apelqvist AA, Gu X, et al. Calcineurin/NFAT signalling regulates pancreatic beta-cell growth and function. Nature 2006; 443(7109):345–349.
5. The Diabetes Control and Complications Trial Research Group. The effect of intensive treatment of diabetes on the development and progression of long-term complications in insulin-dependent diabetes mellitus. N Engl J Med 1993; 329(14): 977–986.
6. Nathan DM, Cleary PA, Backlund JY, et al. Intensive diabetes treatment and cardiovascular disease in patients with type 1 diabetes. N Engl J Med 2005; 353(25):2643–2653.
7. Pambianco G, Costacou T, Ellis D, Becker DJ, Klein R, Orchard TJ. The 30-year natural history of type 1 diabetes complications: The Pittsburgh Epidemiology of Diabetes Complications Study experience. Diabetes 2006; 55(5):1463–1469.
8. Hovind P, Tarnow L, Rossing K, et al. Decreasing incidence of severe diabetic microangiopathy in type 1 diabetes. Diabetes Care 2003; 26(4):1258–1264.
9. Nordwall M, Bojestig M, Arnqvist HJ, Ludvigsson J. Declining incidence of severe retinopathy and persisting decrease of nephropathy in an unselected population of

Type 1 diabetes-the Linkoping Diabetes Complications Study. Diabetologia 2004; 47(7):1266–1272.

10. Finne P, Reunanen A, Stenman S, Groop PH, Gronhagen-Riska C. Incidence of end-stage renal disease in patients with type 1 diabetes. JAMA 2005; 294(14):1782–1787.

11. Venstrom JM, McBride MA, Rother KI, Hirshberg B, Orchard TJ, Harlan DM. Pancreas transplantation decreases survival for patients with diabetes and preserved kidney function. JAMA 2003; 290(21):2817–2823.

12. Liu EH, Siegel RM, Harlan DM, O'Shea JJ. T cell-directed therapies: Lessons learned and future prospects. Nat Immunol 2007; 8(1):25–30.

13. Fioretto P, Steffes MW, Sutherland DE, Goetz FC, Mauer M. Reversal of lesions of diabetic nephropathy after pancreas transplantation [see comments]. N Engl J Med 1998; 339(2):69–75.

14. Luzi L. Pancreas transplantation and diabetic complications. N Engl J Med 1998; 339(2):115–117.

15. Ramsay RC, Goetz FC, Sutherland DE, et al. Progression of diabetic retinopathy after pancreas transplantation for insulin-dependent diabetes mellitus. N Engl J Med 1988; 318(4):208–214.

16. Pearce IA, Ilango B, Sells RA, Wong D. Stabilisation of diabetic retinopathy following simultaneous pancreas and kidney transplant. Br J Ophthalmol 2000; 84(7):736–740.

17. Chow VC, Pai RP, Chapman JR, et al. Diabetic retinopathy after combined kidney-pancreas transplantation. Clin Transplant 1999; 13(4):356–362.

18. Fioretto P, Mauer SM, Bilous RW, Goetz FC, Sutherland DE, Steffes MW. Effects of pancreas transplantation on glomerular structure in insulin-dependent diabetic patients with their own kidneys. Lancet 1993; 342(8881):1193–1196.

19. Wolfe RA, Ashby VB, Milford EL, et al. Comparison of mortality in all patients on dialysis, patients on dialysis awaiting transplantation, and recipients of a first cadaveric transplant. N Engl J Med 1999; 341(23):1725–1730.

20. Bunnapradist S, Cho YW, Cecka JM, Wilkinson A, Danovitch GM. Kidney allograft and patient survival in type i diabetic recipients of cadaveric kidney alone versus simultaneous pancreas/kidney transplants: A multivariate analysis of the UNOS database. J Am Soc Nephrol 2003; 14(1):208–213.

21. Ojo AO, Meier-Kriesche HU, Hanson JA, et al. The impact of simultaneous pancreas-kidney transplantation on long-term patient survival. Transplantation 2001; 71(1):82–90.

22. Reddy KS, Stablein D, Taranto S, et al. Long-term survival following simultaneous kidney-pancreas transplantation versus kidney transplantation alone in patients with type 1 diabetes mellitus and renal failure. Am J Kidney Dis 2003; 41(2):464–470.

23. Robertson RP, Davis C, Larsen J, Stratta R, Sutherland DE. Pancreas and islet transplantation in type 1 diabetes. Diabetes Care 2006; 29(4):935.

24. Fritsche A, Stefan N, Haring H, Gerich J, Stumvoll M. Avoidance of hypoglycemia restores hypoglycemia awareness by increasing beta-adrenergic sensitivity in type 1 diabetes. Ann Intern Med 2001; 134(9 Pt 1):729–736.

25. Diamanatopoulos S, Allende G, Martin-Pagola A, et al. Recurrence of Type 1 Diabetes (T1DR) after simultaneous pancreas–kidney (SPK) transplantation is associated with islet cell autoantibody conversion[abstract]. Acta Diabetol. 2007; 44(Suppl 1):S12.

26. Allene G, Diamanatopoulos S, Ferreira J, Burke GW, Pugliese A. Retrospective assessment of islet cell auto-antobidies in pancreas-organ donors [abstract]. Acta Diabetol. 2007; 44(Suppl 1): S2.

27. Shapiro AM, Lakey JR, Ryan EA, et al. Islet transplantation in seven patients with type 1 diabetes mellitus using a glucocorticoid-free immunosuppressive regimen. N Engl J Med 2000; 343(4):230–238.

28. McAlister VC, Gao Z, Peltekian K, Domingues J, Mahalati K, Macdonald AS. Sirolimus-tacrolimus combination immunosuppression. Lancet 2000; 355(9201): 376–377.

29. Couzin J. Diabetes. Islet transplants face test of time. Science 2004; 306(5693):34–37.

30. Rother KI, Harlan DM. Challenges facing islet transplantation for the treatment of type 1 diabetes mellitus. J Clin Invest 2004; 114(7):877–883.

31. Ryan EA, Paty BW, Senior PA, et al. Five-year follow-up after clinical islet transplantation. Diabetes 2005; 54(7):2060–2069.

32. Shapiro AM, Ricordi C, Hering BJ, et al. International trial of the Edmonton protocol for islet transplantation. N Engl J Med 2006; 355(13):1318–1330.

33. Koh A, Rudnisky C, Tennant M, et al. Stabilization of diabetic retinopathy following clinical islet transplantation [abstract]. Acta Diabetol. 2007; 44(Suppl 1): S28.

34. Bhargava R, Senior PA, Ackerman TE, et al. Prevalence of hepatic steatosis after islet transplantation and its relation to graft function. Diabetes 2004; 53(5):1311–1317.

35. Hirshberg B, Mog S, Patterson N, Leconte J, Harlan DM. Histopathological study of intrahepatic islets transplanted in the nonhuman primate model using edmonton protocol immunosuppression. J Clin Endocrinol Metab 2002; 87(12):5424–5429.

36. Senior PA, Zeman M, Paty BW, Ryan EA, Shapiro AM. Changes in renal function after clinical islet transplantation: Four-year observational study. Am J Transplant 2007; 7(1):91–98.

37. Mohanakumar T, Narayanan K, Desai N, et al. A significant role for histocompatibility in human islet transplantation. Transplantation 2006; 82(2):180–187.

38. Campbell PM, Senior PA, Salam A, et al. High risk of sensitization after failed islet transplantation. Am J Transplant 2007; 7(10):2311–2317.

39. Keymeulen B, Gillard P, Mathieu C, et al. Correlation between beta cell mass and glycemic control in type 1 diabetic recipients of islet cell graft. Proc Natl Acad Sci USA 2006; 103(46):17444–17449.

40. Korsgren O, Nilsson B, Berne C, et al. Current status of clinical islet transplantation. Transplantation 2005; 79(10):1289–1293.

41. Ryan EA, Lakey JR, Paty BW, et al. Successful islet transplantation: Continued insulin reserve provides long-term glycemic control. Diabetes 2002; 51(7):2148–2157.

42. Korsgren O, Lundgren T, Felldin M, et al. Optimising islet engraftment is critical for successful clinical islet transplantation. Diabetologia 2008; 51(2):227–232.

43. Bennet W, Groth CG, Larsson R, Nilsson B, Korsgren O. Isolated human islets trigger an instant blood mediated inflammatory reaction: Implications for intraportal islet transplantation as a treatment for patients with type 1 diabetes. Ups J Med Sci 2000; 105(2):125–133.

44. Moberg L, Johansson H, Lukinius A, et al. Production of tissue factor by pancreatic islet cells as a trigger of detrimental thrombotic reactions in clinical islet transplantation. Lancet 2002; 360(9350):2039–2045.

45. Cabric S, Sanchez J, Lundgren T, et al. Islet surface heparinization prevents the instant blood-mediated inflammatory reaction in islet transplantation. Diabetes 2007; 56(8):2008–2015.
46. Calafiore R, Basta G, Luca G, et al. Standard technical procedures for microencapsulation of human islets for graft into nonimmunosuppressed patients with type 1 diabetes mellitus. Transplant Proc 2006; 38(4):1156–1157.
47. Ghofaili KA, Fung M, Ao Z, et al. Effect of exenatide on beta cell function after islet transplantation in type 1 diabetes. Transplantation 2007; 83(1):24–28.
48. Gale EA. Can we change the course of beta-cell destruction in type 1 diabetes? N Engl J Med 2002; 346(22):1740–1742.

12

Creating an Artificial Pancreas—The Marriage of Insulin Pumps and Glucose Sensors

Bruce Buckingham and Tandy Aye

Department of Pediatric Endocrinology, Stanford Medical Center, Stanford, California, U.S.A.

BACKGROUND

Diabetes is a chronic disease, which currently can be controlled only by constant vigilance. Chronic elevations, and likely fluctuations, of the blood glucose are associated with long-term complications (blindness, kidney failure, heart disease, and lower extremity amputations). Perversely, tight glucose control increases the risk of serious hypoglycemia. Despite insulin infusion pumps and programs that promote intensive diabetes management, the average A1c at major diabetes treatment centers remains higher than 8% (1), which is well above the recommended goal of 7% for adults and for age-adjusted pediatric goals (Table 1). Many factors contribute to this failure: (*i*) the difficulties in correctly estimating the amount of carbohydrates in a meal, (*ii*) missed meal boluses, and (*iii*) anxiety about hypoglycemia resulting in undertreatment, especially overnight. It has always been difficult to achieve compliance with complicated medical regimes, whether it is taking pills three or four times a day or administration of insulin three or more times a day. As long as diabetes treatment demands constant direct intervention, the vast majority of people with diabetes will not meet treatment goals. By taking the patient out of the loop or closing the loop, an "artificial pancreas" would allow the person with diabetes to go about their daily activities without the need to

Table 1 Hemoglobin A1c Goals by Age

Age (yr)	Target range (mg/dL)	HbA1c
0–5	80–200	7.5–8.5%
6–11	70–180	Less than 8%
12–20+	70–150	Less than 7%

constantly remember to check their blood glucose, count carbohydrates, and take insulin multiple times each day.

An artificial pancreas consists of three components: an insulin infusion pump, a continuous glucose sensor, and an algorithm that translates data from the glucose sensor and determines insulin delivery (Fig. 1). The most likely first closed-loop system would use a SQ sensor and insulin infusion pump. However, an implantable system is also feasible. The main difficulties in optimizing a SQ system are (*i*) accuracy of the SQ continuous glucose sensors, (*ii*) lags in interstitial SQ glucose measurements when the glucose is changing rapidly, (*iii*) delays in the onset of insulin action after a SQ injection, (*iv*) prolonged insulin action of 4 to 6 hours following a SQ injection, and (*v*) the lack of algorithm models that exactly mimic islet physiology. Thus, with current technology, a SQ sensor–SQ insulin delivery system does not fully mimic normal beta cell function; however, initial studies indicate that excellent diabetes control can be achieved using such a system on a short-term basis (2).

Before a functional artificial pancreas (AP) will receive FDA approval, clinical safety in an outpatient setting must be demonstrated. The most important safety issue in the short term will be the avoidance of severe hypoglycemic events. Fortunately, when SQ glucose sensors fail, they generally indicate falsely low glucose readings. A falsely low glucose would cause underdelivery of insulin in a closed-loop system, resulting in hyperglycemia and not hypoglycemia. Hypoglycemia can also be avoided by aiming for a slightly higher glucose target. As an example, if the target is set to 120 mg/dL, and the sensor was inaccurate by 50%, glucose values would still be above 60 mg/dL. Current glucose sensors are more accurate above 70 mg/dL (3–5), and since a closed-loop would generally maintain glucose levels above this level, the system would be functioning in a glucose range where sensors have greater accuracy, which is another safety feature to prevent hypoglycemia. As algorithms improve, the amount of time spent above 200 mg/dL can also be progressively decreased. Currently, children with an average A1c of 6.9% spend an average of 6 hours with glucose readings above 200 mg/dL each day (6). With a closed-loop system it should be possible to significantly decrease the time spent in hyperglycemia without increasing hypoglycemia and thereby decrease glycemic variability. Glycemic variability, independent of HbA1c levels, has recently been described as an independent risk factor for diabetic complications (7,8), although this concept is controversial (9).

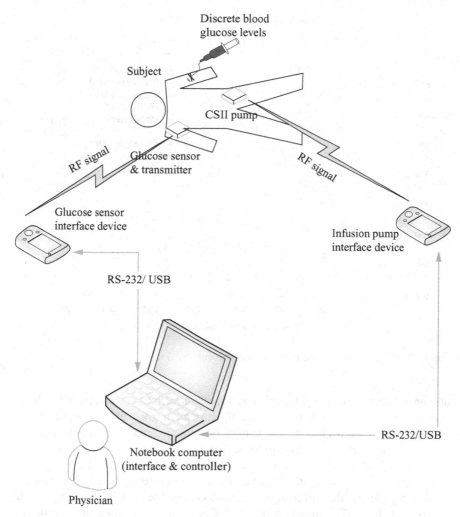

Discrete blood
glucose levels

Subject

CSII pump

RF signal

Glucose sensor
& transmitter

RF signal

Glucose sensor
interface device

Infusion pump
interface device

RS-232/ USB

RS-232/USB

Notebook computer
(interface & controller)

Physician

Figure 1 Schematic diagram of elements for a closed-loop for insulin delivery.

SENSORS

A number of devices and technologies have been proposed for continuous glucose monitoring (CGM), including the use of near-infrared and mid-infrared spectroscopy, erythrocyte scattering, photoacoustic phenomenon, optical coherence tomography, thermo-optical techniques, Raman spectroscopy, and fluorescence measurements (10). The currently available commercially continuous glucose sensors are based on measuring SQ (interstitial) glucose levels. These are electrochemical sensors that use glucose oxidase and measure an electric current generated when glucose reacts with oxygen. They are coated with specialized membranes to make them biocompatible, generating almost no tissue reaction,

Accuracy by glucose concentration

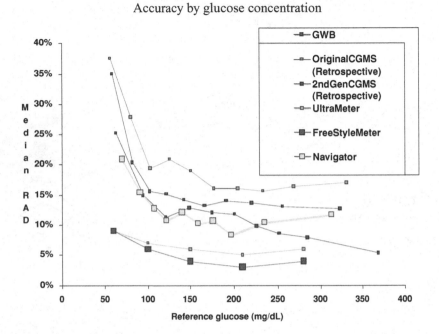

Figure 2   Continuous glucose monitor sensor accuracy.

and providing a barrier to potential cross reactants such as acetaminophen. These sensors are relatively stable and generally provide a good glucose signal for 3 to 7 days. Interstitial glucose is a distinct physiologic space when compared to the blood glucose; when blood glucose levels are changing rapidly, interstitial glucose levels will lag behind blood glucose by about 18 minutes (11). In pigs, the temporal changes in interstitial blood glucose levels correlate better with changes in the CNS glucose than do changes in the blood glucose (11). Perhaps interstitial glucose levels would correlate better with CNS function than do blood glucose levels, though this remains to be determined in humans. Although real-time cCGM is not as accurate as discrete blood glucose monitoring (Fig. 2), CGM values are generally within 15% of the discrete measurement. A discrete blood glucose has been compared to a snapshot and real-time monitoring to a video, where there is less information in each frame but the video provides the added dimension of glucose change over time which the snapshot cannot provide.

The currently available needle-like continuous glucose sensors pass through the skin, so there is always a potential for an infection at the insertion site. Current sensors have a transmitter attached to them once they are inserted. The transmitter provides a source of energy to power the sensor as well as allows transmission of the glucose signal to a receiver by using a radiofrequency signal. These sensors often take from 2 to 10 hours to stabilize to the local interstitial environment before they generate a reasonably accurate glucose signal. Because of the differences in interstitial and blood glucose levels when glucose values are changing rapidly, it is important to calibrate the sensor when blood glucose levels are stable (ideally when changes are ≤ 0.5 mg/dL/min) (12). Unfortunately, when patients enter their first calibration value, they are "blind" to the data from their continuous glucose sensor and their glucose rate of change. After their initial calibration, they are able to "see" their glucose trends and assess their rate of change before entering subsequent glucose values. The calibration system could be significantly improved if sensors internally evaluated the stability of their glucose signal and only asked for calibration values when the glucose signal was stable.

In addition to these safety issues that can be improved upon, there remain multiple factors that affect a patient's use of the sensors. For many patients, the time required for calibration limits their use. Since the tissue reaction to the trauma of the sensor insertion is one variable affecting calibration time, work to reduce these effects may significantly enhance the user's experience. Similarly, because these sensors require a continuous source of power, the transmitter cannot be detached from the sensor for any length of time, or the sensor must be recalibrated. Finally, one of the biggest user issues with these devices has been the adhesive required to secure the sensor and transmitter to the skin. The adhesives can be irritating to some wearers and others will develop a true tape allergy. One of the biggest issues for prolonged sensor wear (greater than 3 days) is maintaining the adhesive. For those who use continuous SQ insulin infusions (CSII; pump), there are two insertion sites (one for the pump cannula and one for the sensor), and two areas for potential tape-related issues. Wearing the tape repeatedly in the same area can temporarily disrupt the usual skin barriers to infection. Future devices may be able to combine a continuous glucose sensor with an insulin infusion set into one platform adhering to the skin.

One way to avoid the topical skin issues associated with adhesives is to implant the sensor. Implanted sensors are attractive to patients since these are not visible, they do not have to insert a needle-like sensor under their skin repeatedly, and these would not interfere with daily activities such as showering, swimming, or exercising. There is one published report of a long-term implanted SQ continuous sensors (13). The sensors were surgically implanted into the abdomen under local anesthesia. Two months after implantation 13 of the 15 implanted sensors were functioning and had a mean absolute relative difference of 25% when compared to YSI (Yellow Springs Instrument Glucose Analyzer; Yellow Spring Instruments, Yellow Springs, OH), glucose levels. As noted above, this difference is considerably higher than the 15% error reported from SQ sensors. For implanted devices to be acceptable, these will probably need to function for at least 1 year once they are implanted and ideally the insertion and removal could be performed in a physician's office and not require a surgical referral. Another approach would be an intravascular continuous glucose sensor. This technology was initially developed by Dr. David Gough (14). A similar technology has been used in clinical trials conducted by MiniMed, Inc. in France (15) and the United States, but no data from these studies have been published. This sensor has about a 20-minute delay in reported glucose levels, which has created difficulties when trying to integrate the sensor information into an AP.

PUMPS

Insulin infusion pumps have been commercially available for almost 30 years (16). Since the initial pumps were developed there have been progressive improvements in their software features, their size, and the insulin infusion sets. Most pumps are attached to the patient using an infusion set catheter. A newer pump (a "patch" or "pod" pump) eliminates the need for infusion set tubing and manual insertion of the infusion set catheter. One such pump is the OmniPod (Insulet Corporation, Bedford, Massachusetts). The software features of the current pumps include the ability to calculate different carbohydrate to insulin ratios and different responses sensitivities for insulin correction doses at different times of the day. They also feature a calculation of residual insulin activity following an insulin bolus. Most pumps can now automatically receive data from a glucose meter (by radiofrequency, infrared, or they have a glucose meter built into the pump) and so glucose values need not be manually entered. Conscientious pump users can often achieve very good glycemic control if they monitor their blood glucose frequently, adjust their insulin doses based on the an accurate assessment of the quantity and type of meals they are eating, and compensate for the effect of physical activity on glucose levels. This may require a prolonged bolus (square wave) for foods, which are gradually absorbed, and often requires a premeal bolus of insulin prior to eating, especially in the morning, and temporary changes in basal infusion rates to account for physical activity. If the user also makes additional adjustments for activity level even better control can be achieved. However, as with all chronic, life-long conditions, the problem is the "human factor" with people remembering to give an insulin bolus before all meals, and knowing the amount of carbohydrate, protein, and fat in the meal, and how rapidly the food will be absorbed. In a review on downloaded pump data at the Barbara Davis Center, 65% of adolescents were missing at least one meal bolus a week and their HbA1c was 0.8% higher than those not missing a meal bolus (17).

A pump with the ability to store and deliver more than one hormone might better mimic islet physiology and its mechanism of glucose control. Even the option of two hormones, for instance the addition of the counterregulatory hormone such as glucagon would be an added countermeasure to prevent hypoglycemia. In fact, Dr. Edward Damiano and Firas El-Khatib have conducted studies using pigs and a dual infusion system and model predictive control (MPC), where small doses of glucagon are given to prevent impending hypoglycemia. They found that glucagon was stable in an insulin infusion pump attached to the pig for at least 7 days (18). The onset of action of SQ glucagon was very rapid, allowing for quick prevention of possible hypoglycemia. This therapy, of course, depends on the patient having adequate glycogen stores. Epinephrine has also been tried in the treatment of hypoglycemia, but was relatively ineffective (19). Amylin, or islet amyloid polypeptide, can also be added to delay gastric emptying resulting in a slower rate of glucose change following a meal, since meals with their rapid rate of change present the greatest challenge to a SQ insulin/SQ sensor closed loop.

Infusion Sets

Currently, infusion sets are generally used for 3 days, whereas continuous glucose sensors are generally functional for 5 to 7 days (5,20). Patients would prefer to have one device attached to their body, which could serve as both the sensor and insulin infusion pump. For both to be merged onto a common platform it would require a longer duration of insulin infusion set function or the ability to insert several infusion sites on or into a common sensor platform. Another proposal is to use microneedle arrays (21) to deliver intradermal insulin. It has not been demonstrated, however, that this produces a more rapid rate of insulin absorption.

Insulin

One of the problems with the current "rapid-acting" insulins is that they are relatively slow for the purposes of a closed loop. The reach half their maximum activity in 20 minutes and do not reach full activity for 45 minutes (22). When this is coupled with a 12- to 30-minute delay in the algorithm detecting the onset of a meal (based on the rate of change of glucose levels), meal delivery of insulin becomes very difficult. This can be partially compensated for by having the patient give a premeal bolus of insulin, but then it is no longer a closed-loop system. Another approach would be to use an insulin with a more rapid onset of action. This can be accomplished by keeping the insulin in a monomeric (instead of hexameric) state. A new insulin developed by Biodel (VIAject^{TM} insulin) keeps the insulin in a monomeric state by chelating zinc, which allows a more rapid onset of action thus reaching peak activity about 10 to 15 minutes earlier than current analog short-acting insulins (23). Other possible solutions would be to change the insulin delivery so that it is provided to a more vascular area or the insulin could be delivered into the peritoneal cavity where some of the insulin would directly be absorbed through the portal circulation. Minimed has developed an implanted insulin pump using U-400 insulin and intraperitoneal insulin delivery. The greatest experience with this infusion system has been in France (24), but there are currently no plans to market this system in the United States.

Algorithms

Control algorithms are, by definition, designed and tuned based on a model of how a system works, ranging from the simple (knowledge of whether a manipulated input increases or decreases the output) to the complex (sets of nonlinear partial differential equations). This range trades off ease of design and implementation and possibly robustness to uncertainty with performance and ability to fine-tune and learn. These trade-offs become increasingly challenging when delays separate action and effect. Currently available insulin pumps use simple algorithms to incorporate current glucose levels into suggestions for bolus doses (the "bolus calculator" or "bolus wizard" features). With the availability of glucose trend from continuous glucose sensors, more sophisticated algorithms can be developed. Perhaps the initial step in integrating the sensor data and the insulin pump is the development of a limited algorithm that would not deliver insulin but could shut off insulin delivery. For instance, Dr. Peter Chase has proposed that patients using an insulin infusion pump could have their insulin infusion stopped for 1 to 2 hours if they have a predicted low blood glucose and do not respond to a hypoglycemic alarm. This would be particularly important overnight, when patients fail to respond to over 70% of alarms (25). Since the pump would not be delivering increased insulin doses based on the sensor glucose value, this approach may have many safety advantages and may be the easiest "partial-closed loop" for the FDA to initially consider for approval.

Another retrospective approach would be to have a computer program review 3 to 6 days of CGM and pump data looking for patterns. This can be done by dividing the day into 3-hour windows, with windows beginning when a meal bolus has been given. Time blocks beyond the meal blocks can be used for adjustment of basal insulin infusion rates. If a patient is using an insulin infusion pump, this can be accomplished by downloading both the sensor and pump information into a common file. If there is a consistent trend seen over multiple days, this could generate a recommendation to the patient to change either a basal rate or a carbohydrate to insulin ratio for a particular meal. These suggested doses would be more accurate than what physicians initially calculate and would allow for testing of algorithms before fully closing the loop.

Finally, a third partial approach to closing the loop would be to have an algorithm incorporated into the insulin infusion pump, which includes glucose rate of change information as well as insulin action profiles into the bolus calculator. This would allow adjustment of meal bolus doses and basal infusion rates based on glucose trend analysis as well as glycemic targets, but the final decision on insulin delivery is done by the user.

To create a fully functional AP there must be an algorithm that determines insulin delivery. Several algorithms have been proposed, including a proportional–intergral–derivative (PID) algorithm (26), MPC (27–29), and adaptive neural networks (30). The first of these models to be tested in humans has been the PID algorithm (2). At each point in time, the controller assesses how far the current glucose is from the desired glucose (proportional), the rate of change in glucose (derivative), and how long the glucose has remained above or below target (integral). In these CRC studies on 10 patients with type 1 diabetes who were on the AP for 30 hours, the PID controller achieved excellent control overnight, but there was mild hyperglycemia following meals, particularly breakfast,and a tendency for hypoglycemia 4 to 6 hours following meal insulin delivery. These issues can be partly addressed by using a feed-forward algorithm, where a partial meal bolus is given 5 to 10 minutes before the meal, but this is no longer a full closed-loop system. The basal rate can also be decreased several hours after a meal to compensate for the insulin onboard from the meal bolus. With extended hyperglycemia, there is an increase in the integral component of insulin delivery. The only way the equation can decrease this component is to have the glucose remain below the target for an equal area "under" the curve as the area of hyperglycemia "over" the curve. To prevent this from happening, constraints can be placed on the insulin infusion rates by using techniques such as "reset windup." Reset windup places a limit on how much insulin can be added to the integral component by either limiting the glucose level the controller can adjust to (e.g., cutoff of 250 mg/dL instead of 400 mg/dL) or by limiting the absolute amount of insulin the integral component can contribute to the insulin delivery (e.g., no more than 1 U/hr when the equation might dictate 2 U/hr) (31).

In MPC, the controller has a model of expected glucose values and responses to insulin, which may vary by time of day (dawn phenomenon), meal events, and changes in insulin sensitivity. At each point in time, the model compares the predicted glucose with the actual glucose and the model is then updated with a new prediction horizon. At each step the model takes into account the previous history of glucose measurements and insulin delivery and model may be updated to learn from discrepancies between actual and predicted values, and then the optimization is repeated. How to best update the model to correct for model mismatch is one of the major challenges to MPC. MPC has been used in a simulated patient (27) and there are some short-term studies in humans (32,33).

It should be noted that MPC is a basic strategy or concept, but any number of model types can be used, with many different methods of performing the optimization. Classic MPC uses a fixed linear model, but there have been many formulations using nonlinear models (34). A nice feature of an optimization-based approach is that different weighting on the control objective can be used depending on whether the glucose is entering hyperglycemia or hypoglycemia condition. Also, multiobjective optimization techniques can be used to rank order the important objective, for example, the highest ranked objective might be to avoid hypoglycemia.

POTENTIAL FUTURE APPLICATIONS OF A CLOSED-LOOP SYSTEM

One of the most promising uses for CGM and a closed-loop system may be in the ICU. Tight glycemic control in the ICU has produced dramatic improvements in morbidity and mortality (35). Sensor that provides glucose information to the patient every few minutes (real-time CGM) has functioned well in an ICU setting even with variable changes in the core body temperature, use of inotropes, and body-wall edema (36). When intravenous glucose infusions are provided at a steady rate, the blood glucose fluctuations associated with oral absorption of meals are absent. In an ICU setting, insulin is delivered intravenously, which significantly improves the pharmacodynamics of insulin delivery in a closed-loop system because it has a more rapid onset of action and a shorter duration of action. The ICU may therefore be one of the initial settings where closed-loop delivery of insulin by using a continuous glucose sensor will be implemented.

Another use would be to prevent glucotoxicity, which is particularly dele-terious to the beta cell around the time of clinical onset of type 1 diabetes and perhaps also at time of islet transplantation. Islet glucotoxicity occurs at the onset of type 1 diabetes and even with type 2 diabetes. When beta cells are stimulated by hyperglycemia, they express increased levels of beta cell antigens (37–43) and are more susceptible to damage by cytokines (44–47). One potential use of a closed-loop system would be at the onset of diabetes to limit glucotoxicity. The effectiveness of this therapy was demonstrated in studies by Shah and Malone; they used a Biostater (Miles Laboratories, Elkhart, IN) for 2 weeks at the onset of diabetes to preserve c-peptide secretion (48). Prevention of glucotoxicity at the time of transplantation could also prolong the life of the transplanted islets.

Strict metabolic control of blood glucose levels should be beneficial in many situations in the future treatment of diabetes. Initial applications will need to be in a research setting with further expansion into ICUs and other inpatient settings. Eventually these studies may provide the basis for the FDA to approve the use of sensor for daily outpatient use.

CONCLUSION

Even with constant vigilance, current diabetes therapy does not prevent the fluc-tuations in blood glucose values. The most motivated patients find it difficult to achieve good control with a hemoglobin A1c ≤7% over multiple years, even with the currently available insulin infusion pumps and CGM systems. A closed-loop insulin delivery system could significantly decrease the patient burden of manag-ing diabetes and should decrease the risks of both hyper- and hypoglycemia.

However, there are multiple factors that will eventually determine the feasi-bility of an ambulatory, outpatient closed-loop system. The system will have to be safe and have a very low incidence of significant hypoglycemia. Currently patients with a HbA1c of 6.8% spend about 15 minutes each day with glucose values ≤50 mg/dL and about 5 minutes each day with glucose values ≤40 mg/dL accord-ing to FreeStyle Navigator CGM readings. These patients had no seizures or loss of consciousness (6). A closed-loop system should do better than this, and there should be no values ≤50 mg/dL for its use to be considered safe.

An initial closed-loop system ready for clinical use may have only limited goals; for example, automatically decreasing or stopping insulin delivery to prevent hypoglycemia rather than aiming for complete normalization of glucose values. Later models will control nocturnal glucose levels and eventually postprandial hyperglycemia. Much of the progress will be based on demonstrating safety of the proposed algorithms, but additional work is needed in making the devices unobtrusive, comfortable, and easy to wear and use.

Following are some of the specific areas for future research:

Device insertion sites:
- What is the physical distance that needs to separate a SQ sensor probe from an insulin infusion catheter?
- Does lipohypertrophy significantly affect sensor performance and insulin action times?
- What is the best depth to place devices?
- Can insulin infusion sets and sensors be placed onto a common platform, and if so, how long can the insulin infusion set function (i.e., are the changes that could be made to the insulin infusion set to prolong infusion set survival)?
- Decreasing the size and weight of sensor and infusion set devices will be critical.

Insulins:
- Can a more rapid onset of action be developed?

Function of control system and algorithms:
- Ability to quickly and correctly identify a meal.
- Ability to determine size of the meal.
- Does a measure of exercise need to be included?
- Detection of sensor failure.
- Detection of infusion site failure.

The user interface:
- Combining the sensor receiver, controller, and algorithm with a transmission system to the pump into one device. Should all transmission be wireless instead of tethered?
- Combining the many devices a patient routinely uses today into one device, i.e., cell phone, music player, glucose meter (for calibration), and AP into one platform.
- The goal is a lightweight, unobtrusive, integrated system that requires minimal input and decisions from the user.

REFERENCES

1. EDIC. Sustained effect of intensive treatment of type 1 diabetes mellitus on development and progression of diabetic nephropathy: The Epidemiology of Diabetes Interventions and Complications (EDIC) study. JAMA. 2003; 290:2159–2167.
2. Steil GM, Rebrin K, Darwin C, et al. Feasibility of automating insulin delivery for the treatment of type 1 diabetes. Diabetes 2006; 55:3344–3350.
3. DirecNet. The accuracy of the CGMS in children with type 1 diabetes: Results of the diabetes research in children network (DirecNet) accuracy study. Diabetes Technol Ther 2003; 5:781–789.

4. DirecNet. Accuracy of the modified continuous glucose monitoring (CGMS(R)) sensor in an outpatient setting: Results from a Diabetes Research in Children Network (DirecNet) Study. Diabetes Technol Ther 2005; 7:109–114.

5. Wilson DM, Beck RW, Tamborlane WV, et al. The accuracy of the FreeStyle Navigator continuous glucose monitoring system in children with type 1 diabetes. Diabetes Care 2007; 30:59–64.

6. DirecNet, Buckingham. Continuous glucose monitoring in children with type 1 diabetes. J Pediatr 2007; 151:388–393.

7. Monnier L, Mas E, Ginet C, et al. Activation of oxidative stress by acute glucose fluctuations compared with sustained chronic hyperglycemia in patients with type 2 diabetes. JAMA 2006; 295:1681–1687.

8. Brownlee M, Hirsch IB. Glycemic variability: A hemoglobin A1c-independent risk factor for diabetic complications. JAMA 2006; 295:1707–1708.

9. Kilpatrick ES, Rigby AS, Atkin SL. The effect of glucose variability on the risk of microvascular complications in type 1 diabetes. Diabetes Care 2006; 29:1486–1490.

10. Khalil OS. Non-invasive glucose measurement technologies: An update from 1999 to the dawn of the new millennium. Diabetes Technol Ther 2004; 6:660–697.

11. Nielsen JK, Djurhuus CB, Gravholt CH, et al. Continuous glucose monitoring in interstitial subcutaneous adipose tissue and skeletal muscle reflects excursions in cerebral cortex. Diabetes 2005; 54:1635–1639.

12. Buckingham BA, Kollman C, Beck R, et al. Evaluation of factors affecting CGMS calibration. Diabetes Technol Ther 2006; 8:318–325.

13. Garg SK, Schwartz S, Edelman SV. Improved glucose excursions using an implantable real-time continuous glucose sensor in adults with type 1 diabetes. Diabetes Care 2004; 27:734–738.

14. Armour JC, Lucisano JY, McKean BD, et al. Application of chronic intravascular blood glucose sensor in dogs. Diabetes 1990; 39:1519–1526.

15. Renard E, Costalat G, Bringer J. From external to implantable insulin pump, can we close the loop? Diabetes Metab 2002; 28:2S19–2S25.

16. Felig P, Tamborlane W, Sherwin RS, et al. Insulin-infusion pump for diabetes. N Engl J Med 1979; 301:1004–1005.

17. Burdick J, Chase HP, Slover RH, et al. Missed insulin meal boluses and elevated hemoglobin A1c levels in children receiving insulin pump therapy. Pediatrics 2004; 113:e221–e224.

18. El-Khatib FH, Jiang J, Gerrity RG, et al. Pharmacodynamics and stability of subcutaneously infused glucagon in a type 1 diabetic Swine model in vivo. Diabetes Technol Ther 2007; 9:135–144.

19. Monsod TP, Tamborlane WV, Coraluzzi L, et al. Epipen as an alternative to glucagon in the treatment of hypoglycemia in children with diabetes. Diabetes Care 2001; 24:701–704.

20. Weinstein RL, Schwartz SL, Brazg RL, et al. Accuracy of the 5-Day FreeStyle Navigator Continuous Glucose Monitoring System: Comparison with frequent laboratory reference measurements. Diabetes Care 2007; 30:1125–1130.

21. Nordquist L, Roxhed N, Griss P, et al. Novel microneedle patches for active insulin delivery are efficient in maintaining glycaemic control: An initial comparison with subcutaneous administration. Pharm Res 2007; 24:1381–1388.

22. Mudaliar SR, Lindberg FA, Joyce M, et al. Insulin aspart (B28 asp-insulin): A fast-acting analog of human insulin: Absorption kinetics and action profile compared with regular human insulin in healthy nondiabetic subjects. Diabetes Care 1999; 22:1501–1506.

23. Steiner SS, Hompesch M, Pohl R, et al. Pharmacokinetics and phrmacodynamics of insulin VIAject and regular human insulin when injected subcutneously directly before a meal in patietns with type1 diabetes. Diabetes 2007; 56:A9.

24. Renard E. Implantable closed-loop glucose-sensing and insulin delivery: The future for insulin pump therapy. Curr Opin Pharmacol 2002; 2:708–716.

25. Buckingham B, Block J, Burdick J, et al. Response to nocturnal alarms using a real-time glucose sensor. Diabetes Technol Ther 2005; 7:440–447.

26. Steil GM, Rebrin K, Janowski R, et al. Modeling beta-cell insulin secretion–implications for closed-loop glucose homeostasis. Diabetes Technol Ther 2003; 5:953–964.

27. Parker RS, Doyle FJ III, Peppas NA. A model-based algorithm for blood glucose control in type I diabetic patients. IEEE Trans Biomed Eng 1999; 46:148–157.

28. Dua P, Doyle FJ III. Model Based Blood Glucose Control for Type 1 Diabetes via Parametric Programming. IEEE Trans Biomed Eng. 2006 Aug; 53(8):1478–1491.

29. Parker RI, Doyle FJ III. Advanced Model Predictive Control (MPC) for Type 1 Diabetic Patient Blood Glucose Control. Proc American Control Conference, 2000:3483–3487.

30. Trajanoski Z, Regittnig W, Wach P. Simulation studies on neural predictive control of glucose using the subcutaneous route. Comput Methods Programs Biomed 1998; 56:133–139.

31. Bequette BW. Process Control: Modeling, Design and Simulation. Upper Saddle River, NJ: Prentice Hall, 2003.

32. Schaller HC, Schaupp L, Bodenlenz M, et al. On-line adaptive algorithm with glucose prediction capacity for subcutaneous closed loop control of glucose: Evaluation under fasting conditions in patients with Type 1 diabetes. Diabet Med 2006; 23:90–93.

33. Plank J, Blaha J, Cordingley J, et al. Multicentric, randomized, controlled trial to evaluate blood glucose control by the model predictive control algorithm versus routine glucose management protocols in intensive care unit patients. Diabetes Care 2006; 29:271–276.

34. Bequette BW. Nonlinear control of chemical processes: A review. Ind Eng Chem Res 1991; 30:1391–1413.

35. van den Berghe G, Wouters P, Weekers F, et al. Intensive insulin therapy in the critically ill patients. N Engl J Med 2001; 345:1359–1367.

36. Piper HG, Alexander JL, Shukla A, et al. Real-time continuous glucose monitoring in pediatric patients during and after cardiac surgery. Pediatrics 2006; 118:1176–1184.

37. McCulloch DK, Barmeier H, Neifing JL, et al. Metabolic state of the pancreas affects end-point titre in the islet cell antibody assay. Diabetologia 1991; 34:622–625.

38. Hao W, Li L, Mehta V, et al. Functional state of the beta cell affects expression of both forms of glutamic acid decarboxylase. Pancreas 1994; 9:558–562.

39. Hagopian WA, Karlsen AE, Petersen JS, et al. Regulation of glutamic acid decarboxylase diabetes autoantigen expression in highly purified isolated islets from *Macaca nemestrina*. Endocrinology 1993; 132:2674–2681.

40. Aaen K, Rygaard J, Josefsen K, et al. Dependence of antigen expression on functional state of beta-cells. Diabetes 1990; 39:697–701.
41. Kampe O, Andersson A, Bjork E, et al. High-glucose stimulation of 64000-Mr islet cell autoantigen expression. Diabetes 1989; 38:1326–1328.
42. Bjork E, Kampe O, Andersson A, et al. Expression of the 64 kDa/glutamic acid decarboxylase rat islet cell autoantigen is influenced by the rate of insulin secretion. Diabetologia 1992; 35:490–493.
43. Bjork E, Kampe O, Karlsson FA, et al. Glucose regulation of the autoantigen GAD65 in human pancreatic islets. J Clin Endocrinol Metab 1992; 75:1574–1576.
44. Mehta V, Hao W, Brooks-Worrell BM, et al. The functional state of the beta cell modulates IL-1 and TNF-induced cytotoxicity. Lymphokine Cytokine Res 1993; 12:255–259.
45. Mellado-Gil JM, Aguilar-Diosdado M. Assay for high glucose-mediated islet cell sensitization to apoptosis induced by streptozotocin and cytokines. Biol Proced Online 2005; 7:162–171.
46. Mellado-Gil JM, Aguilar-Diosdado M. High glucose potentiates cytokine- and streptozotocin-induced apoptosis of rat islet cells: Effect on apoptosis-related genes. J Endocrinol 2004; 183:155–162.
47. Maedler K, Storling J, Sturis J, et al. Glucose- and interleukin-1beta-induced beta-cell apoptosis requires Ca_2 +influx and extracellular signal-regulated kinase (ERK) 1/2 activation and is prevented by a sulfonylurea receptor 1/inwardly rectifying K+ channel 6.2 (SUR/Kir6.2) selective potassium channel opener in human islets. Diabetes 2004; 53:1706–1713.
48. Shah SC, Malone JI, Simpson NE. A randomized trial of intensive insulin therapy in newly diagnosed insulin-dependent diabetes mellitus. N Engl J Med 1989; 320:550–554.

Index

Printed in the United States
by Baker & Taylor Publisher Services